HUMAN ANATOMY

Regional and Clinical

Abdomen and Lower Limb
(Vol. 2)

HUMAN ANATOMY

Regional and Clinical

Abdomen and Lower Limb
(Vol. 2)

A. HALIM

M.B.B.S., M.S., F.I.M.S.A.
Formerly Professor and Head, Department of Anatomy
King George's Medical College, Lucknow, India

W.H.O. Fellow in Medical Education (U.K.)
Fellow, British Association of Clinical Anatomists
Fellow, International Medical Sciences Academy
Ex-member, Academic Council
King George's Medical and Dental Universities

I.K. International Publishing House Pvt. Ltd.

NEW DELHI • BANGALORE

Published by

I.K. International Publishing House Pvt. Ltd.
S-25, Green Park Extension
Uphaar Cinema Market
New Delhi - 110 016 (India)
E-mail: ik_in@vsnl.net

ISBN 978-81-906566-3-4 (Vol. 2)
      978-81-906566-1-0 (Set)

© 2008 I.K. International Publishing House Pvt. Ltd.

Published by Krishan Makhijani for I.K. International Publishing House Pvt. Ltd., S-25, Green Park Extension, Uphaar Cinema Market, New Delhi - 110 016 and Printed by Rekha Printers Pvt. Ltd., Okhla Industrial Area, Phase II, New Delhi - 110 020.

This Volume is Dedicated to

Late Prof. Dharam Narayan

M.S., F.A.M.S.

Formerly Head
Department of Anatomy
King George's Medical College, Lucknow

Preface

The present book encompasses different sub-divisions of anatomy to enable medical students to learn all the relevant aspects of topics like osteology, soft parts, development and clinical application at the same time, since they have been dealt with exhaustively. It is common knowledge that bone carries our anatomy and forms its central part. As such, each topic begins with a brief description of the skeletal framework of the region followed by the description of the surrounding soft parts. The study of soft parts does not merely lie in cramming of relations of structures but it essentially relies on visualization of parts and regions based on dissection and diagrams. Anatomy, if not understood in its proper perspective and only memorised in parts, tends to be forgotten. Anatomy per se is a visual science and the best methods of visual recall of structural interrelationship are simple diagrams. Line diagrams which can be easily reproduced constitute an important feature of the book. Besides, this book is profusely illustrated with diagrams to serve as the reader's delight. Every mutual relationship of soft structures has been explained by well-placed diagrams.

The book also caters to the exam-oriented needs of students. It is widely recognised by the knowledgeable people that anatomy can be made interesting, easy to understand and to assimilate by dealing with its clinical applications. At the end of each topic under the heading Clinical Application, close relationships existing between the regional anatomy and clinical medicine are explained. Thus, the book is meant to be very useful to the students during their clinical years.

It is hoped that the book will be highly useful for students of Human Anatomy.

— A. HALIM

Acknowledgements

First and foremost, I must acknowledge the encouragement which my students gave me in writing these volumes on the Anatomy of the human body incorporating my lecture diagrams. The subject of anatomy by its very nature is a visual one and the best means of visual recall are dissections and simple line diagrams. Originally, the illustrations in this book were drawn by me and then redrawn in an accurate and artistic manner by Late Mr. G. C. Das under my critical supervision. Mr. G.C. Das was a medical artist who served in the Department of Anatomy, King George's Medical College, Lucknow. I count myself most fortunate in having his assistance throughout the preparation of this book. The diagrams in the new edition have been redrawn by Mr. Sunil Dutt who is an eminent medical artist. I am thankful to him for further improving the diagrams.

My sincere thanks are due to the staff of I.K. International Publishing House Pvt. Ltd.

— A. HALIM

Contents

SECTION–I
Abdomen

1. Bones of Abdomen and Pelvis   **1-12**
2. Abdomen: Anterior Abdominal Wall   **13-28**
3. Posterior Abdominal Wall: Muscles, Nerves and Vessels   **29-47**
4. The Peritoneum   **48-64**
5. Abdominal Viscera: Kidneys, Ureters and Suprarenals   **65-76**
6. Gastrointestinal Tract   **77-97**
7. Liver, Extrahepatic Biliary Apparatus, Pancreas and Spleen   **98-114**
8. The Pelvis: Walls, Nerves, Vessels and Floor   **115-124**
9. Pelvic Peritoneum and Pelvic Viscera   **125-158**
10. The Perineum and the Joints of Pelvis   **159-186**

SECTION–II
Lower Limb

11. The Bones of the Lower Limbs   **189-225**
12. Lower Limb—Front of Thigh   **226-245**
13. The Gluteal Region, Back of the Thigh and the Popliteal Fossa   **246-259**
14. Hip Joint   **260-264**
15. Front of the Leg and the Dorsum of the Food   **265-277**
16. Back of the Leg, Knee, Tibiofibular and Ankle Joints   **278-298**
17. Sole of the Foot, Joints and Arches of Foot   **299-314**
18. The Venous and Lymphatic Drainage and Segmental Innervation of Lower Limb   **315-318**

Index   **319-328**

SECTION—I
ABDOMEN

1

Bones of Abdomen and Pelvis

THE LUMBAR VERTEBRAE

The lumbar vertebrae are five in number.

GENERAL FEATURES (FIG. 1.1)

They have :
- massive body, the transverse diameter being more than the anteroposterior,
- absence of foramen transversarium,
- absence of costal facets on body,
- triangular vertebral foramen,
- quadrangular spinous process which projects horizontally backwards being thickened along the posterior and inferior borders,
- concave facets on the superior articular processes which face medially and backwards,
- convex facets on the inferior articular processes which face laterally and forwards,
- thin and long transverse processes (except in 5th lumbar) and
- presence of a small rough elevation, the *accessory process*, on the postero-inferior part of the root of each transverse process.

The fifth lumbar vertebra is atypical; the rest are typical.

ATTACHMENTS AND RELATIONS

BODY

Upper and lower surfaces : These are :
- covered with *articular cartilage*, and
- related to *intervertebral disc.* (Fig. 1.2).

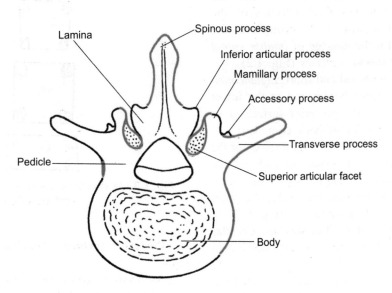

Lamina

Spinous process

Inferior articular process

Mamillary process

Accessory process

Pedicle

Transverse process

Superior articular facet

Body

Fig. 1.1 : Typical lumbar vertebra—superior aspect.

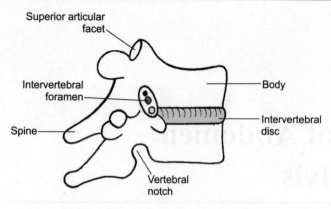

Fig. 1.2 : Lumbar vertebra—lateral view

Upper and lower borders :
- Anteriorly : Attachment of *anterior longitudinal ligament*.
- Lateral to above : Origin of *psoas major* and its *tendinous arch* (Fig. 1.5).
- Posteriorly : Attachment of *posterior longitudinal ligament*.

Anterior surface : (Fig. 1.5)
- Area around midline : Attachment of *anterior longitudinal ligament*.
- On either side of above : Attachment of *crura of diaphragm* (right crus on L_1-L_3 and left on L_{1-2}).
- Further laterally : Related to *lumbar arteries* (under the tendinous arch of psoas major). (Fig. 1.5)

PEDICLES : These are short but thick. The superior vertebral notches are shallow but the inferior ones are deep. With corresponding vertebral notches of the vertebrae above and below they complete the intervertebral foramina for the passage of *lumbar spinal nerves* and *branches of lumbar arteries* (Fig. 1.2).

LAMINAE : These are broad and short. *Ligamentum flava* is attached to the upper border and to the lower half of the anterior surface. The posterior surface gives attachment to the *deep muscles* of back (Fig. 1.6).

VERTEBRAL CANAL : The vertebral foramen of the first lumbar vertebra lodges the *conus medullaris* (the terminal part of the spinal cord) and the *spinal meninges*; those of the remaining lumbar vertebrae lodge the *filum terminale, couda equina* and the *meninges* (Fig. 1.7).

ARTICULAR PROCESSES : The superior articular processes are farther apart than the inferior ones but in the fifth lumbar vertebra the reverse is the case while in the fourth the distances are almost equal. The articular surfaces face laterally. The posterior border of each

superior articular process shows a rough elevation called the *mamillary process* (Fig. 1.1). It gives attachment to the *multifidus* and *medial intertransverse* muscles.

SPINOUS PROCESS : It is short, rectangular and almost horizontal. The tip gives attachment to the *posterior lamella of thoracolumbar fascia* on either side of the midline and to the *supraspinous ligament* in the midline; the sides to *erector spinae, multifidus* and other *deep muscles* of back (Fig. 1.17).

TRANSVERSE PROCESS : Each transverse process is thin and elongated. A small rough elevation is present on the postero-inferior aspect of the root. This is called the *accessory process*.

Tip : Attachment of *middle lamella of thoracolumbar fascia*. In addition, the tip of the first lumbar transverse process gives attachments to the *medial* and *lateral arcuate ligaments* (Fig. 1.2).

Anterior surface : It presents a nearly vertical ridge about its middle (Fig. 1.2).
- On the ridge: Attachment of *anterior lamella of thoracolumbar fascia*.
- Lateral to ridge : Insertion of *quadratus lumborum*.
- Medial to ridge : Origin of *psoas major*.

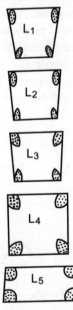

Fig. 1.3 : Dotted areas represent articular processes of lumbar vertebrae.

Posterior surface : Attachment of *deep muscles* of back.

Accessory process : Attachment of *medial intertransverse* muscle.

Upper and lower borders : Attachment of *lateral intertransverse* muscle.

CHARACTERISTICS OF THE FIFTH LUMBAR VERTEBRA : These are (Fig. 1.4).

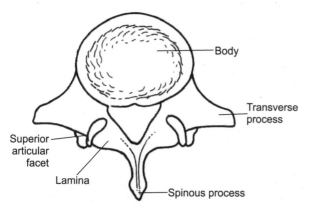

Fig. 1.4 : Fifth lumbar vertebra.

• Strong and stout transverse processes connected to the whole of the pedicle and partly to the body as well.

• The distance between the inferior articular processes is equal to or more than that between the superior articular process (Fig. 1.3).

• The body is much deeper anteriorly than posteriorly (due to the lumbosacral angle).

In addition to other attachments, the tip and the lower part of the anterior surface of the transverse processes of the firth lumbar vertebra give attachment to the *iliolumbar ligament.*

THE SACRUM

GENERAL FEATURES (FIG. 1.8, 1.9 & 1.10)

FORMATION : The sacrum is formed by the fusion of five sacral vertebrae but it may consist of six. Sometimes the coccyx is also fused with it.

GENERAL FORM : It is wedge shaped and placed between the two hip bones, the base of the wedge being directed superiorly and the apex inferiorly.

ANATOMICAL POSITION : The bone lies at an angle with the fifth lumbar vertebra so that the ventral surface looks forwards and downwards (Fig. 1.10).

SURFACES : It possesses a *base* an *apex*, a *pelvic* or *ventral*, a *dorsal*, and *two lateral surfaces* and encloses a canal, the *sacral canal.*

Base : It is formed by the upper surface of the first sacral vertebra.

The **anterior portion of the central part** represents the body which is large, lumbar in type (tranverse diameter being greater than the anteroposterior). It has an anterior projection called the *promontory.* The body is covered with articular cartilage and is related to the

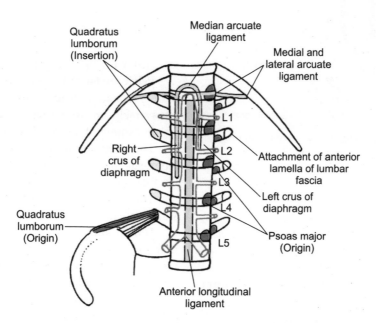

Fig. 1.5 : Ventral aspect of the lumbar part of vertebral column.

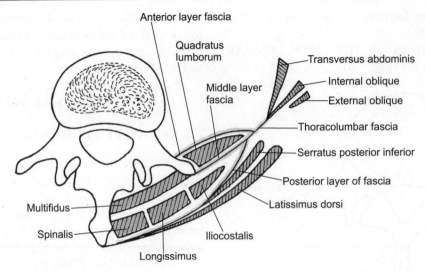

Fig. 1.6 : Relations of spines, pedicles, laminae and transverse processes of lumbar vertebrae.

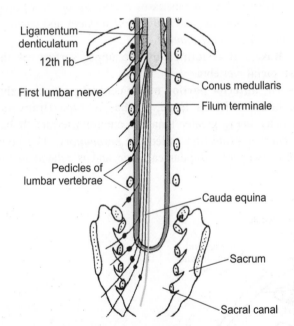

Fig. 1.7 : Contents of the vertebral canal of the lumbar region and of sacral canal.

intervertebral disc which is specially thick anteriorly causing the *lumbosacral angle (sacrovertebral angle)* which measures about 210°. The anterior and posterior surfaces of the body give attachment to the *anterior* and *posterior longitudinal ligaments*.

The **posterior portion of the central part** represents the vertebral arch of the first sacral vertebra. The pedicles are directed backwards and laterally while the *laminae* are directed backwards medially and

downwards so that the *vertebral foramen* is triangular in shape. The *superior articular processes* projecting upwards bear concave articular facets for articulation with the inferior articular processes of the fifth lumbar vertebra. The lateral aspect of each process is rough and corresponds to the mamillary process.

The rest of the base on either side of the body is known as the **ala** and is formed by the fusion of the transverse process and costal element of the primitive vertebra. The ala can be subdivided into a smooth medial part and a rough lateral part.

Apex : The apex represents the inferior surface of the body of the fifth sacral vertebra and articulates with the body of the coccyx. Sometimes, however, the latter is fused with the sacrum.

Pelvic surface : It is directed downwards and forwards and is concave from above downwards as well as transversely but to a slight extent.

It exhibits **4 pairs of anterior sacral foramina**.

The **median area between the sacral foramina** represents the anterior surfaces of the sacral vertebrae and the four transverse ridges in between indicate their fusion.

The surface lateral to the sacral foramina on each side, represents a fusion of the costal elements.

Dorsal surface : The dorsal surface in the midline is raised to form the median sacral crest which represents the fused spinous processes.

On either side of the median sacral crest and in line with the articular processes of the first sacral vertebra is present a tuberculated ridge forming the **intermediate sacral crest**. It represents the fused articular processes

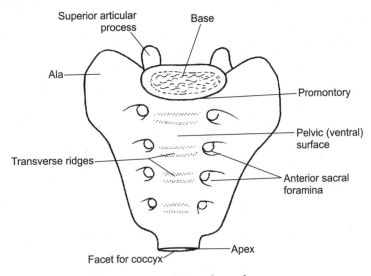

Fig. 1.8 : The pelvic surface of sacrum.

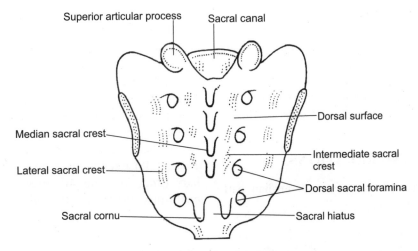

Fig. 1.9 : The dorsal surface of sacrum.

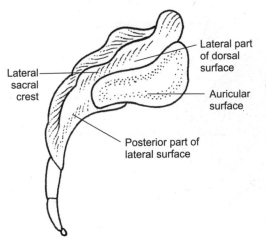

Fig. 1.10 : The three constituents of lateral surface of sacrum.

and the tubercles are called *articular tubercles*. The area between the median and intermediate sacral crests represents the *fused laminae*.

Lateral to the intermediate sacral crest are 4 pairs of dorsal sacral foramina representing the dorsal parts of the intervertebral foramina.

Lateral to the dorsal foramina, on each side is another tuberculated crest, the **lateral sacral crest**, which represents the fused transverse processes. The tubercles are called *transverse tubercles*.

Sacral canal : The upper end of the dorsal surface of the bone in the midline shows a V-shaped opening which leads into the sacral canal. The canal represents the vertebral foramina of the sacral vertebrae.

The lower end of the sacral canal opens out through

a U-shaped opening of the dorsal surface of the bone. It is known as the **sacral hiatus**. The hiatus is caused by the failure of the laminae of the 5th sacral vertebra to unite. The free ends of the hiatus are known as the **sacral cornua** and represent the inferior articular processes of the 5th sacral vertebra.

Lateral surface : It includes the lateral part of the dorsal surface (lateral to the lateral sacral crest) and the lateral surface proper of the bone and represents a fusion of the transverse and costal elements.

The **anterior portion of the surface** in its upper part upto a variable extent of the 3rd piece of sacrum is occupied by the **auricular surface** which is covered with articular cartilage and articulates with the hip bone to form the sacro-iliac joint.

The **posterior part of the surface** upto the lower limit of the auricular surface gives attachment to the *interosseous* and *dorsal sacro-iliac ligaments*.

The **lower part of the surface** is a thin border and provides attachments to the *coccygeus* muscle, *sacrospinous* and *sacrotuberous ligaments* and *gluteus maximus* muscle in that order from before backwards.

The **anterior and inferior margins of the auricular surface** give attachment to the *anterior sacro-iliac ligament*.

ATTACHMENTS AND RELATIONS

The ala can be subdivided into a smooth median part and a rough lateral part.

Smooth area : It is related to the *lumbosacral trunk* medially and *iliolumbar vessels* laterally. The *sympathetic trunk* crosses the bone medial to the lumbosacral trunk while the *obturator nerve* is lateral to the iliolumbar vessels (Fig. 1.11).

Rough area : Gives origin to part of the *iliacus* muscle anteriorly and attachment to the *lumbosacral* and *anterior (ventral) sacro-iliac ligaments* posteriorly.

Both areas are covered by the *psoas major* muscle.

Pelvic surface : The 4 pairs of anterior sacral foramina give exit to the *anterior primary rami of the upper four sacral nerves* and entry to the *lateral sacral arteries* (Fig. 1.11).

The median area between the sacral foramina (Fig. 1.12) is related the *median sacral artery*. On each side, just medial to the sacral foramina, is related the *sympathetic trunk*. The upper two and half pieces of the bone are related to the *peritoneum* and the root of the *pelvic mesocolon* (sympathetic trunks and median sacral artery intervening). The lower two and half pieces are related to the *posterior surface of the rectum* but the *superior rectal artery* intervenes up to a variable level.

The **surface lateral to the sacral foramina**, (Fig. 1.11). The *lateral sacral vessels* are related along the long axis of the bone just lateral to the anterior sacral foramina. The *piriformis* muscle takes origin from the bars of bone between the 1st and 2nd, 2nd and 3rd and 3rd and 4th foramina and from the area lateral to these bars (2nd, 3rd and 4th pieces of sacrum). On the piriformis muscle lie the *lumbosacral trunk* and the

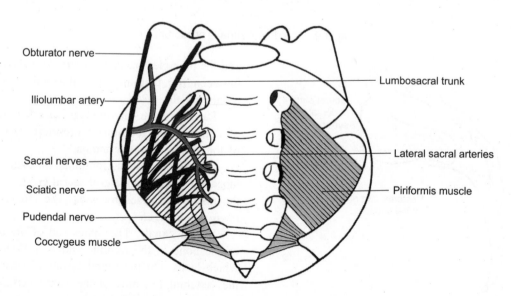

Fig. 1.11 : Relations of the lateral area of the pelvic surface of sacrum.

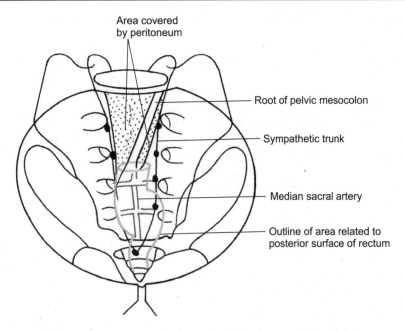

Fig. 1.12 : Relations of median area of sacrum between the sacral foramnia.

ventral primary rami of the upper three sacral nerves. The muscle and the nerves are covered by the *fascia of piriformis* which is attached to the bone just medial to the anterior sacral foramina. On the fascia lie the *branches of internal iliac artery* and *corresponding veins.*

Dorsal surface : In the midline the (Fig. 1.13) **median sacral crest** gives attachment to the *erector spinae* muscle and *posterior layer of thoracolumbar fascia.*

4 pairs of dorsal sacral foramina representing the dorsal parts of the intervertebral foramina which give exit to the *dorsal rami of the upper four sacral nerves.*

The *erector spinae* muscle takes origin in a U-shaped

manner from the lateral and median sacral crests, the horizontal limb of the U corresponding to a line passing just above the 4th dorsal foramen. The area enclosed by the U gives origin to the *multifidus* muscle.

Sacral canal (Fig. 1.7) : It contains the *filum terminale, cauda equina* and the *meninges of the spinal cord.* Of the meaninges, the pia mater forms a close investment for the filum terminale throughout the canal but the dura and arachnoid form a close investment only below the level of the lower border of the 2nd sacral vertebra. Above this level, they are separated from the filum and the pia mater by the *subarachnoid space.* Hence the subdural and the subarachnoid spaces end at the lower border of the 2nd sacral vertebra.

Each cornu of the sacral hiatus gives attachment to the *intercornual ligament* which connects it to the corresponding coccygeal cornu. The sacral hiatus gives exit to the *filum terminale* invested by the dura, arachnoid and pia and to the *fifth sacral* and *coccygeal nerves.*

Each *fifth sacral nerve*, after it comes out of the sacral hiatus, passes under the intercornual ligament and divides into the anterior and posterior primary rami.

Each *coccygeal nerve*, after it comes out of the sacral hiatus, curves around the coccygeal cornu.

Lateral Surface (Fig. 1.10)

The **anterior portion of the surface** in its upper part

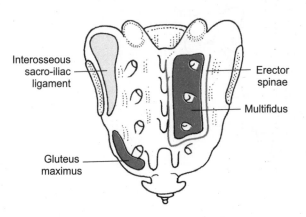

Fig. 1.13 : Attachments on dorsal surface of sacrum.

upto a variable extent of the 3rd piece of sacrum is occupied by the **auricular surface** which is covered with articular cartilage and articulates with the hip bone to form the sacro-iliac joint.

The **posterior part of the surface** upto the lower limit of the auricular surface gives attachment to the *interosseous* and *dorsal sacro-iliac ligaments* (Fig. 1.14).

The **lower part of the surface** is a thin border and provides attachments to the *coccygeus* muscle, *sacrospinous* and *sacrotuberous ligaments* and *gluteus maximus* muscle in that order from before backwards (Fig. 1.13).

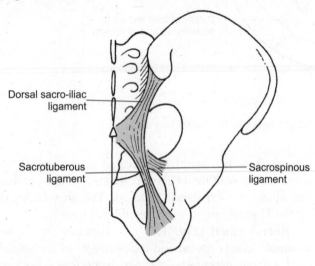

Fig. 1.14 : Attachments of dorsal surface of sacrum

The **anterior and inferior margins of the auricular surface** give attachment to the *anterior sacro-iliac ligament*.

SEX DIFFERENTIATION : This has medicolegal importance.

1. The sacrum is shorter and wider in females.
2. The concavity of sacrum is deeper in females.
3. The auricular surface occupies the upper three sacral segments in both the sexes but is less extensive in females.
4. The sacral index is greater in females.

$$\text{Sacral index} = \frac{\text{Breadth of sacrum at base}}{\text{Length of sacrum}} \times 100$$

N.B. : The sacral index is the most important criterion.

Variations

* The sacrum may consist of six pieces due to:
  - an inclusion of the 5th lumbar vertebra or
  - an extra piece of sacrum or
  - an inclusion of the coccyx in which case the intercornual ligament is ossified.
* The dorsal wall of the sacral canal may be partially wanting due to a lack of fusion of the laminae.

THE COCCYX

The coccyx, triangular in shape, is formed by the fusion of four rudimentary vertebrae but the number may be three or five. The bone has a base, a tip and pelvic and dorsal surfaces (Fig. 1.8).

BASE : The base is formed by the upper surface of the body of the first coccygeal vertebra. It possesses an *oval articular facet* for the apex of the sacrum. Dorsilateral to the facet, on each side, is an upward projection, the *coccygeal cornu*, which articulates with the corresponding sacral cornu and gives attachment to

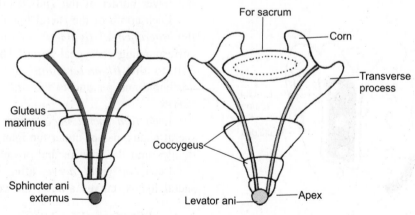

Coccyx: Dorsal surface   Coccyx: Pelvic surface

Fig. 1.15 : Coccyx: Pelvic and dorsal surfaces

the *intercornual ligament*. A lateral projection on each side of the body represents a rudimentary transverse process. It may fuse with the inferolateral angle of the sacrum in which case the sacrum possesses five foramina.

PELVIC SURFACE : It gives attachment to the *ventral sacrococcygeal ligament* just below the base and origin (on each side) to the *levator ani* and *coccygeus* muscles.

DORSAL SURFACE : It has the following attachments.

On each side : *Gluteus maximus* muscle (origin).

At the tip : *Sphincter ani externus*.

Median area : *Dorsal sacrococcygeal ligaments* and *filum terminale*.

THE BONY PELVIS

The word pelvis literally means a basin. Anatomically, it signifies the articulated bony structure comprising the two hip bones, the sacrum and the coccyx. It is situated at the lower end of the verteberal column which it supports and rests on the heads of the femora or in other words, the lower limbs.

POSITION OF PELVIS IN ERECT POSTURE (ANATOMICAL POSITION) : The pubic tubercles and the anterior superior iliac spines lie in the same vertical plane and the pubic symphysis is in the midline. Held in this position, the concavity of the sacrum faces downwards and forwards while the pelvic surface of pubic symphysis faces upwards and backwards.

PARTS OF PELVIS : It is divided into false (greater) and true (lesser) pelvis.

False pelvis : It is the part above and in front of the linea terminales (arcuate line of the ilium at the sides and the pecten pubis and the pubic crest in front) and the sacral promontory behind. Regionally, it is a part of the abdomen.

True pelvis : It is that part of the pelvis which lies below and behind the false pelvis. It is formed by parts of the hip bones (a part of ilium and the whole of ischium and pubis), the sacrum and the coccyx. The term 'pelvis' denotes the true pelvis.

ANATOMICAL AND OBSTERICAL PELVIS : As stated above, the anatomical pelvis includes the coccyx but in obstetrics the coccyx is ignored because of its mobility.

TRUE PELVIS : It has an inlet, a cavity and an outlet.

Inlet (Fig. 1.16) : Also known as the *pelvic brim*, it is bounded by the sacral promontory, anterior borders of the alae of the sacrum, linea terminales, pubic tubercles, pubic crests and the symphysis pubis in that order from behind forwards. Viewed from above, the inlet (synonym : *superior pelvic aperture*) looks heart-shaped because of the forward projection of the sacral promontory.

Cavity : It is a curved canal whose posterior wall is more than 10 cm long while the anterior wall is only 5 cm. It is bounded above and behind by the pelvic surface of the sacrum and coccyx, laterally by the pelvic surfaces of the ischium and part of the ilium

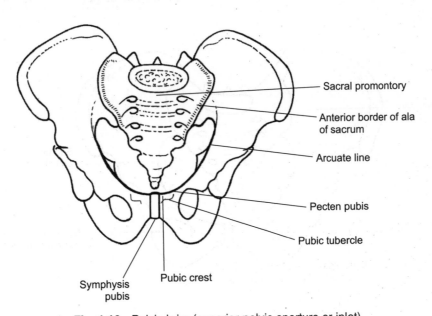

Fig. 1.16 : Pelvic brim (superior pelvic aperture or inlet)

and below and in front by the pubic rami and the symphysis pubis.

Outlet (Fig. 1.17) : Also known as the *inferior pelvic aperture*, it is roughly diamond shaped but is irregular in outline. It is bounded posteriorly by the tip of coccyx, laterally by the ischial tuberosities and anteriorly by the ischiopubic rami. The irregularities are caused by the greater and lesser sciatic notches which are converted into greater and lesser sciatic foramen by the sacrotuberous and sacrospinous ligaments in the recent state. The boundaries mentioned above are those of the *anatomical outlet*. The coccyx, because of its mobility, is ignored while considering the *obstetrical*

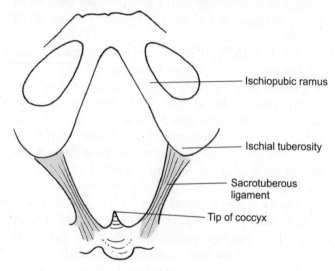

Fig. 1.17 : Inferior pelvic aperture.

outlet. Hence the posterior boundary is considered to be formed by the tip (apex) of the sacrum.

TILT (INCLINATION) OF THE PELVIS ON THE TRUNK (Fig. 8.1) : The pelvis in erect posture lies obliquely in relation to the trunk. The *plane of the pelvic inlet* (plane passing through the upper border of the symphysis pubis and the sacral promontory) forms an angle of about 60 degrees with the horizontal. The *plane of the pelvic outlet* (plane passing through the lower border of the symphysis pubis and the tip of the coccyx) forms an angle of 15 degree approximately. The former is of more practical interest because a greater inclination may give rise to obstetric complications.

The *axis of the inlet* which is a line drawn at right angles to the plane of the inlet at its centre is directed backwards and downwards. On projection it passes through the umbilicus and the middle of the coccyx. The *axis of the outlet* is directed downwards and very slightly backwards. The *axis of the pelvic cavity* is a curved line corresponding to the curvature of the pelvic surface of the sacrum and coccyx and is at right angles to a series of planes placed between the plane of the inlet and that of the outlet.

Functions of Pelvis

1. Weight transmission.
2. Locomotion.
3. Resistances to compressive forces.
4. Provision for muscular attachments.
5. Protection of pelvic viscera (secondary function).

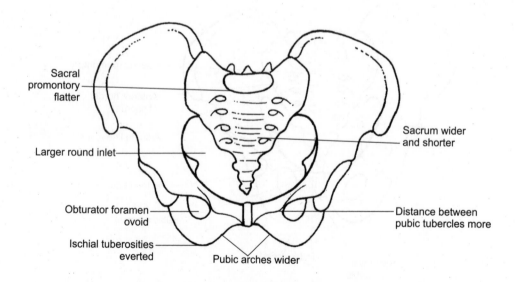

Fig. 1.18 : Female pelvis.

SEX DIFFERENCES IN ADULT PELVIS

	Female (Fig. 1.18)	Male (Fig. 1.19)
Inlet	Larger, bean-shaped/round because	Smaller, heart-shaped because
	1. Sacral promontory flatter	1. Sacral promontory more prominent
	2. Pubic tubercles wider apart	2. Pubic tubercles closer
Cavity	Wider and shallower because	Narrower and deeper because
	1. Pubic symphysis shorter	1. Pubic symphysis wider
	2. Sacrum wider and shorter, flatter in the upper part but sharply curved lower down.	2. Sacrum narrow and curved evenly
	3. Sciatic notches wider	3. Sciatic notches narrow
	4. Ischial spines less projecting inwards	4. Ischial spines more projecting inwards
	5. Distance between pubic tubercles more	5. Distance between pubic tubercles less
Outlet	Larger because	Smaller because
	1. Pubic arches wider (subpubic angle about a right angle)	1. Pubic arches narrower (subpubic angle about 60°)
	2. Ischial tuberosities and spines everted	2. Ischial tuberosities and spines inverted
	3. Coccyx more mobile	3. Coccyx less mobile
Ischiopubic rami	Less everted	More everted
Obturator foramen	Triangular	Ovoid/Oval
Preauricular sulcus	More constant and prominent	Less constant and less prominent
Auricular surface of sacrum	Occupies upper two segments and a small part of third	Occuppies upper two segments and a large part of third
Base of sacrum	Ratio between the transverse width of facet for fifth lumbar vertebra and that of the entire base of sacrum is more than 1 : 2	1 : 2 or less
Curvature of anterior surface of sacrum	1. Deeper	1. Shallower
	2. Less uniform	2. More uniform
	3. Upper part relatively flat with a sharp forward bend at level of middle of third sacral segment	
Sacral index	Greater	Less
$\left[\dfrac{\text{Breadth of base of sacrum}}{\text{Length of sacrum}} \times 100 \right]$		

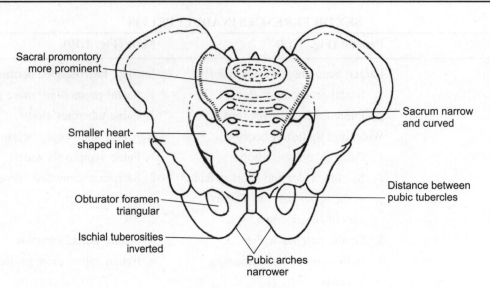

Sacral promontory more prominent

Sacrum narrow and curved

Smaller heart-shaped inlet

Distance between pubic tubercles

Obturator foramen triangular

Ischial tuberosities inverted

Pubic arches narrower

Fig. 1.19 : Male pelvis.

WEIGHT TRANSMISSION : The weight of the trunk reaches the lowest lumbar vertebra from where it is transmitted to the base of the sacrum. It then passes through the upper three sacral segments at which level the weight is divided into two halves (in case of standing posture with both feet planted firmly on the ground). Each half of the weight is transmitted across one sacro-iliac joint along the corresponding iliopectineal line to the femoral head. In the sitting posture the weight passes through the ilium to the ischial tuberosities.

2

Abdomen: Anterior Abdominal Wall

INTRODUCTION

Abdomen is the lower part of the trunk, thorax being the upper part. The diaphragm separates the two parts. Many abdominal viscera, although in the abdominal cavity and not in the thoracic cavity, are protected by the ribcage since the diaphragm arches upwards within the skeleton of the thorax.

The abdomen is divided into **abdomen proper** and **pelvis**. **Perineum,** the lowermost region of the trunk, is separated from the pelvic cavity by the pelvic diaphragm which forms the floor of the true pelvis.

ANTERIOR ABDOMINAL WALL

Bony Framework

The anterior abdominal wall extends from the inferior thoracic aperture (thoracic outlet) above to the inlet of the pelvis below.

- The thoracic outlet (Fig. 2.1) is bounded in front by the xiphoid process and on each side by the lower six costal

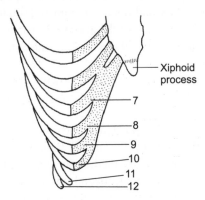

Fig. 2.1: The bony framework of the anterior abdominal wall: The thoracic outlet above

cartilages. The inlet of the pelvis (Fig. 2.2) is bounded in front by the pubic symphysis, the superior margin of the pubis, the anterior margin of the ilium and on each side of the iliac crest.
- To understand the inlet, it is necessary to understand the osteology of the hip bone first.

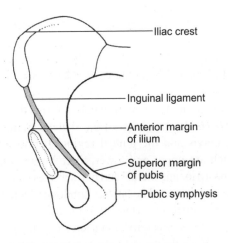

Fig. 2.2: The bony framework of the anterior abdominal wall: The inlet of pelvis below

The Hip Bone (Fig. 2.3)

The hip bone is a large, flat bone of irregular shape which articulates with the sacrum and with its fellow of the opposite side to form the bony pelvis. It also articulates with femur which is the bone of thigh in lower limb. Only those features of the bone which are concerned with the anatomy of abdomen and pelvis are described below.

The hip bone or innominate bone has three parts, the **ilium, pubis** and **ischium** which meet at the acetabular cavity which is a cup-shaped depression on the lateral surface. The ilium forms the upper part of the acetabulum

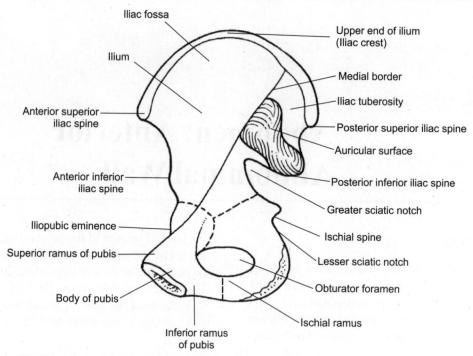

Fig. 2.3: Hip bone: The ventral aspect of the right hip bone showing general features

and the fan-shaped bone above it. The pubis constitutes the anterior part of the acetabulum and the part of the bone associated with it. The rest of the bone forms the ischium.

The *ILIUM* forms most of the skeletal framework of the false pelvis and the gluteal region. It possesses two ends which are upper and lower, three border which are anterior, posterior and medial and two surfaces named lateral or gluteal and medial. The latter is subdivided into the iliac fossa and sacropelvic surface by a medial border.

Upper end is expanded and seen from the top it is S-shaped. It is limited anteriorly and posteriorly by projections termed **anterior** and **posterior superior iliac spines** and is divisible into ventral and dorsal segments, the former forming the anterior two-thirds of it. The ventral segment is bounded by outer and inner lips enclosing between them an intermediate area. The outer lip exhibits a projection, about 5 cm behind the anterior superior iliac spine, known as the **tubercle of the iliac crest**. The dorsal segment possesses lateral and medial sloping surfaces separated by a prominent ridge.
- Lower end forms a part of the acetabulum.
- Anterior border extends between the anterior superior iliac spine and the acetabulum. Just above the latter it is marked by a rough projection, the **anterior inferior iliac spine**.

- Posterior border is longer and irregularly curved. It begins at the **posterior superior iliac spine** and then runs downwards and forwards to terminate at a small **posterior inferior iliac spine**. It then proceeds horizontally forwards and then turns abruptly downwards and backwards to form the **greater sciatic notch**. Lastly it becomes continuous with the posterior border of ischium.
- Medial border is present on the medial surface and separates the **iliac fossa** from the **sacropelvic surface**. Rough and indistinct in the upper part, it becomes sharp where it forms the anterior boundary of the sacral articular surface and finally smooth and rounded where it forms the iliac part of the **arcuate line** (boundary line between the true and false pelvis). It ends at the **iliopubic eminence**.
- Lateral surface of ilium is also known as gluteal surface since it gives attachment to the major muscles of the gluteal region.
- Medial surface is divided into iliac fossa and sacropelvic surface. **Iliac fossa** is the smooth hollowed out anterior and upper part of the medial surface limited by the anterior border in front, medial border behind and the ventral part of the iliac crest above. It forms the lateral wall of the false pelvis. **Sacropelvic surface** forms the

lower and posterior part of the medial surface and is bounded below and behind by the posterior border, above and in front by the medial border and above and behind by the dorsal segment of the iliac crest.

Sacropelvic surface is divided into three areas:
(i) Iliac tuberosity is the area below the iliac crest giving attachment to various ligaments, (ii) Auricular surface situated below and in front of the iliac tuberosity articulating with the sacrum, and (iii) Pelvic surface is the smooth area in front of and below the auricular surface forming a part of the true pelvis.

The *PUBIS* forms the anterior part of the hip bone. It has a body which articulates with the pubis of the opposite side to form the symphysis pubis, a superior ramus which is directed upwards and backwards to meet the ilium and ischium at the acetabulum and an inferior ramus which runs backwards, downwards and laterally to meet the ramus of the ischium and constitutes the ischiopubic ramus.

The anteroposteriorly flattened body forms the anterior wall of true pelvis. The rounded upper border of the body known as the **pubic crest** ends laterally in a blunt projection termed the **pubic tubercle** which gives attachment to the medial end of the inguinal ligament and ascending limb of the loops of cremaster muscle. The pubic crest has anterior and posterior borders which enclose a surface and meet at the pubic tubercle. The anterior border of the pubic crest gives attachment to the anterior wall of the **rectus sheath** and the **conjoint tendon**. The surface gives origin to lateral head of **rectus abdominis** and **pyramidalis** laterally. Medially, it is related to the medial head of **rectus abdominis** (Fig. 2.12).
• The sharp border of the superior ramus which runs from the **pubic tubercle** to the arcuate line is known as **pectineal line**. Together with the pubic crest, it forms the pubic part of the arcuate line. Pelvic surface of the superior ramus is bounded above by the pectineal line and below by its inferior border.

The **ISCHIUM** forms the lower and posterior part of the hip bone and consists of a body and ramus. The ramus extends upwards, forwards and medially from the lower part of the body, forms the lower boundary of the obturator foramen and meets the inferior ramus of the pubic to form the **ischiopubic ramus**. The pelvic surface of the body is bounded in front by the margin of the obturator foramen and behind by its posterior border which is a continuation of the posterior border of ilium and runs first downwards and backwards to complete the lower margin of the **greater**

sciatic notch. The posterior border forms a projection termed the **ischial spine** below which it forms the **lesser sciatic notch**.

Obturator foramen is a gap in the hip bone. It is bounded above and in front by the superior ramus and body of the pubis, medially and below by the ischiopubic ramus, behind by the body of ischium and above by the inferior margin of the acetabulum. It is large and oval in the male but smaller and triangular in the female. In the recent state it is closed by the **obturator membrane** except superiorly where there is a gap known as the **obturator canal**.

Superficial Fascia

Midway between the umbilicus and pubis the superficial fascia is condensed on its deep surface to form a membranous layer. So it has two layers in this part of the anterior abdominal wall.
• A fatty layer (**Camper's fascia**) and a membranous layer (**Scarpa's fascia**) Fig. 2.4.

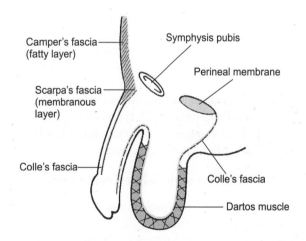

Fig. 2.4: Anatomy of the fascial layers of the anterior abdominal wall

• **Superficial fatty layer** (Camper's fascia) has a variable amount of fat. It contains the superficial blood vessels, nerves, lymphatics and is continuous with the superficial fascia of the rest of the body but is especially fatty in the abdomen. Over the pubis it continues as the superficial layer of the superficial perineal fascia. Just below the superficial inguinal ring it gives place to the **dartos muscle** of the scrotum which contains smooth muscle fibres. There is no subcutaneous fat in the penis or scrotum.

- **Deep membranous layer** (Scarpa's fascia) is a fibrous layer (Fig. 2.5). It is present only on the anterior abdominal wall. It is disposed as follows:
- **Superiorly:** It fades away midway between the pubis and umbilicus above.

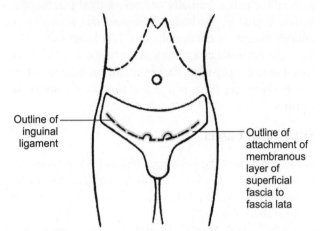

Fig. 2.5: Scarpa's membranous fascia is like front half of a pair of underwear

- **Laterally:** It fades away in the lumbar region.
- **Inferiorly:** In the lateral part it passes over the inguinal ligament into the upper thigh, where it is attached to the fascia lata just below and parallel to the inguinal ligament (Fig. 2.6).
- In the intermediate position it passes downwards over the front of the pubis as a flattened funnel-shaped extension and changes its name to **Colle's fascia** (deep layer of superficial perineal fascia).

Colle's Fascia (Superficial Perineal Fascia)

Just below the superficial inguinal ring, the Scarpa's fascia is known as Colle's fascia (Fig. 2.4). In the perineum it covers the penis only up to the glans, gives a fascial covering to the scrotum under the dartos muscle; it then covers the muscles in the superficial compartment of the perineum.

Attachments

- **Superiorly:** Continuous with the fascia of scarpa.
- **Inferiorly:** Attached to the posterior border of the urogenital diaphragm.
- **Laterally:** Attached to the conjoined ischiopubic ramus.
- **Medially:** Continuous with its fellow of the opposite side.

    The extent of the Scarpa's and Colle's fascia can be compared to only the front of a half of a pair of underpants as they are present only on the anterior abdomen and perineum.

CLINICAL APPLICATION

- Scarpa's fascia contains fibrous tissue which may provide support for sutures during wound closure of the abdomen.
- In rupture of urethra in the perineum the urine is extravasated under Colle's fascia and due to arrangement of the fasciae extends as follow:
- Downwards it can extend to the lower border of the urogenital diaphragm as here the Colle's fascia fuses with the base of the diaphragm.
- Laterally it extends up to the combined ischiopubic rami because of the attachment of Colle's fascia there.
- Upwards it extends over the penis and scrotum because they are covered by Colle's fascia.
- It then extends upwards alongside the spermatic cord onto the anterior abdominal wall because Colle's fascia is continuous with the Scarpa's fascia without any attachment to pubis.
- Urine collects under the Scarpa's fascia and extends down over the inguinal ligament, until it is held up by the attachment of Scarpa's fascia to fascia lata. This attachment does not allow the urine to enter the thigh.

Cutaneous Nerves (Fig. 2.6)

The skin of the anterior abdominal wall is supplied by the ventral rami of lower six thoracic nerves and first lumbar

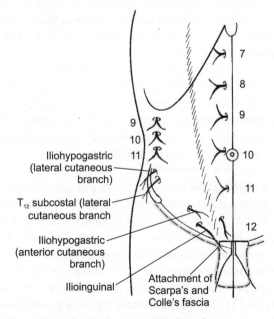

Fig. 2.6: Anterior abdominal wall: Cutaneous nerves and attachment of membranous layer of superficial fascia

nerve. They have anterior and lateral cutaneous branches arranged in anterior and lateral series.

In the anterior series, which appear close to the midline, are the anterior cutaneous branches of lower five intercostal nerves (T_7 to T_{11}) and the **subcostal** (T_{12}) and **iliohypogastric** (L_1) and also terminal part of the **ilioinguinal** (L_1) nerves. T_{10} is at the level of umbilicus and T_{12} ends by supplying the skin of pubis. The iliohypogastric (L_1) appears 2.5 cm above the superficial inguinal ring and the ilioinguinal (L_1) emerges through the ring to supply the skin over the femoral triangle.

In the lateral series are the lateral cutaneous branches of the lower three intercostal (T_9 to T_{11}) and the subcostal (T_{12}). The lateral cutaneous branch of L_1 crosses the iliac crest to supply the superolateral part of the buttocks.

Cutaneous Arteries (Fig. 2.7)

There are three superficial and three deep arteries in the anterior abdominal wall.
- Superficial arteries are branches of the femoral artery and supply skin and superficial fascia below the umbilicus:
  - Superficial external pudendal runs medially to supply the skin of the scrotum **(or labium majus)** and penis.
  - Superficial epigastric runs superomedially, across the inguinal ligament, up to the umbilicus.
  - Superficial circumflex iliac runs towards the anterior superior iliac spine.

Apart from these there are small arteries that accompany the lateral cutaneous branches of the thoracic nerves. They are derived from the posterior intercostal arteries. The small arteries which accompany the anterior cutaneous nerves are derived from the superior and inferior epigastric arteries which are within the rectus sheath.
- Deep arteries are three in number:
  - Superior epigastric arises from the internal thoracic artery and enters the rectus sheath at its upper end.
  - Inferior epigastric is a branch of the external iliac entering through the lower end of the rectus sheath.
  - Deep circumflex iliac arises from the external iliac immediately above the inguinal ligament and ascends to the anterior superior iliac spine.

Superficial Lymphatics (Fig. 2.8)

A divide line surrounds the body at the level of the umbilicus. Lymphatics draining the skin above the line enter the axillary nodes. Those below the umbilicus enter the inguinal nodes. There are no lymph nodes in the abdominal wall to correspond to the intercostal nodes of the thoracic wall.

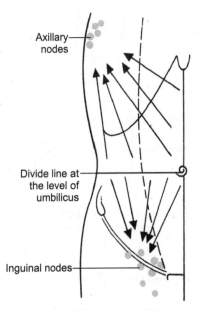

Fig. 2.8: Anterior abdominal wall: Superficial component of the lymph system – drainage of the skin of right quadrants and its watersheds

CLINICAL APPLICATION

A malignant melanoma of skin situated at the level of umbilicus may spread to lymph nodes in both axillae and inguinal regions as the drainage of the abdominal wall is in quadrants.

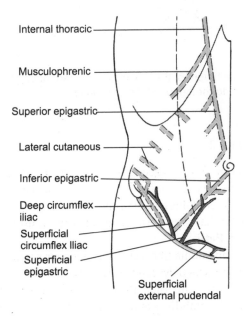

Fig. 2.7: Anterior abdominal wall: Superficial and deep arteries

MUSCLES OF THE ANTERIOR ABDOMINAL WALL

The muscles of the anterior abdominal wall are arranged mainly in three concentric sheet-like layers, the fibres of which run in different directions thus increasing the strength of this wall (Fig. 2.9). From without inwards, these are the **external** and **internal oblique** and **transversus abdominis**. On either side of the median plane there is a longitudinal strap-like muscle, the **rectus abdominis**. In general, each of the sheet-like muscle consists of muscle fibres laterally and aponeurosis medially. The aponeuroses interlace in the median plane to form a dense zone of connective tissue extending from the xiphoid process to the pubic symphysis. It is called **linea alba** due to its white appearance.

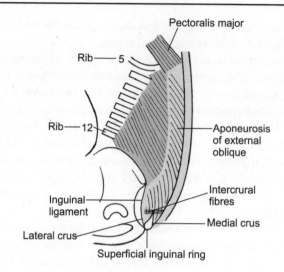

Fig. 2.10: External oblique: Side view showing origin from lower eight ribs. The last slip presents a free margin

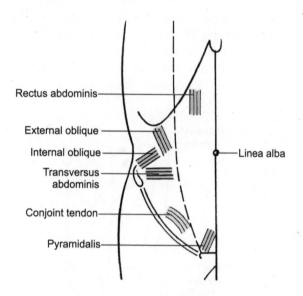

Fig. 2.9: Muscles of anterior abdominal wall and the direction of their fibres

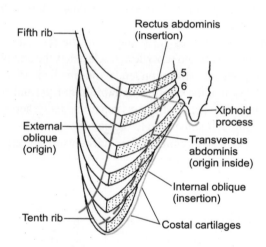

Fig. 2.11: Attachment of the muscles of anterior abdominal to the bones of thoracic outlet

External Oblique (Fig. 2.10)

It forms the outer layer of the abdominal wall musculature and has fibres which run downwards, forwards and medially. The muscle layer becomes aponeurotic at approximately the midclavicular line.

Origin (Fig. 2.11)

- By eight digitations one from each of the lower eight ribs just lateral to their anterior extremities. Laterally the upper interdigitate with serratus anterior and the lower with those of latissimus dorsi.

Insertion (Fig. 2.12)

- The posterior fibres descend almost vertically to get inserted into the anterior half of the iliac crest. The free posterior border of this part of the muscle with latissimus dorsi and the iliac crest form the boundaries of **lumbar triangle of Petit**.
- The upper and middle fibres end in an aponeurosis along an angled line which descends vertically from the ninth costal cartilage and then turns laterally along the line joining the umbilicus and the anterior superior iliac spine.

It is disposed of as follows:
- Medially it forms the anterior wall of the rectus sheath, by running superficial to rectus abdominis and the aponeurosis of internal oblique and transversus abdominis (Fig. 2.18). Finally it gets inserted into the pubic crest and tubercle and linea alba by decussating with the fibres of contralateral aponeurosis.
- The lower margin of the aponeurosis between the anterior superior iliac spine and pubic tubercle rolls under to form the inguinal ligament (Poupart).

There are three structures at the medial end of inguinal ligament (Fig. 2.12):
- Lacunar or Gimbernat's ligament: It is a triangular, horizontal, fibrous structure which lies in the angle between the medial end of the inguinal ligament and the pectineal line of pubis.
- Pectineal ligament (ligament of Cooper): The lateral free edge of Gimbernat's ligament extends laterally along the pectineal line to form the Cooper's ligament.
- Reflected part of the inguinal ligament: It is the part which passes upwards and medially from the medial end of the inguinal ligament behind the medial crus of the superficial ring and the spermatic cord (in the male) or round ligament (in the female) to the linea alba.

About 7.5 cm above and lateral to the pubic tubercle there is a triangular opening in the aponeurosis known as the **superficial inguinal ring**. Here the aponeurosis splits into two crurae.
- The lateral crus inserts into the pubic tubercle, with some tendinous fibres reflected to the superior ramus of pubis as the lacunar ligament **(Gimbernat's)**.
- The medial crus inserts into the pubic symphysis.
- Intercrural fibres strengthen the apex of the superficial ring.

The superficial inguinal ring transmits the spermatic cord in the male or the round ligament of the uterus in the female. It is the medial end of a canal in the anterior abdominal wall lying above the medial half of the inguinal ligament and known as **inguinal canal**.

Internal Oblique (Fig. 2.13)

It is the intermediate layer of abdominal wall musculature. Its fibres pass upwards and inwards at right angles to the fibres of external oblique thereby crossing each other like the limbs of the letter X.

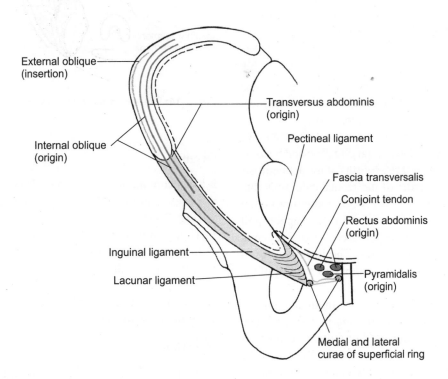

Fig. 2.12: The lower abdominal collar to show the attachment of muscle layers on iliac crest, inguinal ligament and pubic crest

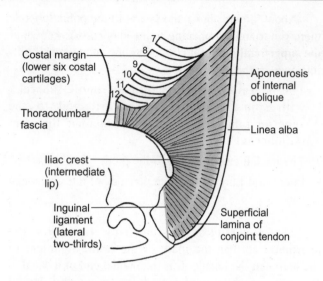

Fig. 2.13: Internal oblique:Side view showing origin

In the male the spermatic cord passes through the internal oblique muscle and carries a covering with it into the scrotum. This consists of fibromuscular tissue constituting the **cremasteric fascia** and **cremaster muscle**. The muscle fibres are in loops and by their contraction pull up the spermatic cord and the testis and help to support them. Cremaster muscle is supplied by the genital branch of the genitofemoral nerve.

Transversus Abdominis (Fig. 2.14)

It forms the innermost layer of the abdominal musculature. The fibres run in a horizontal direction towards its aponeurosis.

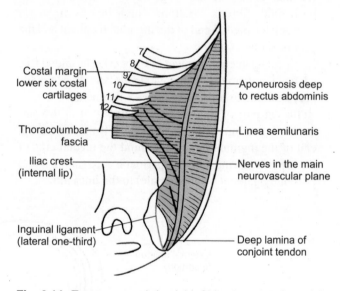

Fig. 2.14: Transversus abdominis: Side view showing origin

Origin (Fig. 2.12)

It has a continuous fleshy origin which from behind forwards is as follows:
- Entire vertical extent of the thoracolumbar fascia.
- Intermediate area of the anterior two-thirds of the iliac crest.
- Lateral two-thirds of the upper grooved surface of the inguinal ligament.

Insertion (Fig. 2.13)

- Upper fibres which arise from the thoracolumbar fascia run upwards along the costal margin to gain attachment to the inner aspect of the lower three ribs.
- Intermediate fibres which arise from the iliac crest curve in an upward, forward and medial direction and become aponeurotic. The upper three-fourths of the aponeurosis splits at the lateral border of the rectus abdominis into two laminae which enclose the rectus abdominis before merging with the linea alba (Fig. 2.18). The upper limit of attachment of this part of the muscle is to the seventh, eight and ninth costal cartilages. The lower fourth of the aponeurosis does not split and passes in front of the rectus abdominis.
- Lowermost fibres that arise from the inguinal ligament arch over the inguinal canal forming its roof and then curve behind the spermatic cord or around ligament of uterus to join the lower aponeurotic fibres of the transversus abdominis to gain attachment to the **pubic crest pectin pubis** thus, forming the **conjoint tendon** of insertion (Fig. 2.15).

Origin

It has a continuous fleshy origin from:
- Inner aspects of the lower six costal cartilages (Fig. 2.11).
- Thoracolumbar fascia between the twelfth rib and the iliac crest (Fig. 2.14).
- Anterior two-thirds of the inner lip of the iliac crest (Fig. 2.12).
- Lateral one-third of the upper grooved surface of the inguinal ligament (Fig. 2.12).

Insertion

The fibres travel towards the median plane and approximately at the linea semilunaris, the muscle fibres cease and the layer becomes aponeurotic.

- Upper three-fourths of the aponeurosis passes behind the rectus abdominis to join the posterior lamina of the internal oblique (Fig. 2.18 b).
- Intermediate portion of the aponeurosis passes in front of the rectus abdominis (Fig. 2.18 c).
- Lowermost part contributes in the formation of the conjoint tendon which is inserted into the pubic tubercle and pubic crest (Fig. 2.15).

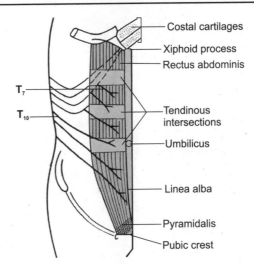

Fig. 2.16: The rectus abdominis: Note that it is widest at its origin the nerves pass from the thoracic wall to the abdominal wall along the homologous intermuscular plane to enter posterior to rectus abdominis

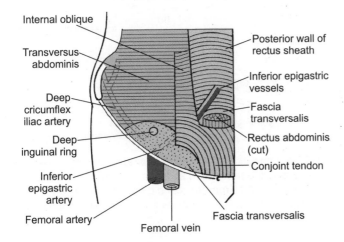

Fig. 2.15: Schematic diagram to explain the formation of the conjoint tendon, the position of the deep inguinal ring and the inferior epigastric artery

The nerves of the abdominal wall run on its superficial surface which is the neurovascular plane.

Rectus Abdominis (Fig. 2.16)

Rectus abdominis lies in the paramedian plane enclosed in a fibrous sheath called the **rectus sheath**. Its fibres run vertically between the pubis and thorax. It is strap-like, widest at its origin and has usually three transverse tendinous intersections which are:
- At the level of the umbilicus.
- Just below the xiphoid process.
- Midway between these two.

Occasionally there may be another intersection between the umbilicus and pubis. These intersections are attached to the anterior layer of the rectus sheath but not to the posterior layer. They indicate the segmental origin of the rectus abdominis.

Origin (Fig. 2.12)

It has two heads:
- Lateral head from the lateral part of pubic crest.

- Medial head from the superior ligament of symphysis pubis.

Insertion (Fig. 2.11)

The two heads unite to ascend to their insertion into:
- A horizontal line extending from the anterior surface of xiphoid process and across the 5th , 6th and 7th costal cartilages.

Pyramidalis

- It is a small triangular muscle lying in front of the lower part of the rectus abdominis.

Origin (Fig. 2.12)

- Superior ligament of pubic symphysis and ;
- Adjoining pubic bone.

Insertion

Ascending medially it is inserted into:
- The linea alba between symphysis pubis and umbilicus.

RECTUS SHEATH

Walls

They are formed by the fusion of the aponeurosis of the external oblique, internal oblique and transversus abdominis muscles, as they approach the lateral border of rectus abdominis muscle. It has an anterior wall and a posterior wall. The posterior wall (Fig. 2.17) is deficient above the

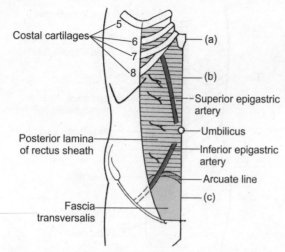

Fig. 2.17: The bed of rectus abdominis: The posterior rectus sheath is deficient above and below. Above it is replaced by costal cartilages and below by fascia transversalis. The epigastric vessels and the nerves run behind the muscle. Levels (a), (b) and (c) indicate the levels of section of Fig. 1.18

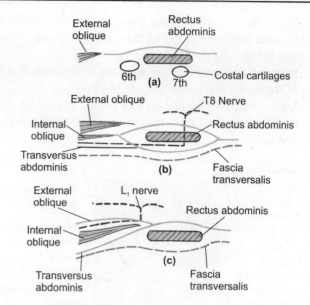

Fig. 2.18: Formation of the rectus sheath and course of nerves shown by the transverse sections: (a) Above the costal margin. (b) From the xiphoid process to a point midway between the umbilicus and the pubic symphysis. (C) Below the level midway between umbilicus and pubic symphysis.

subcostal margin and below the **arcuate line (of Douglas)** which is the lower extent of the posterior wall midway between the umbilicus and pubic symphysis.

- Above the costal margin (Fig. 2.18 a):
- Anterior wall is thin and is formed solely by the aponeurosis of external oblique.
- Posterior wall is deficient and the muscle rests on 5th, 6th and 7th costal cartilages.
- Anywhere from the xiphoid process to a point midway between the umbilicus and the pubic symphysis (Fig. 2.18b).

Anterior wall is formed by the anterior lamella of the internal oblique aponeurosis blending with the aponeurosis of external oblique.

Posterior wall is formed by the posterior lamella of internal oblique aponeurosis blending with the aponeurosis of transversus abdominis.

- Below the level midway between umbilicus and pubic symphysis (Fig. 2.18 c).
  - Anterior wall is thickest as it is formed by the fusion of the aponeurosis of all the three flat muscles of the abdominal wall.
  - Posterior wall is deficient and so the rectus abdominis lies directly on fascia transversalis which separates it from extraperitoneal tissue and parietal peritoneum. The lower free edge of the posterior wall of rectus sheath formed by this transition is known as the **arcuate line or semicircular fold (of Douglas).**

Contents

- **Two muscles:**
  - Rectus abdominis.
  - Pyramidalis.
- **Two arteries:**
  - Superior epigastric.
  - Inferior epigastric.
  - **Superior epigastric** is a branch of internal thoracic artery and enters by crossing the upper border of transversus abdominis and runs vertically downwards.
  - **Inferior epigastric** is a branch of the lower end of the external iliac just above the inguinal ligament. It runs upwards and medially in the extraperitoneal tissue along the medial margin of deep inguinal ring. It pierces the fascia transversalis just at the lateral border of rectus abdominis and enters the rectus sheath. After crossing the arcuate line it runs upwards.

These arteries anastomose on the posterior wall of the sheath.

- Terminal parts of the lower five intercostal and subcostal nerves. They enter the rectus sheath by piercing its posterior wall. Within the rectus sheath they lie in front of the epigastric arteries pierce the rectus muscle and the anterior wall of the rectus sheath to come out as their anterior cutaneous branches which supply the skin of the anterior abdominal wall (Fig. 2.6).

Nerve Supply of Muscles of Anterior Abdominal Wall

* Lower five intercostal and subcostal nerves.
* Iliohypogastric and ilioinguinal nerves.

The main part of these nerves and the ascending branch of the deep circumflex iliac artery lie in the neurovascular plane which is between the internal oblique and transversus abdominis muscles (Fig. 2.14).

Action of the Muscles of Anterior Abdominal Wall

* To protect and retain the abdominal viscera in the abdominal cavity.
* To assist the emptying of hollow viscera during defalcation, micturition, parturition and vomiting by increasing the intra-abdominal pressure by contracting with the diaphragm and pelvic floor.
* To push the diaphragm upwards in deep expiration, in sneezing and coughing.

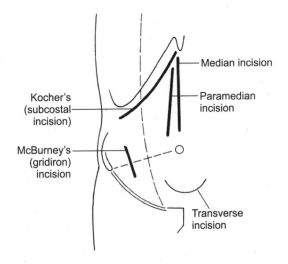

Fig. 2.19: Abdominal incisions

* To help in the movements of vertebral column e.g.,:
  - Flexion when getting up from lying down position.
  - Extension of the trunk in upright position.
  - Rotation of trunk to one side, the internal oblique of that side and the external oblique of opposite side contract simultaneously.

CLINICAL APPLICATION

The arrangement of the muscles of the anterior abdominal wall is used by surgeons when planning incisions. The muscles are split in the direction of their fibres, rather than cut across. The incision traverses muscle rather than fascia, as the scar left in the peritoneum is best protected by muscle.

* The nerve supply to the lateral abdominal muscles forms a network so incision through one or two nerves, produces no ill-effects.
* The segmental nerve supply to rectus abdominis has little cross communication and damage to its nerves is avoided.
* The important abdominal incisions (Fig. 2.19) can be classified as follows on the basis of:

(a) *Dividing no muscle*

Median or midline incision is made through the linea alba. As it passes through fibrous tissue only, it provides a comparatively bloodless rapid approach to the abdominal cavity.

Paramedian incision is made 3 to 4 cm lateral and parallel to the midline. The anterior wall of the rectus sheath is opened, the rectus is displaced laterally and not cut as the intercostal and subcostal nerves run horizontally and enter the posterior surface of the muscle from lateral side. The posterior sheath and the peritoneum are then incised. The incision has the advantage that, on suturing the peritoneum, the rectus slips back into place to cover and protect the peritoneal scar.

(b) *Dividing muscles*

Transrectus incision, in this incision the rectus abdominis is split in the midline and not displaced laterally as in paramedian incision. The disadvantage is that the muscle medial to the incision is deprived of its innervation and undergoes **atrophy** if the incision is made more than 1 cm from the medial border as the rectus receives its nerve supply from the lateral side at its back about its middle.

Right subcostal (**Kocher's**) incision is a right sided incision running parallel and 2 to 5 cm below the costal margin commencing from the midline. It is used for approaching the gall bladder and its ducts. The rectus sheath and the muscle are divided almost transversely. The cut edges of the rectus retract very little because of the tendinous intersections above and below.

Oblique lumbar incision in line from the tip of the 12th rib to half way between the umbilicus and the pubis gives good exposure of kidney and other laterally situated structures. These incisions through the lateral abdominal muscles do not damage the nerve supply and heal without weakness.

Lower abdominal transverse incision **(Pfannenstiel's)** is commonly used for approach to pelvic viscera. It is made 3 cm above the pubic symphysis transversely dividing the two recti.

(c) *Splitting muscles*

McBurney's gridiron incision to approach appendix is an oblique incision at right angle to the line joining the anterior superior iliac spine and the umbilicus. It is centred on the junction of the lateral and middle third of this line (McBurney's point). This skin incision is parallel to the fibres of the external oblique which is split or cut in line with the fibres. The internal oblique and transversus are then split at right angles to the opening in the external oblique, that is, in line of their fibres. This gives access to the abdominal cavity without dividing the fibres of the muscles. On closing the incision, these muscles snap together again, leaving a virtually undamaged abdominal wall.

Inguinal Canal

Inguinal canal is an oblique passage in the lower part of the anterior abdominal wall, immediately above the medial half of the inguinal ligament, through which the spermatic cord in the male and around ligament of the uterus in the female take their course. It is 4 cm long and passes downward, forward and medially. At its lateral end is the deep (internal) inguinal ring and at the medial end is the superficial (external) inguinal ring.

Deep (internal) Inguinal Ring (Fig. 2.20)

Fascia transversalis, which is an inner layer of connective tissue that enwraps the abdominal cavity and supports the peritoneum, is attached below to the inguinal ligament except in the region of the femoral sheath. The **deep inguinal ring** is an interruption in this fascia formed by the embryonic extension of the processus vaginalis through the abdominal wall and subsequent passage of the testes through the transversalis fascia during the descent of the testes into the scrotum.

This ring is circular in shape and lies 2.5 cm above the midpoint of the inguinal ligament immediately lateral to the

inferior of epigastric artery. The spermatic cord drags from it a covering which forms the internal spermatic fascia.

Superficial (External) Ring (Fig. 2.23)

It is a triangular opening in the external oblique aponeurosis and lies immediately above and medial to the pubic tubercle. The apex points upwards and laterally. The base is the lateral part of the pubic crest. It has two borders or crurae. The lateral crus is curved and is attached to pubic tubercle. The medial is straight and is attached to the pubic crest near the symphysis (Fig. 2.12). As the spermatic cord traverses the opening, it carries the **external spermatic fascia** from the margins of the ring.

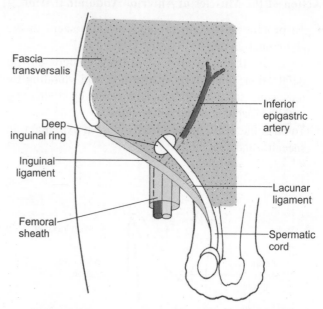

Fig. 2.20: Reconstruction of inguinal canal:Fascia transversalis. The internal lining of the transversus abdominis is attached below to the inguinal ligament except in the region of femoral sheath. It bounds the deep inguinal ring which is about 2.5 cm above the midinguinal point. The inferior epigastric artery runs medially and the upwards medial to deep ring the lacunar ligament is attached posterior to pectineal line. Fascia transversalis forms the posterior wall of the inguinal canal throughout its full length

Boundaries (Fig. 2.24)

Anteriorly

- External oblique aponeurosis covers the full length of the canal. (Fig. 2.23)
- Internal oblique (fleshly inguinal fibres) in the lateral half (Fig. 2.22).

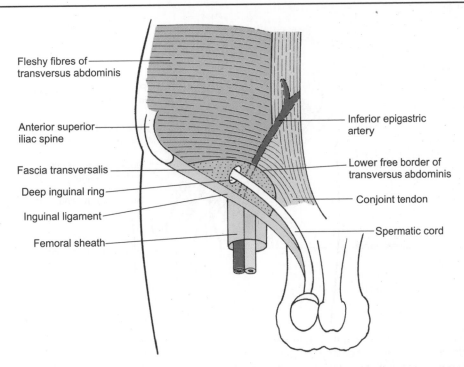

Fleshy fibres of transversus abdominis

Anterior superior iliac spine

Fascia transversalis

Deep inguinal ring

Inguinal ligament

Femoral sheath

Inferior epigastric artery

Lower free border of transversus abdominis

Conjoint tendon

Spermatic cord

Fig. 2.21: Reconstruction of inguinal canal: Front view of transversus abdominis after reflection of internal oblique. The whole length of the canal is exposed. The conjoint tendon forms the posterior boundary of the medial half of the canal

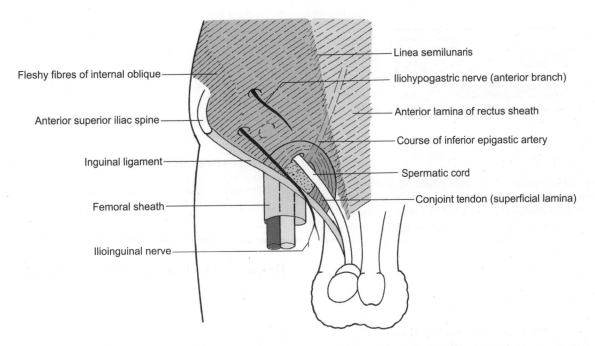

Fleshy fibres of internal oblique

Anterior superior iliac spine

Inguinal ligament

Femoral sheath

Ilioinguinal nerve

Linea semilunaris

Iliohypogastric nerve (anterior branch)

Anterior lamina of rectus sheath

Course of inferior epigastic artery

Spermatic cord

Conjoint tendon (superficial lamina)

Fig. 2.22: Reconstruction of inguinal canal: Front view of internal oblique after reflection of external oblique. Only the lateral half of the anterior wall of the canal is formed by the internal oblique. Note that the ilioinguinal nerve after lying between the transversus abdominis and internal oblique muscles pierce the latter below and anterior to the point at which the iliohypogastric nerve passes through this muscle. The nerve then accompanies the spermatic cord in the medial part of the inguinal canal

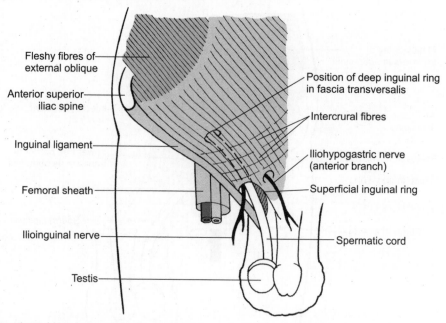

Fig. 2.23: Reconstruction of inguinal canal: Front view of external oblique showing the superficial ring and the ilioinguinal nerve and the structures of the cord emerging from it. The aponeurosis of external oblique forms the anterior wall of the canal in its full length. Note that the anterior branch of the iliohypogastric nerve pierces the aponeurosis of the external oblique muscle above the superficial ring to terminate in the skin of the pubic region

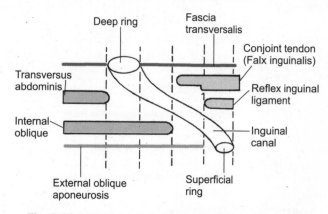

Fig. 2.24: Inguinal canal: Schematic representation of structures forming the anterior and posterior walls. Note that the weakness in any part of the anterior wall is compensated by the strengthening of the posterior wall

Posteriorly

- Fascia transversalis covers the full length of the canal (Fig. 2.20)
- Conjoint tendon in the medial half (Fig. 2.21)
- Reflex inguinal ligament in the medial one-fourth.

Note that the weakness in the anterior wall is compensated by the strengthening of posterior wall and vice versa.

Roof

- Arched lower fleshy fibres of the internal oblique and transversus abdominis (Figs. 2.21 and 2.22).

Floor

- Upper grooved surface of the medial half of the inguinal ligament (Fig. 2.21).
- Abdominal surface of the lacunar ligament **(Gimbernat's)** (Fig. 2.12).

Contents of Inguinal Canal

- Spermatic cord in male and round ligament of uterus in female.
- Ilioinguinal nerve.
- Vestige of processus vaginalis (in male).

Defensive Mechanism of Inguinal Canal

The canal is potentially weak. In response to increased intra-abdominal pressure, this weakness is prevented by the following factors:
- Oblique direction of the canal.
- Protection of the deep ring anteriorly by the double-layered lateral end of the anterior wall of the canal formed by the internal oblique and the aponeurosis of the external oblique. The lowest fibres of the transversus abdominis

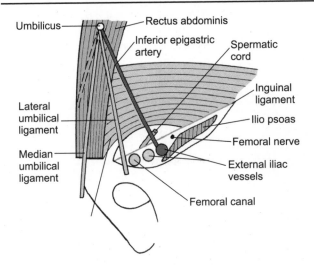

Fig. 2.25: Inguinal (Hesselbach's) triangle: Posterior surface of lower part of anterior abdominal wall showing the boundaries of the triangle

muscle which possibly by descending during contraction close the deep inguinal ring.

- Protection of the superficial ring posteriorly by the two layers of the conjoint tendon and the fascia transversalis.
- Apposition of the anterior and posterior walls in a manner that the weak parts of the anterior wall are strengthened by the strong parts of the posterior wall and vice versa.
- Sphincteric control of the canal by the arched lower fibres of internal oblique and transversus abdominis which descend on the canal like a shutter.

All the above mechanisms come into play when there is a tendency for herniation due to increased intra-abdominal pressure as during straining or coughing.

INGUINAL TRIANGLE (HESSELBACH'S)

It is a triangular area on the back of the lower part of the anterior abdominal wall lateral to the rectus abdominis.

Boundaries

- **Medially:** Outer border of the rectus abdominis.
- **Laterally:** Inferior epigastric artery.
- **Inferiorly:** Inguinal ligament.

It is covered by fascia transversalis, extraperitoneal tissue and peritoneum. It is divided into medial and lateral halves by the **lateral umbilical ligament** (obliterated umbilical artery). The medial part is strengthened by the **conjoint tendon** while the lateral part is relatively weak.

CLINICAL APPLICATION

A hernia is a protrusion of the contents of a cavity through a defect in its wall. Inguinal hernia is a protrusion through a defect above the inguinal ligament. There are two main varieties:
- Indirect.
- Direct.

INDIRECT INGUINAL HERNIA (FIG. 2.26)

It is so classified as it takes an indirect route, offered by the inguinal canal, by passing through the deep ring, traversing the canal and emerging through the superficial ring to enter the scrotum. The protrusion is of abdominal contents varying from extraperitoneal tissue to a pouch or sac of peritoneum containing greater omentum or

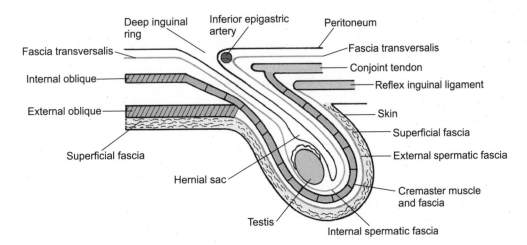

Fig. 2.26: Oblique inguinal hernia with its coverings

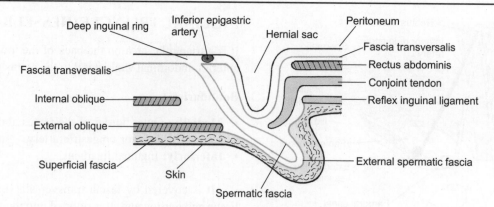

Fig. 2.27: Direct inguinal hernia with its coverings.

intestine. The inferior epigastric artery is medial to the sac. Since, the canal is smaller in the females, this hernia is rare in them.

The hernia sac is covered by:
- Skin.
- Superficial fascia.
- External spermatic fascia from external oblique aponeurosis.
- Cremaster muscle and fascia from internal oblique (only in males).
- Internal spermatic fascia from fascia transversalis.
- Extraperitoneal tissue.

DIRECT INGUINAL HERNIA

Direct inguinal hernia leaves the inguinal triangle through its outer or inner part and is therefore lateral direct or medial direct. It is so named as it pushes directly forwards. It occurs usually in old age. The opening in fascia transversalis lies directly opposite the superficial ring and the examining finger passes straight back through that opening and not in an oblique direction as in indirect hernia. This hernia does not descend into the scrotum.

Lateral direct hernia is more common as the lateral part of the inguinal triangle is relatively weak. The neck of the hernial sac is medial to the inferior epigastric artery.

The coverings of the hernial sac in direct hernia are (Fig. 2.27):
- Skin.
- Superficial fascia.
- External spermatic fascia.
- Cremaster muscle and fascia (only in males in the lateral direct hernia) conjoint tendon (in the medial direct hernia).
- Transversalis fascia.
- Extraperitoneal tissue.

3

Posterior Abdominal Wall: Muscles, Nerves and Vessels

BONY FRAMEWORK (FIG. 3.1)

It is formed by:
- The lumbar part of the vertebral column. The body of T_{12} is not part of the wall but is included for reference.
- The twelfth rib.
- The ala of the sacrum.
- The iliac crest of the hip bone.
- The iliac fossa of the hip bone.
- The pelvic brims.
- The lumbar part of the vertebral column.

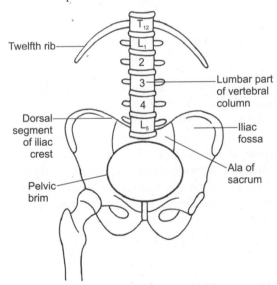

Fig. 3.1: Posterior abdominal wall: Bony framework

The lumbar vertebrae are somewhat rectangular in anterior view. They increase in width and height from above down as each body is to be stronger than the one above as it has to carry more weight.

On the anterior surface, on the area around midline, is the attachment of anterior longitudinal ligament. Lateral to this from the upper and lower borders is the origin of psoas

major and its tendinous arches. Right crus of the diaphragm is attached to the bodies of L_1, L_2, and L_3 and the left crus to the bodies of L_1 and L_2 on either side of the anterior longitudinal ligament.

The transverse processes project from the upper parts of the sides of the bodies. The tip gives attachment to the **middle lamella of thoracolumbar fascia**. In addition, the tip of the L_1 transverse process gives attachment to the **medial** and **lateral arcuate ligaments**. The anterior surface presents a nearly vertical ridge about its middle to which is attached the **anterior lamella of lumbodorsal fascia**. Lateral to the ridge is the insertion of **quadratus lumborum** and medial to it is the origin of **psoas major**.

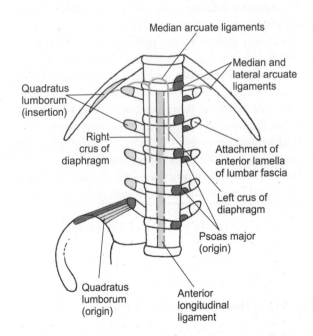

Fig. 3.2: Ventral aspect of the lumbar part of vertebral column: Origin and insertion of quadratus lumborum are shown on right side and origin of psoas major on the left side

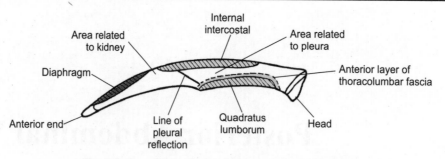

Fig. 3.3: Twelfth rib: Right side showing attachments

The intervertebral discs are thicker in the lumbar region than elsewhere and contribute more than one-third of the length of the lumbar part of the column. Lateral parts give origin to psoas major starting from the one between T_{12} and L_1 above to the one between L_4 and L_5 vertebrae.

THE TWELFTH RIB (Fig. 3.3)

The twelfth rib has the following identifying features:
- Head has only one facet for articulation with the body of twelfth thoracic vertebra.
- Neck, tubercle, angle and costal groove are absent.
- Pointed anterior end instead of a cup-shaped depression.

The shaft possesses inner and outer surfaces, upper and lower borders and anterior and posterior ends.

The inner surface which takes part in the formation of posterior abdominal wall has following attachments:
- **Quadratus lumborum** muscle is inserted in the lower part of medial half of inner surface.
- **Anterior layer of thoracolumbar fascia** is attached above the insertion of the quadratus lumborum.
- **Diaphragm** arises from the anterior one-fourth of the inner surface close to the upper border.
- **Internal intercostal muscle** of the eleventh interspace is inserted into the middle two-fourth of the inner surface close to the upper border.
- **Costodiaphragmatic recess of the pleura** is related to the medial half of the inner surface.
- **Kidney,** with fat intervening is related to the lateral half of the surface.

The Ala of the Sacrum (Fig. 3.4)

The sacrum is formed by the fusion of five sacral vertebrae. It is wedge-shaped and placed between the two hip bones, the base of the wedge being directed upwards and the apex

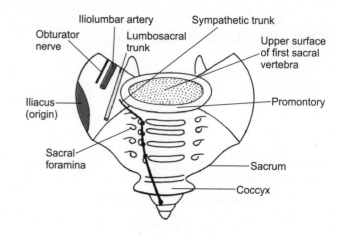

Fig. 3.4: The ala of sacrum

downwards. It possesses a base, an apex, a pelvic or ventral surface, a dorsal and two lateral surfaces and encloses a canal, the sacral canal.

Base is formed by the upper surface of the first sacral vertebra. It has an anterior projection called the **promontory**. The wing-shaped upper surface of the lateral part is known as the **ala**. The ala can be subdivided into a smooth medial part and a rough lateral part. The smooth medial area is related to nerves and vessels and the rough lateral area gives origin to a part of iliacus muscle. Both areas are covered by the psoas major muscle.

The Iliac Crest (Fig. 3.5)

The upper end of ilium is known as iliac crest. It is expanded and seen from the top it is S-shaped. It is limited anteriorly and posterioly by projection termed **anterior** and **posterior superior iliac spines** and is divisible into ventral and dorsal segments, the former forming the anterior two-thirds and the latter posterior one-third. The dorsal segment is hidden from view by the ala of the sacrum. The ventral segment

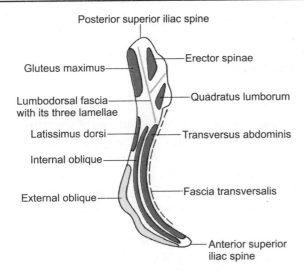

Fig. 3.5: Attachments of the ventral and dorsal segments of iliac crest. Erector spinae and gluteus maximus are attached to dorsal segment while rest of the muscles are attached to ventral segment

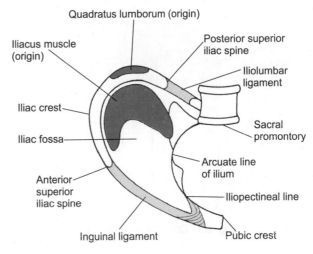

Fig. 3.6: Iliac fossa and the pelvic brim

Pelvic brim separates the **false pelvis** above and in front from the **true pelvis** below and behind. Regionally the false pelvis is a part of the abdomen.

is bounded by outer and inner lips, enclosing between them an intermediate area which gives attachment to the three flat muscles of the anterior abdominal wall. The dorsal segment has two sloping surfaces separated by a well-defined ridge which terminates in the posterior-superior iliac spine.

The inner lip of the ventral segment gives origin to **quadratus lumborum,** a muscle of posterior abdominal wall, in its posterior one-third. The **anterior** and **middle lamella of thoracolumbar fascia** encloses the quadratus lumborum and are attached to the bone hare. Traced posteriorly the attachment of the middle lamella passes between the attachments of quadratus lumborum and erector spinae which is attached to the medial slope of the dorsal segment. The anterior two-thirds of the inner lip gives origin to transversus abdominis and on its inside to fascia transversalis of the anterior abdominal wall.

The Iliac Fossa and the Pelvic Brim (Fig. 3.6)

The iliac fossa is the smooth hollowed out anterior and upper part of the medial surface of the bone limited by the anterior border in front, medial border behind and the ventral part of the iliac crest above. Margin adjoining the iliac crest gives attachment to **fascia iliaca. Iliacus muscle** arises from upper two-thirds of the surface.

The pelvic brim is formed by **linea terminalis** at the sides and front and **sacral promontory** behind. Each linea terminalis includes the arcuate line of ilium (smooth and rounded part of its medial border), pecten pubis (iliopectineal line) and pubic crest.

MUSCLES OF POSTERIOR ABDOMINAL WALL

The posterior abdominal wall is formed by the following muscles:
- Quadratus lumborum.
- Psoas major and psoas minor.
- Iliacus.
- Diaphragm whose posterior part with its crurae also forms part of the posterior abdominal wall.

Quadratus Lumborum (Fig. 3.7)

Origin (Fig. 3.6)

- Iliolumbar ligament which attaches the tip and lower and front part of the transverse process of L_5 vertebra to the crest of ilium immediately in front of the sacro-iliac joint. It is continuous above with the thoracolumbar fascia.
- Iliac crest—posterior one-third of the inner lip of ventral segment.

It lies on the middle lamella of thoracolumbar fascia which is attached to the tips of lumbar transverse processes (Fig. 3.8). The anterior layer of fascia covers the quadratus lumborum and is attached medially to the vertical ridge on the anterior aspects of the lumbar transverse processes. Lateral to quadratus lumborum the three layers of the fascia form a zone of dense connective tissue extending from the iliac crest to the twelfth rib.

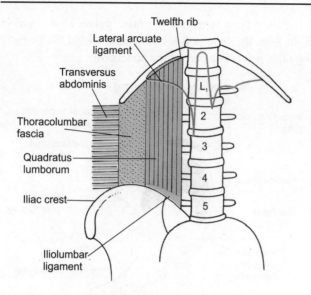

Fig. 3.7: Quadratus lumborum

Insertion (Fig. 3.2)

*   Tips and lower margins of L_1 to L_4 transverse processes.
*   Medial half of the lower border of twelfth rib.

Nerve Supply

*   Ventral rami of T_{12}, L_1, L_2 and L_3 nerves.

Action

*   Lateral flexor of lumbar vertebral column when acting on one side.
*   Flexor of vertebral column when acting together.

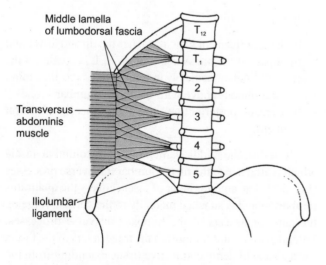

Fig. 3.8: The middle lamella of thoracolumbar fascia

*   Fixes the last rib for the contraction of diaphragm during respiration.

Psoas Major (Fig. 3.9)

Origin (Fig. 3.2)

*   Medial part of the anterior surfaces of the transverse processes of the lumbar vertebrae by five fleshy slips.
*   Anterolateral surfaces of the intervertebral discs and the adjacent margins of the T_{12} and all lumbar vertebral bodies. The highest slip from T_{12} and L_1 vertebrae lies above the lateral lumbocostal arch and therefore, is in the lowest part of the posterior mediastinum.
*   A series of fibrous arches at the concave middle sides of the bodies of upper lumbar vertebrae.

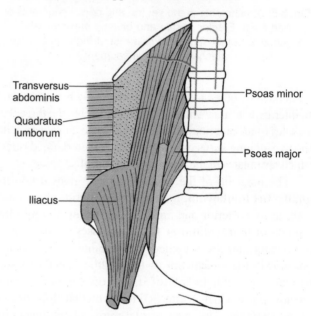

Fig. 3.9: Psoas major and minor and iliacus muscles

Insertion

Lesser trochanter of femur by a strong tendon which passes deep to the inguinal ligament. On its lateral aspect the tendon is joined by fibres of iliacus. Psoas major overlies the medial part of quadratus lumborum.

Nerve Supply

Roots of the lumbar plexus (L_1 to L_3) supply it. The lumbar plexus is situated within the muscle.

Action

*   Flexion of the thigh.

- Medial rotation of thigh till the long axis of femur crosses the long axis of the muscle, then onward it produces lateral rotation.

Psoas Minor (Fig. 3.9)

When present, it has the following attachments:

Origin

- Lateral aspect of the intervertebral disc between T_{12} and L_1 vertebrae and adjacent margins of these vertebrae.

Insertion

- Middle of the arcuate line and;
- Iliopubic eminence.

Nerve Supply

- L_1 fibres.

Iliacus (Fig. 3.9)

Origin (Fig. 3.6)

- Upper half or more of the hollow of the iliac fossa upto the inner lip of the iliac crest.
- Anterior sacroiliac ligament by encroaching across the sacroiliac joint.
- Ala of sacrum.

Insertion

Lateral border of the tendon of psoas major by fibres which converge downwards and medially.

Shaft of femur in a linear fashion in front of and below the lesser trochanter.

Nerve Supply

- Femoral nerve (L_2 and L_3) in the iliac fossa.

Diaphragm (Fig. 3.10)

It is a dome-shaped musculotendinous partition which closes the thoracic outlet thereby separating the abdominal cavity from the thoracic cavity. It is flat in the centre but elevated as domes on each side. The most convex part is called the **cupola**. The right cupola is higher in level than the left and reaches upto the level of the fifth rib.

It has lumbar, costal and sternal parts attached to the circumference of the outlet.

Origin

Lumbar part

By two crurae arising from the anterolateral aspects of upper three lumbar bodies. The right crus from all the three bodies, the left from the upper two.

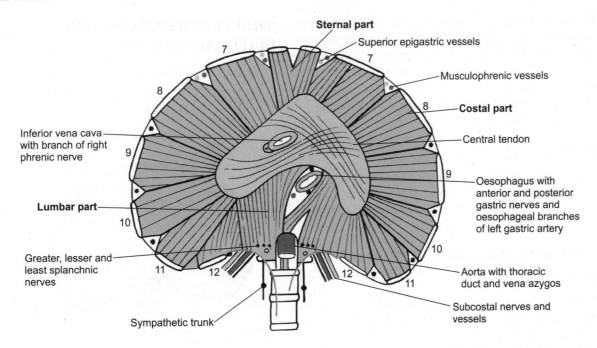

Fig. 3.10: The diaphragm: Abdominal aspect (numbers indicate the corresponding ribs and the intervening intercostal nerves and vessels)

From the paired **medial** and **lateral arcuate ligaments** and from the **median arcuate ligament** which is formed by the meeting of the tendinous crurae in the midline at the level of the disc between T_{12} and L_1, in the shape of a pointed arch. The **medial arcuate ligaments** (medial lumbocostal arches) are tendinous bands which stretch across the psoas muscle and extend from the body of L_1 vertebra to its transverse process. The **lateral arcuate ligaments** (lateral lumbocostal arches) are also tendinous bands which stretch across the quadratus lumborum muscle and extend from the transverse process of L_1 vertebra to the lower border of twelfth rib.

Costal part

Inner surface of the lower six costal cartilages by fleshy slips which interdigitate with transversus abdominis.

Sternal part

Back of the xiphoid process by two slips.

Insertion

Central tendon receives the insertion of the three parts. It is somewhat crescentic, with right and left leaves and a small anterior leaf (trifoliate).

Nerve Supply

- Phrenic nerve (C_3 to C_5 mainly C_4). It is the only motor nerve to the diaphragm. In addition, it also sends sensory fibres to the central part of the diaphragm.
- Lower five intercostal and subcostal nerves furnish sensory fibres to the peripheral parts of the diaphragm. The crurae are said to receive sensory innervation from the upper lumbar nerves.

Action

- It is the main muscle of respiration and acts alternately with abdominal and pelvic floor muscles.
- In expulsive phenomena, like vomiting or defaecation, it acts along with abdominal and pelvic floor muscles.

MAIN OPENINGS IN THE DIAPHRAGM
(Figs. 3.10.and 3.11)

- **Vena caval opening,** in the central tendon between its right and median leaves, is situated at the level of T_8 vertebra. It transmits:
  - Inferior vena cava.
  - Right phrenic nerve.

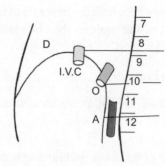

Fig. 3.11: Vertebral levels of the main openings in the diaphragm

- **Oesophageal opening,** formed by the fibres of right crus which ascend up and cross the midline to embrace the lower end of oesophagus and decussate beyond it, is situated at the level of T_{10} vertebra. It transmits:
  - Oesophagus.
  - Oesophageal branches of the left gastric artery and corresponding veins.
  - Anterior and posterior gastric nerves.
- **Aortic opening,** which is an osseoaponeurotic opening in the shape of a pointed arch between the median arcuate ligament and the disc between T_{12} and L_1 vertebrae. It transmits:
  - Aorta.
  - Thoracic duct.
  - Vena azygos.

SMALLER OPENINGS IN THE DIAPHRAGM (Fig. 3.10)

- Interval between the sternal fibres and costal fibres from the seventh rib (Larrey's space) conducts:
  - Superior epigastric vessels.

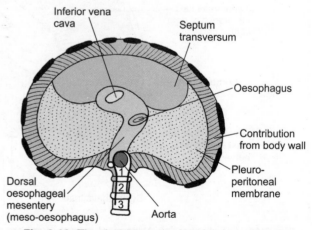

Fig. 3.12: The development of diaphragm: Several contributions to form the definitive diaphragm

- Intervals between the adjoining costal slips give passage to:
  - Lower five intercostal nerves and vessels.
- Behind the lateral arcuate ligament:
  - Subcostal nerve and vessels.
  - Quadratus lumborum muscle.
- Behind the medial arcuate ligament:
  - Sympathetic trunk.
  - Psoas major muscle.
- Small openings in the crura:
  - Greater, lesser and least splanchnic nerves.
  - Descending intercostal lymph trunks.

Development (Fig. 3.12)

The diaphragm develops in the cervical region along with the heart. The mesodermal basis is derived from four component parts:
- **Septum transversum** forms the region of central tendon.
- **Body wall** mesoderm forms the peripheral part.
- **Dorsal oesophageal mesentery** forms the crurae.
- **Pleuroperitoneal membranes,** which close the primitive communication between the pleural and peritoneal cavities, form the parts between the crura and the costal origins.

This mesodermal basis is invaded by the descending mass of muscle fibres developed principally from the fourth and partly from the third and fifth cervical myotomes thereby retaining the motor nerve supply from C_3 to C_5 and accounting for the long course of the phrenic nerve.

CLINICAL APPLICATION

- Sensation from the larger central region is carried by the phrenic nerves to segments C_3 to C_5 of the spinal cord. Irritation of the diaphragmatic pleura or diaphragmatic peritoneum is referred to the shoulder region referred via supraclavicular nerves (C_3, C_4).
- Sensation from the peripheral region is supplied by the intercostal nerves. Pain from the periphery of the diaphragm is referred to the costal margin of the abdominal wall.
- Irritation of the phrenic nerve can cause spasmodic contraction of the diaphragm resulting in hiccup.
- Damage to the phrenic nerve paralyses one side of the diaphragm which becomes immobile and can be observed during screening.

- Certain weak areas result in the diaphragm due to developmental defects and are sites of hernia. These hernia are 8 to 10 times more common on the left than on the right side and occur through:
  - Sternocostal hiatus or triangle (**foramen of Morgagni**) which is the area of penetration of the diaphragm by the superior epigastric vessels between the xiphoid and costal origins anteriorly.
  - Lumbocostal triangle (**foramen of Bochdalek**) located posteriorly between costal and lumbar origins (region of pleuroperitoneal canal). The area may be nonmuscular, with only two layers of serous membrane separating the thoracic from the abdominal cavity.
  - Congenitally large **oesophageal hiatus** due to failure of development of muscle around the oesophageal hiatus. There is prolapse of cardio-oesophageal junction or part of the fundus of stomach into the thorax. It is called **hiatus hernia**.

THE NERVES OF THE POSTERIOR ABDOMINAL WALL

Somatic nerves of the posterior abdominal wall innervate the abdominal musculature and convey sensation from the skin and parietal peritoneum.

Lumbar Plexus (Fig. 3.13)

The lumbar plexus is formed from the ventral rami of nerves L_1 to L_4. As the ventral rami emerge from the intervertebral **foramina,** they are covered by psoas major muscle and it is within the substance of that muscle that the divisions and unions which constitute the plexus take place. As a result the branches of the plexus appear either at the edges of psoas major or on its anterior surface.
- L_1 gives off upper, larger branch and a lower smaller branch:
  - The upper, larger branch divides into the **iliohypogastric** and **ilioinguinal nerves** which emerge at the lateral border of psoas.
  - The lower, smaller branch joins a branch of L_2 to form the **genitofemoral nerve** which pierces the psoas major at the level of L_3 vertebra to descend on its anterior surface.
- L_2 to L_4 divide into a ventral and dorsal divisions:
  - The dorsal divisions join to form the **femoral nerve** which emerges at the lateral border of psoas and lies between it and the iliacus.

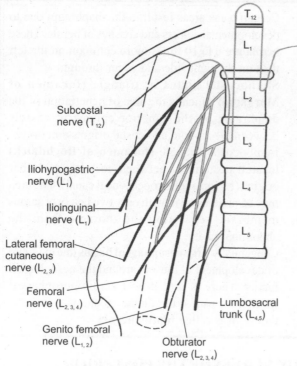

Fig. 3.13: The lumbar plexus

– The ventral divisions form the **obturator nerve** which emerges from the medial border of the psoas and enters the pelvis over the ala of sacrum.
• Dorsal divisions of L_2 and L_3 give origin to the **lateral femoral cutaneous nerve** which is associated with the femoral nerve. It runs across the iliacus and enters the thigh by passing under the inguinal ligament.
• Dorsal divisions of L_2 and L_3 give origin to the **accessory obturator nerve** which is associated with the obturator nerve. It is present only in 30% of individuals. It emerges from the medial border of the psoas muscle.
• L_4 gives a large branch which joins the ventral ramus of L_5 to form the **lumbosacral trunk,** which descends across the ala of sacrum to join the sacral plexus.

Course of the Nerves of Lumbar Plexus (Fig. 3.14)

• **The iliohypogastric nerve** (L_1) after emerging from the lateral side of the psoas muscle runs within the musculature of the abdominal wall. Its iliac branch is sensory to the upper gluteal region. Its hypogastric branch is motor to the internal oblique and transversus

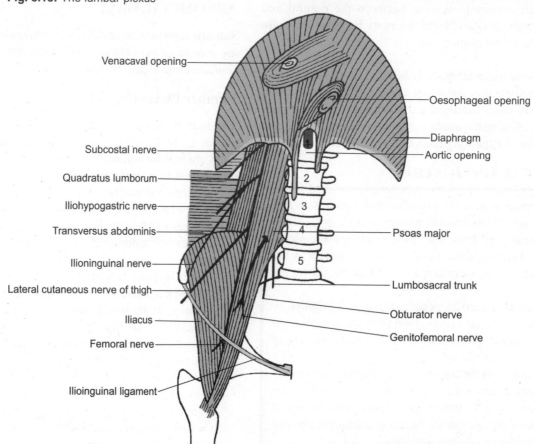

Fig. 3.14: Course of nerves of lumbar plexus on the posterior abdominal wall

abdominis muscles and sensory to the skin overlying the pubis.

- The **ilioinguinal nerve** (L_1) after emerging from the lateral border of the psoas muscle runs parallel to the iliohypogastric nerve. It covers a somewhat lower territory. It is motor to internal oblique and transversus abdominis muscles and sensory to upper medial part of the thigh, the root of the penis or mons pubis and the anterior scrotum or superior portion of the labia majora. Its terminal branch accompanies the spermatic cord through the superficial inguinal ring.

- The **genitofemoral nerves** (L_1 and L_2) emerge anterior to the psoas muscle and runs along its anterior surface. The genital branch is motor to the cremaster muscle and sensory to the anterior scrotum or superior portion of the labia majora. Its femoral branch passes into the thigh beneath the inguinal ligament, medial to the psoas muscle. This branch is sensory to the anterior superior aspect of the thigh.

- The **lateral femoral cutaneous nerves** (L_2 and L_3) emerge lateral to the psoas muscle, runs across the iliac fossa and passes beneath the inguinal ligament close to the anterior superior iliac spine. It is sensory to the lateral aspect of the thigh.

- The **femoral nerves** (L_2 to L_4) emerge from the lateral border of the psoas major muscle then lies in the deep groove between the iliacus and psoas. It supplies both these muscles then stays in the groove as it passes beneath the inguinal ligament.

- The **obturator nerves** (L_2 to L_4) emerge from the medial border of the psoas major muscle crosses the pelvic brim and then enters the thigh through the obturator foramen.

- The **lumbosacral trunks** (L_4 and L_5) are a large connector joining the lumbar plexus with the sacral plexus.

CLINICAL APPLICATION

- The iliohypogastric nerve provides the afferent and efferent limbs for the abdominal reflex in which stroking of the lower anterior abdominal wall produces a rippling of the underlying abdominal muscles.
- The iliohypogastric and ilioinguinal nerves may be damaged during an **appendectomy**. The proximity of the ilioinguinal nerve to the McBurney's incision

may injure the nerve and paralyse its branch to the conjoint tendon. This may predispose to a direct inguinal hernia, because of the laxity of the muscles supplied by these nerves.
- The skin and muscles of lower anterior abdominal wall are supplied by spinal nerve L_1. The inguinal ligament lies at about dermatome L_1. Pain in the inguinal region L_1 may have a local origin e.g., an inguinal hernia, or may be referred from irritated L_1 roots or from a ureter (T_{11}-L_2) that is blocked by a ureteric calculus.
- Genitofemoral nerve provides the afferent and efferent limbs of the **cremaster reflex** in men, whereby stroking the anteromedial aspect of thigh produces elevation of the testes within the scrotum by the contraction of cremaster muscle. The femoral branch is sensory to the anterior superior aspect of the thigh and provides the afferent limb of the reflex, while the genital branch which is motor to the cremaster muscle is the efferent limb.
- Lateral femoral cutaneous nerves (L_2 and L_3) supplies skin lateral to the genitofemoral nerve in the thigh. Pressure on this nerve can cause an uncomfortable burning sensation in the lateral femoral area (**meralgia paraesthetica**).
  The nerve can be injected near the anterior superior iliac spine to produce local anaesthesia for obtaining a skin graft.

Sympathetic Nerves

The lumbar sympathetic system comprises:
- The **lumbar sympathetic trunk** connecting the sympathetic ganglia.
- Branches of communication to and branches of distribution from the ganglia.
- Sympathetic innervation of all abdominal viscera is provided by the lower thoracic and upper lumbar segments of the spinal cord.
  Sympathetic nerves contain visceral afferents and efferents.

Lumbar Sympathetic Trunks (Fig. 3.15)

The lumbar sympathetic trunks are the downward continuation of the thoracic sympathetic trunks and they enter the abdomen by passing behind the medial arcuate ligaments. They run downward along the medial border of

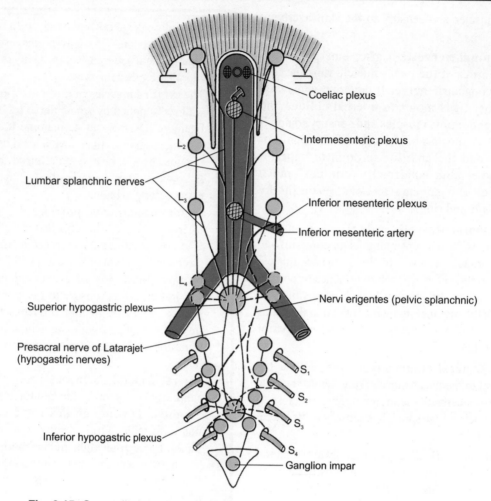

Fig. 3.15: Sympathetic and parasympathetic nerves on the posterior abdominal wall

the psoas major in the groove between it and the vertebral bodies. Both the trunks lie in front of the lumbar vessels.

The lumbar part of the trunk usually carries four ganglia upon it. All the ganglia lie on the vertebral bodies. The first occupies a variable position to the crus of the diaphragm. It may be in front of, or in the substance of, or just behind the crus.

Only the upper lumbar ganglia receive white rami, which bring to the trunk preganglionic fibres. All ganglia give off gray rami communicates to the ventral rami of lumbar nerves. The upper lumbar ganglia give medial branches that are the lumbar splanchnic nerves. These nerves contain preganglionic visceral efferent fibres that relay in the aortic ganglia after the lumbar splanchnic nerves join the aortic plexus, which they help to form.

Prevertebral Ganglia (Figs. 3.15 and 3.16)

Sympathetic fibres innervating the abdominal viscera do not synapse in the paravertebral ganglia of sympathetic chain but synapse instead in the prevertebral ganglia which lie deeper in the abdomen, generally around major blood vessels. Prominent examples of prevertebral ganglia are:
- **Coeliac.**
- **Superior mesenteric.**
- **Inferior mesenteric.**

After entering the abdomen through the diaphragm, the thoracic splanchnic nerves communicate with each other in front of the aorta, giving rise to the aortic plexus. This plexus is augmented by lumbar splanchnic nerves, which feed preganglionic fibres to the plexus. The coeliac, superior and inferior mesenteric plexuses are offshoots of the aortic plexus. Before entering these plexuses preganglionic sympathetic fibres relay in ganglia which are located near the origins of their respective arteries. After synapsing on these prevertebral ganglia, sympathetic fibres spread along complex plexuses (usually surrounding major

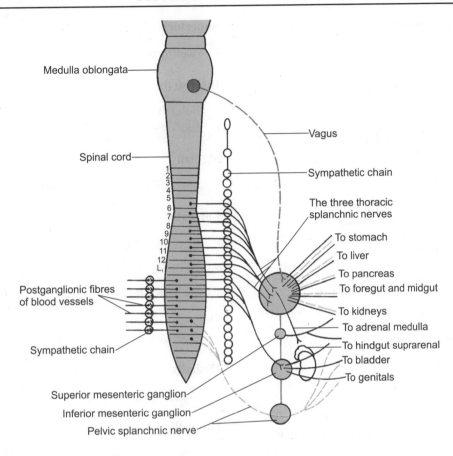

Medulla oblongata

Spinal cord

Vagus

Sympathetic chain

The three thoracic splanchnic nerves

To stomach

To liver

To pancreas

To foregut and midgut

To kidneys

To adrenal medulla

To hindgut suprarenal

To bladder

To genitals

Postganglionic fibres of blood vessels

Sympathetic chain

Superior mesenteric ganglion

Inferior mesenteric ganglion

Pelvic splanchnic nerve

Fig. 3.16: Scheme to show the distribution of the autonomic fibres to abdominal and pelvic viscera

blood vessels) to their target organs. The aortic plexus below the origin of inferior mesenteric artery, continues down into the pelvis and is known as superior hypogastric plexus.

- **Coeliac ganglia,** one on either side of the coeliac artery, are found between the two suprarenal glands. Each ganglion receives preganglionic sympathetic fibres from the **greater and lesser splanchnic nerves** which reach their respective ganglion after piercing the corresponding crus of the diaphragm. The two ganglia are connected by a plexus of nerve fibres known as **coeliac plexus** which is reinforced by the posterior gastric nerve a continuation of right vagus nerve. From this plexus arise other subsidiary plexuses such as the **phrenic, hepatic, splenic, superior and inferior mesenteric and intermesenteric (aortic) plexuses.**
- **Superior mesenteric ganglia** lie on each side of the origin of superior mesenteric artery and may unite below the artery to form an unpaired ganglion.
- **Aorticorenal ganglion,** frequently is identifiable, a

little lower down, lying close to the origin of renal artery.

- **Inferior mesenteric ganglion** is embedded in the inferior mesenteric plexus and may be difficult to find.

PARASYMPATHETIC NERVES
(Figs. 3.15 and 3.16)

The parasympathetic innervation of the foregut and midgut is furnished by the vagi; that of the hindgut, by the pelvic splanchnic nerves derived from S_2-S_4 segments of the spinal cord. Synaptic relay of parasympathetic efferents occurs in small intramural or enteric ganglia of the organs they serve. Parasympathetic fibres of the vagal origin commingle with the sympathetic fibres in the aortic plexus and its offshoots. The vagi enter the abdomen with the oesophagus and their branches join the aortic plexus in the coeliac region.

Visceral afferents of both parasympathetic and sympathetic systems run along with the efferent fibres of each system. The sympathetic afferent ascend through the splanchnic nerves, the sympathetic chains and white rami communicates into the spinal nerves. Parasympathetic afferents from the foregut and midgut ascend with the vagus; those from the hindgut descend to pelvic splanchnic nerves located in the pelvis.

FASCIAE OF THE POSTERIOR ABDOMINAL WALL (FIG. 3.17)

Each muscle of the posterior abdominal wall is covered by a dense fascia. They provide a firm fixation for the peritoneum and retroperitoneal viscera.

Diaphragmatic fascia

The **transversalis fascia,** which clothes the inner surface of the transversalis muscle, is continued onto the lower surface of the diaphragm as the **diaphragmatic fascia.**

Fascia of Quadratus Lumborum (Fig. 3.17)

Lumbar part of the thoracolumbar fascia has three layers which enclose two compartments. Quadratus lumborum occupies the anterior compartment between the anterior and middle layers. Erector spinae, a muscle of the back, fills the posterior compartment between the middle and posterior layers. The attachment of the layers enclosing the quadratus lumborum is as follows:

Anterior layer

Superiorly (Fig. 3.3)

- Lower border of twelfth rib. It is thickened above to form the lateral arcuate ligament which gives rise to the diaphragm.

Inferiorly (Fig. 3.2.)

- Iliolumbar ligament.
- Adjoining part of iliac crest.

Medially (Fig. 3.2)

- Front of the roots of lumbar transverse processes.

Laterally

- Blends with the middle layer.

Middle layer (Fig. 3.8)

Superiorly

- Twelfth rib.

Inferior]ly

- Iliolumbar ligament.
- Iliac crest.

Medially

- Tips of lumbar transverse processes.

Laterally

- Blends with both anterior and posterior layers along the lateral border of erector spinae.

Psoas Sheath (Fig. 3.17)

The psoas major is covered by a fascial sleeve called the **psoas sheath**. It has following attachment:

Medially

- Bodies of lumbar vertebrae.

Laterally

- Fuses with the anterior lamella of the lumbodorsal fascia in the upper part and with the fascia iliaca in the lower part.

Inferiorly

- Passing deep to the femoral artery blends with the tendon of the muscle in the thigh.

Superiorly

- Upper border of the sheath is free and thickened to form the medial arcuate ligament from which is the origin of diaphragm.

Iliac Fascia

The iliacus muscle is covered by a strong fascia which is attached to the iliac crest and inguinal ligament close to the attachment of fascia transversalis. Behind the external iliac vessels it contributes to the formation of the posterior wall of **femoral sheath,** the anterior wall of which is formed by fascia transversalis.

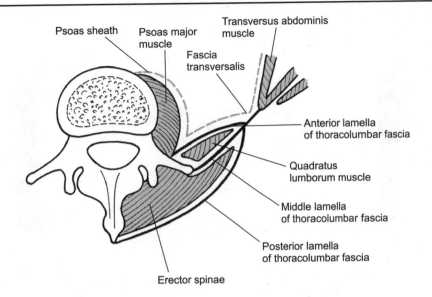

Fig. 3.17: Fasciae of the posterior abdominal wall

CLINICAL APPLICATION

The upper part of the psoas sheath is a funnel-shaped orifice which is held open by the attachments of the medial arcuate ligament and communicates with the posterior mediastinum. Pus from a tuberculous infection of the lumbar vertebrae in abdomen or thoracic vertebrae in posterior mediastinum passes laterally into the psoas sheath **(psoas abscess)**. Pus then tracks down under the inguinal ligament into the femoral triangle where it produces a swelling behind and on each side of the femoral vessels.

THE VESSELS ON POSTERIOR ABDOMINAL WALL

THE ABDOMINAL AORTA

The abdominal aorta enters the abdomen via the aortic opening between the diaphragmatic crurae at the lower border of T_{12}. Through this opening, the vena azygos and thoracic duct pass upwards. It continues downward and ends slightly to the left of the median plane by dividing opposite the body of L_4 into right and left common iliac arteries.

Relations

Posterior (Fig. 3.18)

- Upper four lumbar vertebrae and intervening intervertebral discs.
- Anterior longitudinal ligament.
- Left lumbar veins (Fig. 3.25).

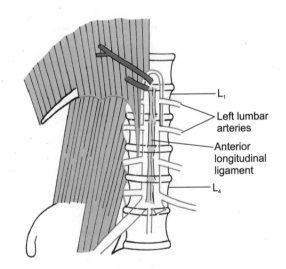

Fig. 3.18: Extent and posterior relations of abdominal aorta

Right lateral (Figs. 3.19. (a) and (b))

- Right crus of diaphragm and right coeliac ganglion.
- Cisterna chyli and vena azygos near the diaphragm.
- Inferior vena cava.

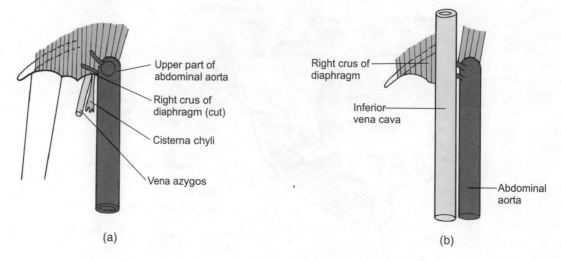

Fig. 3.19: Right lateral relation of abdominal aorta (a and b)

Left lateral (Fig. 3.20 a)

- Left crus of diaphragm and left coeliac ganglion.
- Sympathetic trunk.
- Inferior mesenteric vessels.
- Duodenojejunal flexure.
- Fourth part duodenum.

Anterior from above downwards (Figs. 3.20 (a) and (b))

- Median arcuate ligament.
- Body of pancreas.
- Splenic and left renal veins, the latter separates it from origin of superior mesenteric artery.
- Third part of duodenum.
- Left gonadal vein.
- Coils of small intestine.

Branches (Fig. 3.21)

The branches of the abdominal aorta may be considered unpaired and paired.

Unpaired branches

These may be regarded as arteries of the primitive gut, from above downward they are at the levels indicated:
- Coeliac trunk (to foregut) (T_{12}).

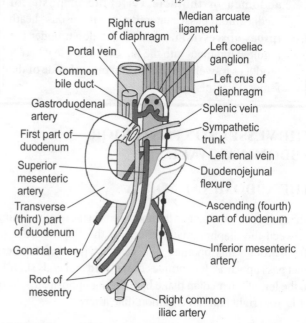

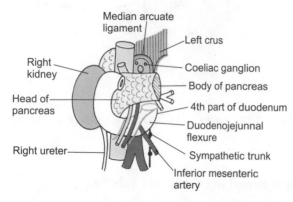

(a) Left lateral relations of aorta and right lateral and anterior relations of inferior vena cava.

(b) Anterior relations of aorta and anterior and left lateral relations of inferior vena cava.

Fig. 3.20: Relations of aorta and inferior vena cava

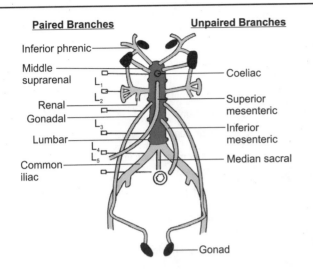

Fig. 3.21: Branches of abdominal aorta with their vertebral level of origin

- Superior mesenteric (to midgut) (L_1)
- Inferior mesenteric (to hindgut) (L_3).
- Median sacral (L_4).

Paired branches

- Inferior phrenic (T_{12})
- Middle suprarenal (L_1)
- Renal (L_1)
- Gonadal (testicular or ovarian) (L_2)
- Lumbar (L_1 to L_4)
- Common iliac (L_4).

Course of Unpaired Branches (Fig. 3.22)

Coeliac Trunk

It is a short trunk arising anteriorly from the abdominal aorta at the level of T_{12} vertebra as the aorta enters the abdomen. The coeliac ganglia hug its sides and the coeliac plexus surrounds it. It supplies the foregut derivatives which include the abdominal part of oesophagus, the stomach, the duodenum down to the entry of the common bile duct, the spleen, liver and portions of the pancreas.

Superior Mesenteric Artery

It arises at the level of L_1 vertebra. It supplies the midgut derivatives which extend from the opening of the common bile duct into the duodenum to the proximal two-thirds of transverse colon. It passes downwards, forwards and to the right towards the right iliac fossa.

Inferior Mesenteric Artery

It arises from the aorta opposite L_3 vertebra. It supplies hindgut derivatives which include left one-third of transverse colon, descending colon, sigmoid colon, rectum and the anal canal. It runs downwards to the left and continues in the pelvis as superior rectal artery.

Median Sacral Artery

It arises from the back of the aorta, 2.5 cm above its bifurcation. It represents the terminal part of aorta. It runs down on the middle of sacrum upto the coccyx.

Course of Paired Branches (Fig. 3.22)

Inferior Phrenic Arteries

They arise at the level of the coeliac trunk, from the postero-lateral aspects of the aorta and ascend on the diaphragm, deep to the inferior vena cava on the right and to the oesophagus on the left. They supply the inferior surface of the diaphragm.

Middle Suprarenal Arteries

They arise at the level of the superior mesenteric artery on each side and supply the suprarenal glands.

Renal Arteries

They arise at the lower part of L_1 vertebra. Each is largely hidden by its vein. The right renal artery is longer and crosses behind the inferior vena cava. They supply the kidneys.

Gonadal Arteries (Testicular or Ovarian)

They arise opposite the L_2 vertebra. They pass in front of the ureter. The right also passes in front of the inferior vena cava. They take a long course to enter the gonads.

Lumbar Arteries

They are four paired branches. They hug the lumbar ventral bodies and pass deep to the fibrous arches of the psoas major deep to the sympathetic trunk. The upper two on the right pass deep to the cisterna chili, vena azygos, and the right crus, the latter separating them from the inferior vena cava.

Common Iliac Arteries

These are large terminal branches. Each inclines laterally on the psoas major. Opposite the sacral promontory

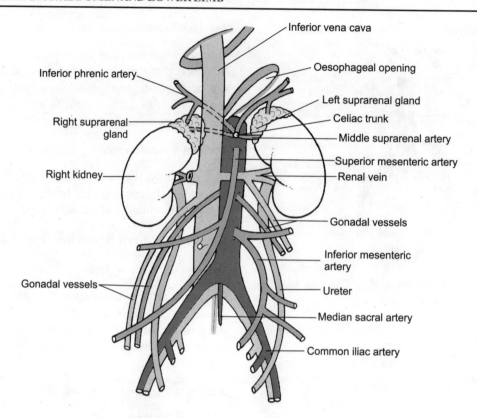

Fig. 3.22: Course of the branches of abdominal aorta

and anterior to the sacroiliac joint, it bifurcates into external and internal iliac arteries. The external iliac inclines toward the lateral edge of psoas and the internal iliac turns down into the pelvis in front of the sacroiliac joint.

THE INFERIOR VENA CAVA

The inferior vena cava is formed at the level of the lower border of L_5 vertebra on the right side of the midline by the union of the two common iliac veins. It lies to the right side of the aorta along the anterior aspect of the vertebral bodies and ascends upwards to enter the thoracic cavity through the opening in the central tendon of the diaphragm situated at the level of T_8 vertebra. After a short intrathoracic course, it pierces the pericardium to open in the right atrium of the heart at the level of the 6th costal cartilage.

Posterior Relations

Posterior relations from below upwards are (Fig. 3.23):
- Bodies and discs of lower three lumbar vertebrae.
- Right lumbar arteries.

- Right sympathetic trunk.
- Right renal artery.
- Right crus of diaphragm.
- Right suprarenal gland (medial half).
- Right middle suprarenal artery.
- Right inferior phrenic artery.

Anterior Relations

Anterior relations from below upward (Fig. 3.20):
- Right common iliac artery.
- Coils of small intestine.
- Root of mesentery containing superior mesenteric vessels.
- Third part of duodenum.
- Head of pancreas.
- First part of duodenum from which it is separated by portal vein, common bile duct and the gastroduodenal artery (Fig. 3.24).
- Foramen epiploicum which separates the inferior vena cava from the right free margin of lesser omentum and its contents (Fig. 3.24).
- Right lobe of liver.

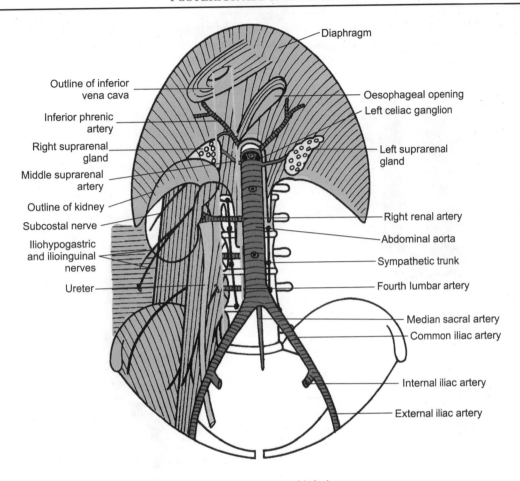

Fig. 3.23: Posterior relations of inferior vena cava

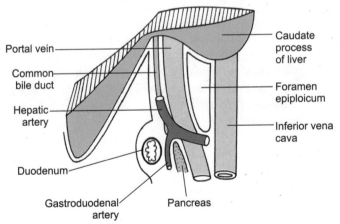

Fig. 3.24: Foramen epiploicum and structures in lesser omentum are anterior relations of inferior vena cava

On right side (Fig. 3.20 a)

- Right ureter.

- Medial border of right kidney.
- Right phrenic nerve in the vena caval opening.

On left side (Fig. 3.20 b)

- Aorta in the lower part.
- Right crus of diaphragm and right coeliac ganglion in the upper part.

Tributaries (Fig. 3.25)

These are:

- Right and left common iliac veins.
- Lumbar vein (four pairs).
- Right gonadal vein (testicular or ovarian).
- Right and left renal veins.
- Right suprarenal vein.
- Right inferior phrenic vein.
- Right and left hepatic veins.

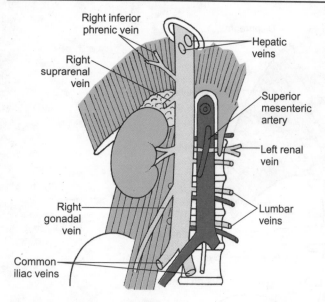

Fig. 3.25: The tributaries of the inferior vena cava (Note that the left renal vein is clipped by the superior mesenteric artery)

CLINICAL APPLICATION

- Aortic aneurysm usually results from atherosclerosis in older age groups. It is a dangerous clinical condition since a rupture of the aneurysm is usually fatal.
- A large tumour from the structures in anterior relationship with the aorta e.g., pancreas or stomach, may transmit the pulsations of the aorta and may be mistaken as an aneurysm.
- The lumbar veins are connected with vertebral venous plexuses. These veins and plexuses are not provided with valves and hence the blood can flow in both directions depending on the pressure changes. Through these veins and similar veins in the pelvis, metastases from pelvis can spread to the vertebral column or the brain. Cancer of prostate is an example.
- When the vena cava is obstructed blood may enter the portal system where there are connections between it and veins that drain into the inferior vena cava.

LYMPHATICS OF POSTERIOR ABDOMINAL WALL

The lymph glands of the abdomen are arranged in two large groups:
- The **parietal,** lying behind the peritoneum, on the posterior abdominal, in relation to the large blood vessels.

- The **visceral,** which lie along the visceral arteries and are dealt with in connection with the lymph drainage of the various viscera.

Parietal Nodes

The main lymph nodes lie in chains alongside the main arteries from which they derive their names (Fig. 3.26):
- The **iliac nodes** lie alongside the external iliac, common iliac and internal iliac arteries. They are named after the artery on which they lie.

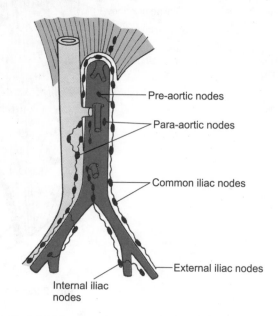

Fig. 3.26: Parietal lymph nodes on posterior abdominal wall

The **external iliac nodes** receive the lymphatic vessels from the lower limb as well as the buttocks and the external genitalia via the inguinal lymph nodes which also receive deep lymph vessels from the anterior abdominal wall below the umbilicus. They drain into the common iliac nodes which also receive the vessels from the internal iliac nodes of the pelvis.
- The **aortic** or **lumbar nodes** consist of glands which are named according to their position in relation to the aorta.
- **Pre-aortic nodes** lie in front of the aorta and lie around the origins of the coeliac, superior mesenteric and inferior mesenteric arteries and are named after these blood vessels. They receive lymph vessels from the portions of the gut supplied by the corresponding artery i.e., foregut, midgut and hindgut regions. They are drained by a single lymph vessel, the **intestinal trunk** which enters the **cisterna chyli.**
- **Para-aortic** which lie on the right and left side of the

aorta in relation to the origins of the paired branches of the aorta. The common iliac nodes drain into them.

They also receive lymphatic vessels from the posterior and lateral abdominal wall, the kidneys and suprarenals; the gonads (testes or ovaries); the ovaries, the uterine tubes and the fundus of uterus in the female.

The efferents of the para-aortic glands unite to from a single trunk on each side, the **right and left lumbar lymph trunks,** which unite to form the **cisterna chyli**.

CISTERNA CHYLI (FIG. 3.27)

The **intestinal lymph trunk** and the two **lumbar lymph trunks** join to form a dilated sac known as **cisterna chyli**. The descending intercostal lymph trunks which receive lymph vessels from the lower intercostal spaces pierce the corresponding crus of the diaphragm to join the cisterna chyli.

Cisterna chyli is 5 cm long and only 4 mm wide. Its relations are:

Anteriorly

- Right crus

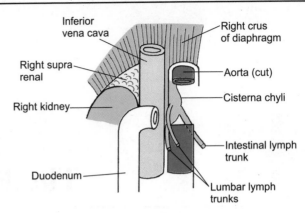

Fig. 3.27: The cisterna chyli

Posteriorly

- Bodies of L_1 and L_2 vertebrae.
- Upper two right lumbar arteries.
- Vena azygos.

The cranial end of cisterna chyli narrows to from the **thoracic duct** which passes through the aortic opening of the diaphragm lying on the right side of the aorta, between the aorta and the vena azygos.

4

The Peritoneum

INTRODUCTION

The peritoneum, like the pleura or the serous pericardium, forms a closed serous sac. It consists of two subdivisions:
- **Parietal peritoneum.**
- **Visceral peritoneum.**

The **parietal peritoneum** clothes the anterior and posterior abdominal walls, the under surface of the diaphragm and the cavity of the pelvis. The **visceral peritoneum** is the continuation of parietal peritoneum, which leaves the peritoneal wall to invest some viscera partly or other completely. All organs lie outside the peritoneum, although if they invaginate it, they can become almost wholly covered by peritoneum and then get connected to the peritoneum lining the body wall by a double fold of peritoneum called **mesentery** or **ligament**.

The survey of the peritoneal cavity can be best understood by the elementary developmental considerations.

Developmental Events

- The mesoderm in the developing embryo gets cavitated on either side with a resulting paired cavity viz., coelom and a median septum enclosing the endodermal tube. The septum is called **ventral** and **dorsal mesentery** (Fig. 4.1).
- The **ventral mesentery** in the distal part gets broken and has a free margin. The coelom thus becomes a single continuous cavity. Different parts of the adult from head to pelvis can be visualized on the embryo (Fig. 4.2).
- Endodermal tube dilates to form the stomach and the liver cords which sprout from the foregut invade the ventral mesentery which can be called the ventral mesogastrium (ventral mesentery of the foregut (Fig. 4.3).

Fate of Ventral Mesogastrium (Fig. 4.3)

- The ventral mesogastrium at this stage is the septum

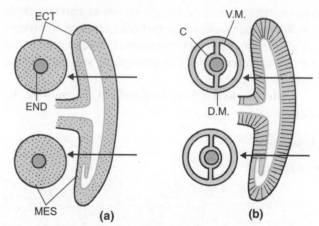

Fig. 4.1: The development of peritoneum: (a) The embryo in sagittal and transverse section showing the three primary germ layers (ECT = Ectoderm, END = Endoderm, MES = Mesoderm). (b) Cavitation of mesoderm with a resulting paired cavity viz., coelom and a median septum enclosing the endodermal tube (C = Coelom, DM = Dorsal mesentery, VM = Ventral mesentery)

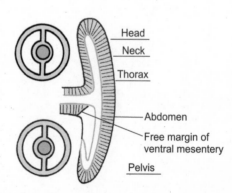

Fig. 4.2: Coelom becomes a single continuous cavity with the breaking of the distal part of ventral mesentery which gets a free margin. Different parts of the adult from head to pelvis can be visualized

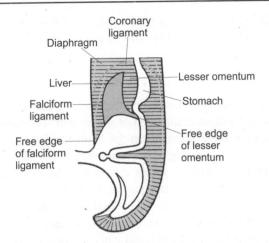

Fig. 4.3: Fate of ventral mesogastrium: Endodermal tube dilates to form stomach and liver bud grows into ventral mesogastrium dividing it into three parts

transversum, a wedge-shaped block of mesoderm ventral to the foregut.

- The development of liver in the ventral mesogastrium divides it into three parts viz.,
  - **Falciform ligament** and **coronary ligaments** between the body wall and the liver.
  - The **lesser omentum** between the liver and the lesser curvature of the stomach.
  - The **visceral peritoneal covering of the liver (Glisson's capsule)** (Fig. 4.3.)
- With the rotation of stomach the plane of lesser omentum changes from sagittal to coronal.
- The lesser omentum has along its free edge the bile duct, hepatic artery and portal vein. The falciform ligament supports the umbilical vein along its inferior edge. Posterosuperiorly the coronary ligament retains the liver in contact with the portion of the diaphragm that is derived from septum transversum.

Fate of Dorsal Mesogastrium (Fig. 4.4)

- The attachment of the dorsal mesogastrium to the foregut defines the greater curvature of the stomach and the future medial border of the duodenum, both of which at this stage face posteriorly.
- The dorsal mesogastrium contains the spleen and the pancreas.
- The developing spleen divides the dorsal mesogastrium into three parts. The part above it forms the **gastrophrenic ligament** which connects the stomach

with the diaphragm. The part below it gives rise to **greater omentum** and **transverse mesocolon** which hangs down into the more caudal part of the peritoneal cavity. The middle part is divided by spleen into three parts viz., an anterior part, the **gastrosplenic ligament** between the greater curvature of stomach and spleen, a middle part forming the **covering of spleen** and a posterior portion the **lienorenal ligament** between the spleen and the dorsal midline attachment of the mesogastrium (Fig. 4.4). The lienorenal ligament comes to lie parallel to the surface of the left kidney and contains the pancreas and the splenic vessels.

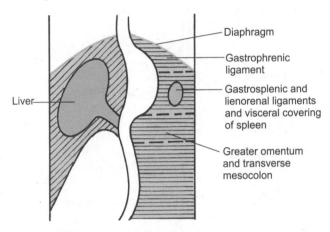

Fig. 4.4: Fate of dorsal mesogastrium: It is divided into three parts by the developing spleen which further divides second part into another three parts

- Destabilisation of dorsal mesogastrium occurs due to the rotation of stomach and duodenum, which takes place along their longitudinal axis, in a manner that turns their original right surface posteriorly. The dorsal mesogastrium is invaded by the cavity of the **right pleuroperitoneal canal** causing the spleen to bulge into the **left pleuroperitoneal canal** and aiding the stomach in pointing its greater curvature to the left. From the right side of the dorsal mesogastrium a **pneumatoenteric recess** excavates, dorsal to the liver, towards the right lung bud (Fig. 4.5). A **pancreaticoenteric recess** excavates from right to left behind the stomach. A **hepatoenteric recess** thins and expands the lesser omentum. Confluences of these recesses form the early **omental bursa.** The parietal attachment of the dorsal mesogastrium is altered and from attachment to the midline of the dorsal abdominal wall, it now sweeps from the oesophageal orifice downwards and to the left across the diaphragm and the upper pole of the left

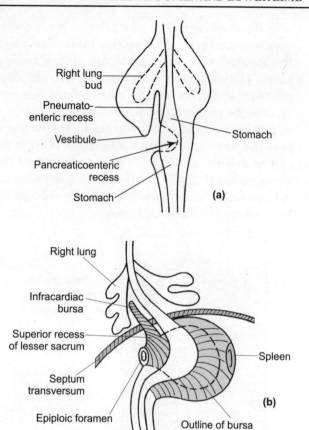

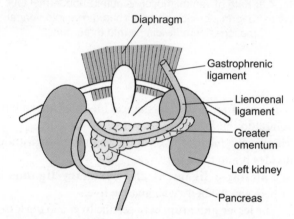

kidney, it then moves to the right until it reaches first part of duodenum (Fig. 4.6). It grows downward with the greater omentum.

Fate of Mesoduodenum (Fig. 4.7)

- The duodenum is formed by the most caudal part of the foregut and the cranial part of the midgut. The junction between these segments in the adult lies immediately distal to the opening of the hepatopancreatic duct. As it grows in length, it forms a C-shaped loop, with the rotation of stomach it is pushed to the right side of the midline. Gradually the mesoduodenum fuses with the dorsal body wall thus rendering the duodenum (except the most proximal and distal parts) retroperitoneal.

Fig. 4.5: Destabilisation of dorsal mesogastrium to create the omental bursa: (a) Formation of the omental bursa. Arrow passes dorsal to the stomach into the bursa. (b) The increase in the size of stomach to the left is a factor towards the formation of lesser sac

Fig. 4.6: The attachments of dorsal mesogastrium to posterior abdominal wall after the creation of omental bursa. As the omental bursa enlarges to the left, part of the greater sac is obliterated in front of the left kidney

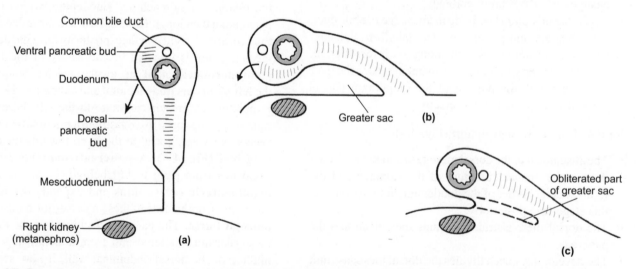

Fig. 4.7: Fate of mesoduodenum: (a) As the duodenum falls to the right, carrying with it the pancreas. (b) Part of greater sac behind the pancreas becomes obliterated. (c) Duodenum undergoes rotation through 90° so that its ventral surface is directed to the right

Fate of Common Dorsal Mesentery of Midgut and Hindgut

The midgut forms the duodenum (beyond the hepatopancreatic ampula), the jejunum, the ileum, the caecum, the appendix, the ascending colon and the right two-thirds of the transverse colon.

- The midgut forms a loop convex forward. Ventrally it is in communication with the yolk sac through the **vitelline duct**. The whole loop remains suspended from the dorsal body wall by the short dorsal mesentery in which the artery of the midgut, namely, the superior mesenteric artery is contained. The loop grows so rapidly that the intraembryonic coelom is too small to hold it, so that part of the loop is extruded into the extraembryonic coelom in the umbilical cord, forming a temporary physiological umbilical hernia (Fig. 4.8).
- The upper end of the midgut and its lower end i.e., the junction of midgut and hindgut are fixed to the posterior abdominal wall by condensed parts of dorsal mesentery known as **superior** and **inferior retention bands**. Thus, a flexure is formed where the midgut and hindgut join. This is known as **colic angle**. Thus, the two fixed points of midgut loop are, quite close together, forming the **duodenocolic isthmus**. The artery of the midgut loop (superior mesenteric) runs from the aorta to the apex of

the extruded gut to which is attached the obliterated vitello-intestinal duct. The midgut loop and its mesentery still lie in the sagittal plane. The part of the gut in front of the artery is the **prearterial segment** and the part behind is the **postarterial segment**.

- During the fifth week, the bud for the caecum and appendix appears on the postarterial segment of the loop.
- Rotation of midgut loop takes place in three stages:

First stage takes place between the fifth and tenth week. The superior mesenteric artery is considered the axis of rotation. The prearterial segment is pushed down and to the right due to the growth of liver which exercises pressure on the base of this segment. Consequently the postarterial segment moves upwards and to the left. The ends of the midgut loop thereby rotate through 90° in an anticlockwise direction completing the first stage of rotation (Fig. 4.9).

Second stage of rotation occurs at the tenth to eleventh week and is marked by the return of the midgut to the abdomen. About the beginning of the tenth week the midgut loop returns to the abdominal cavity from the umbilical cord. The gut being too bulky to be returned en masse, it retreats in a definite order, commencing with the prearterial portion. The superior mesenteric artery is stretched like a

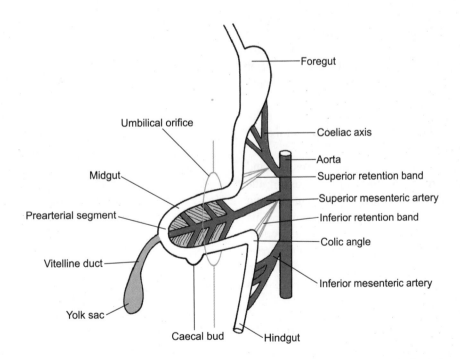

Fig. 4.8: Physiological umbilical hernia: Herniation of U-loop of midgut before commencement of rotation. Dorsal mesentery suspending the gut from the posterior abdominal wall, is not shown

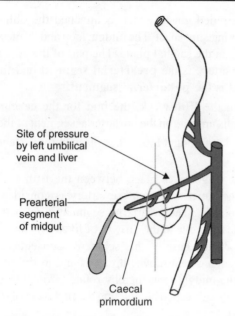

Fig. 4.9: First stage of rotation: The postarterial segment of the midgut loop moves upwards and to the left through 90° in an anticlockwise direction, while the prearterial segment moves down and to the right due to pressure exerted by the left umbilical vein and liver

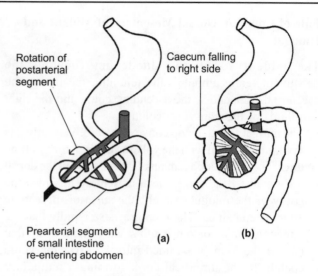

Fig. 4.10: Second stage of rotation: (a) The prearterial segment descends into the left side of peritoneal cavity and the duodenum is placed behind the superior mesenteric artery. (b) The postarterial segment passes upwards and to the right carrying the caecum into the right side of peritoneal cavity

cord from commencement to termination. The prearterial limb passes behind the superior mesenteric artery and to the right of the future descending colon (a hindgut derivative) and its mesentery displacing it to the left from its midline position. This component of rotation carries the future horizontal portion of the duodenum behind the superior mesenteric artery and lays it across the vertebral column, placing the duodenojejunal junction and all of the prearterial segment of the loop into the left side of the coelom, (Fig. 4.10 a). The duodenum becomes fixed in this position quite early in the process of rotation.

The postarterial segment of the loop returns last and reduces, passing upward and to the right and crossing the proximal end of the prearterial segment at the point of origin of the superior mesenteric artery from the aorta. This component of rotation lays the future transverse colon across the descending portion of the duodenum and carries the caecum into the right side of the peritoneal cavity (Fig. 4.10 b). The net result of the second stage of rotation involving 180° rotation is as follows:

- The duodenum crosses behind the upper part of the superior mesenteric artery.
- The transverse colon crosses in front of the same part of this vessel.

- The descending colon is pushed to the left.
- The caecum is on the right side.
- The coils of small intestine lie from left upper to right lower parts of the abdomen.

It is to be noted that the midgut loop rotates on the axis of superior mesenteric artery through 270° from its

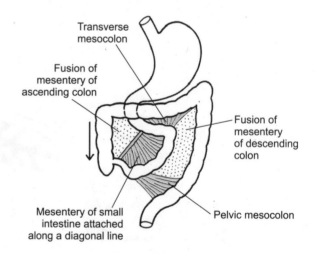

Fig. 4.11: Third stage of rotation: The caecum descends to the right iliac fossa and there is fixation of gut in its definitive arrangement

original sagittal plane, 90° is done in first stage and 180° in the second stage.

Third stage of rotation. This stage lasts from the eleventh week until shortly after birth. The following events, mainly the efficient fixation of the gut, take place:

- The caecum descends to the right iliac fossa (Fig. 4.11).
- Fusion of the mesentery of the ascending and descending, colons to the posterior parietal peritoneum, shown dotted (Figs. 4.11 and 4.12 d).
- Fusion of the mesentery of jejunum and ileum to the parietal peritoneum across a diagonal line that slopes from the duodenojejunal flexure to the ileocaecal junction located in the right iliac fossa (Figs. 4.11 and 4.12 d).
- Fusion occurs between the visceral peritoneum of the transverse colon and the upper layer of the primitive transverse mesocolon on the one hand and the posterior (returning) layer of the greater omentum on the order (Figs. 4.12 a, b and c).

The hindgut forms the left third of the transverse colon, the descending colon, the sigmoid colon, the rectum, the upper part of the anal canal and certain urogenital organs.

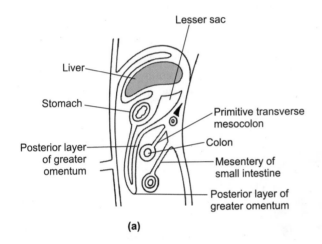

(a)

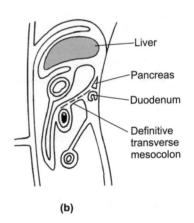

(b)

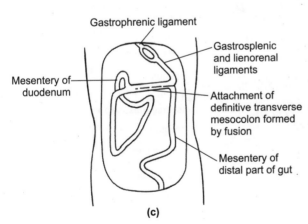

(c)

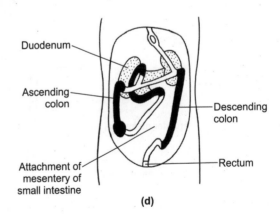

(d)

(a), (b) & (c) Sagittal section views to show formation of transverse mesocolon.

(d) Shows retroperitonealisation of duodenum, ascending colon and descending colon.

Fig. 4.12: Events during the third stage of rotation of gut

CLINICAL APPLICATION

- If the physiological hernia of the midgut loop persists until after birth, the condition of **exampholas** exists. The whole midgut loop or only the caecum or ileum may lie in the sac at the umbilicus at birth.
- The small intestine may twist around the superior mesenteric artery, obstructing the intestine or compressing its blood supply. This results in the condition known as **volvulus**. Clockwise, rather than normal anticlockwise, withdrawal of the midgut loop into the abdominal cavity (reversed rotation) causes **situs inversus viscerum** in which the visceral positions are a mirror image of normal.
- **Meckel's diverticulum** is a persistent remnant of the vitelline duct and is present on the antimesenteric border of the ileum. It occurs 2 feet (62 cm) from the ileocaecal valve, is found in 2 per cent of persons and is 2 inch (5 cm) or more in length. It has the calibre of ileum. A long diverticulum predisposes to obstruction.
- The caecum may fail to descend and may be subhepatic in position.

The adult arrangement and mode of reflection of peritoneum can be clearly understood if the peritoneum is traced vertically as well as transversely.

The Arrangement of Peritoneum in a Longitudinal Section (Fig. 4.13)

The peritoneum of abdominal cavity is best understood by following it in a longitudinal section of the abdomen in a midplane. The peritoneum lines the anterior abdominal wall and passes onto the inferior surface of the diaphragm from which it is reflected onto the upper surface of the liver. It passes onto the anterior and inferior surfaces of the liver into a fissure on the inferior surface and leaves the liver to continue downwards as the anterior layer of the **lesser omentum.** It passes onto the anterior surface of the

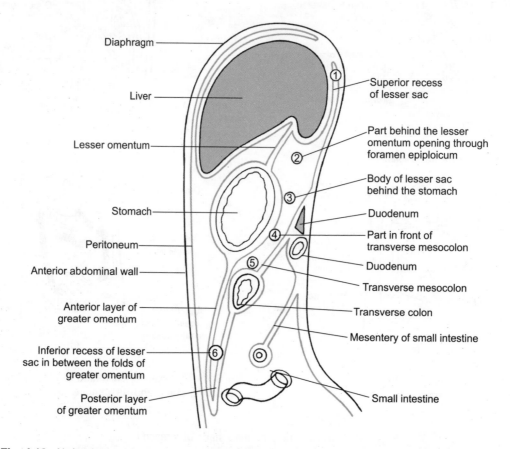

Fig. 4.13: Abdominal cavity in sagittal section showing the extent, parts and anterior and posterior walls of the lesser sac

stomach. At the inferior border of stomach, the peritoneum passes downwards for a considerable distance as the anterior layer of the **greater omentum** and then turns upwards on itself to form the posterior layer of the greater omentum. This layer continues upward behind the transverse colon as the posterior layer of the **transverse mesocolon,** which is the mesentery of colon and reaches the posterior abdominal wall at about the level of the middle of pancreas. The posterior layer of transverse mesocolon continues downwards on the posterior abdominal wall and leaves it to form the **mesentery of the small intestine**. The inferior layer of this mesentery returns to the abdominal wall and after passing downward lies in front of the rectum in the pelvis.

The main part of the peritoneal cavity is known as **greater sac**. The greater sac has a diverticulum passing to the left from the upper part of its posterior wall. This diverticulum is much smaller than the main cavity and is known as the **lesser sac** or the **omental bursa**. The peritoneum of the lesser sac lies behind the stomach. The opening into the lesser sac, known as the **epiploic foramen,** is above the duodenum between it and the liver. The lesser sac extends upwards behind the liver as the **superior recess** and downward for a variable distance into the greater omentum as the **inferior recess**. The anterior layer of the lesser sac forms the posterior layer of lesser omentum. The posterior layer of the lesser sac fuses with the posterior layer of the greater omentum and may be regarded as the upper or anterior layer of the transverse mesocolon.

THE ARRANGEMENT OF PERITONEUM IN TRANSVERSE SECTIONS

The reflection in the transverse direction is different at three levels.

1. At the Level of Foramen Epiploicum (Fig. 4.14)

The parietal peritoneum lining the anterior abdominal wall when traced to the right continues with the visceral peritoneum on the posterior abdominal.

It covers the anterior aspect of the right kidney, the inferior vena cava and the aorta and part of the anterior surface of the left kidney. The peritoneum then leaves the kidney and passes to the hilum of the spleen as the anterior layer of the **lienorenal ligament**. From the hilum of spleen it is reflected onto the greater curvature of the stomach as the posterior layer of the **gastrosplenic ligament**. The visceral peritoneum covers the posterior surface of the stomach and leaves the greater curvature to form the posterior layer of **lesser omentum**. On the right, the lesser omentum has a free border and here the peritoneum folds around the common bile duct, hepatic artery and portal vein. The free border of the lesser omentum forms the anterior margin of the **foramen epiploicum (Winslow's).** The peritoneum then forms the anterior layer of the lesser omentum and then covers the anterior surface of the stomach. At the greater curvature the peritoneum leaves the stomach, forming the anterior layer of the **gastrosplenic ligament** reaches the hilum of the spleen and then covers

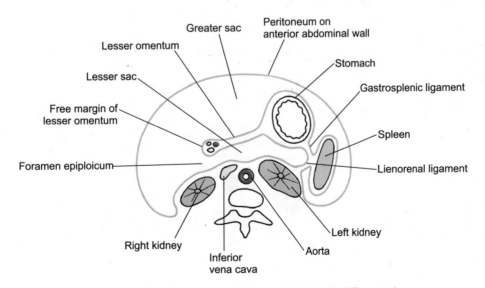

Fig. 4.14: T.S. at foramen epiploicum at the level of T_{12} vertebra

the surfaces of the spleen to reach the hilum again. From the hilum of the spleen it is reflected backward to the posterior abdominal wall, forming the posterior layer of the **lienorenal ligament**. It covers part of the anterior aspect of left kidney and sweeps around the left side of the lateral abdominal wall to reach the anterior abdominal wall.

2.   A T.S. just below the Foramen Epiploicum. At the Level of First Lumbar Vertebra (Fig. 4.15)

There is no continuity between the peritoneum of the greater sac and the lesser sac. The peritoneum of the **greater sac** after lining the anterior and lateral abdominal wall on the right side covers the anterior surface of the right kidney and passes onto the anterior surface of the stomach from where the anterior layer of greater omentum cover the colon and is then continued on the anterior abdominal wall. The peritoneum lining, the interior of the lesser sac at this level covers the posterior surface of the stomach anteriorly and the structures on the posterior abdominal wall that form the **stomach bed** viz., the pancreas, upper pole of right kidney, transverse colon.

3.   A T.S. just below the Umbilicus at the Level of the Fourth Lumbar Vertebra (Fig. 4.16)

The peritoneum on the posterior abdominal wall in the region of aorta and inferior vena cava is reflected as the mesentery whose two layers enclose the small intestine. Laterally, the peritoneum covers the ascending and descending colons, forming medial and lateral **paracolic gutters** on each side and then passes forward to line the anterolateral abdominal wall. The **greater omentum** is present in front of the coils of small intestine. The **omental bursa** is present between its anterior and posterior layers.

PERITONEAL CAVITY

The peritoneal cavity is a potential space that exists between the parietal and visceral layers of peritoneum. It is practically empty excepting for a thin film of lymph-like fluid which serves to lubricate the adjoining surfaces of the viscera and prevents friction during movements. Although organs appear to be inside the peritoneal cavity, they are really extraperitoneal. They have invaginated into the closed sac of peritoneum and lie within it with a layer of peritoneum covering them and separating them from the cavity.

The peritoneal cavity is divided by the pelvic brim into a part within the lesser pelvis and the part within the abdomen proper (Fig. 4.17). Peritoneal reflections divide the abdominal cavity into a **greater sac** and a **lesser sac**. The greater sac is the main part of the cavity that extends from the diaphragm into the pelvis. The **lesser sac,** also known as **omental bursa** is a diverticulum of the greater sac, which forms a potential space mainly behind the stomach and the lesser omentum. It is confined largely to the left side of the upper abdomen and communicates to the right with the greater sac through a passage known as the **epiploic foramen**.

Greater Sac

This sac is the main part of the peritoneal cavity and extends from the diaphragm to the pelvic floor. It is opened by incisions of the abdominal wall and into this sac protrude all the viscera. The **gastrocolic ligament,** the fusion of the greater omentum and transverse mesocolon, divides the greater sac into:
(i)   A supracolic compartment.
(ii) An infracolic compartment.

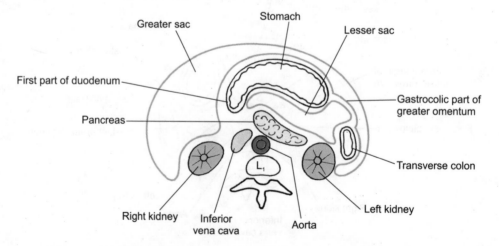

Fig. 4.15: T.S. just below the foramen epiploicum at the level of L₁ vertebra

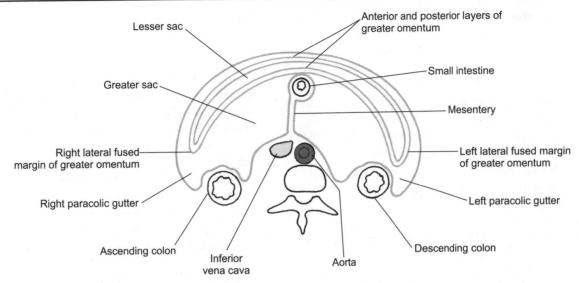

Fig. 4.16: T.S. below the umbilicus at the level of L4 vertebra

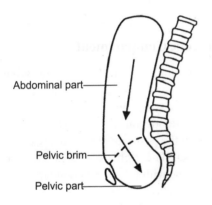

Fig. 4.17: Divisions of the peritoneal cavity and their direction

The Supracolic Compartment (Fig. 4.18)

Anteriorly has the costal margin of the thoracic cage below the diaphragm and the anterior abdominal wall. Posteriorly lies the lesser omentum, stomach and the greater omentum. **Falciform ligament** a fold of peritoneum passing from the anterior abdominal wall and the abdominal surface of the diaphragm to the anterior and inferior surface of the liver, partly divides the supracolic compartment into right and left parts.

- The oesophagus and stomach are in the left upper part below the diaphragm.

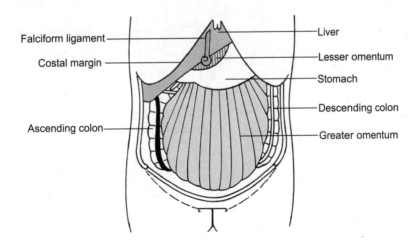

Fig. 4.18: The supracolic compartment of greater sac seen after reflection of the anterior abdominal wall along with the layer of parietal peritoneum

- The **greater omentum** is attached to the convexity leading from the oesophagus around the greater curvature of stomach to the first part of duodenum. To the left it consists of the **gastrophrenic ligament** and of the continuous layers of **gastrosplenic** and **lienorenal ligaments** and to the right, it consists of the **gastrocolic omentum**. The gastrocolic omentum is the part of greater omentum which passes between the transverse colon and the greater curvature of stomach.

- The **lesser omentum** is attached below to the right side of abdominal oesophagus, lesser curvature and pylorus of stomach and the first inch of duodenum. Its upper attachment passes from the oesophageal opening across the diaphragm to the right, behind the liver, to the left of inferior vena cava, so across the under surface of the liver. From the right side of the porta hepatis down to the first inch of duodenum, the right edge of lesser omentum is free, its anterior and posterior layers joining each other. The two layers of the lesser omentum separate at the lesser curvature of stomach to clothe its anterior and posterior walls and reunite at the greater curvature to continue downwards as greater omentum.

- The liver lies in the upper right part of the peritoneal cavity below the diaphragm. The two layers of lesser omentum traced upwards from their attachment to the liver, separate to clothe that viscus and reunite above it to become attached to the diaphragm and the anterior abdominal wall, constituting the **triangular, coronary** and **falciform ligaments of the liver** (Fig. 4.20).

The Infracolic Compartment (Fig. 4.19)

When the greater omentum and transverse colon are turned up, the infracolic compartment of the peritoneal cavity is exposed. The lower layer of transverse mesocolon, which divides the greater sac into supracolic and infracolic compartments, comes into view. It is attached transversely across the posterior abdominal wall. On the right it is attached across the descending part of the duodenum and ends over the lower pole of the right kidney at the right colic flexure. On the left, it ends over the lower pole of the left kidney at the left colic flexure. This part of the cavity has the following divisions:

- Right infracolic compartment.
- Left infracolic compartment.
- Right paracolic recess (gutter)
- Left paracolic recess (gutter)
- Peritoneal fossae in the regions of:
    - Duodenojejunal flexure (Fig. 4.21).
    - Iliocaecal junction (Fig. 4.22).
    - Pelvic mesocolon (Fig. 4.23).

Right Infracolic Compartment

The oblique attachment of the **root of mesentery** divides the infracolic compartment into right and left parts. This attachment begins at the duodenojejunal flexure, crosses the third part of duodenum and slopes downwards across the structures on the posterior abdominal wall to end in the right iliac fossa. The right infracolic compartment is triangular in shape with following boundaries:

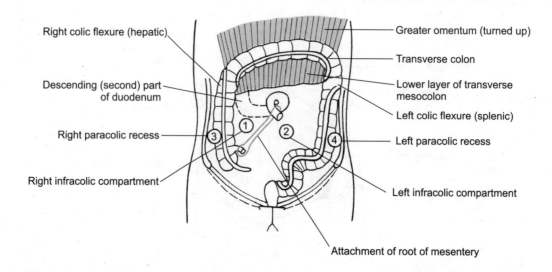

Right colic flexure (hepatic)

Descending (second) part of duodenum

Right paracolic recess

Right infracolic compartment

Greater omentum (turned up)

Transverse colon

Lower layer of transverse mesocolon

Left colic flexure (splenic)

Left paracolic recess

Left infracolic compartment

Attachment of root of mesentery

Fig. 4.19: The infracolic compartment of greater sac seen when the greater omentum is turned up

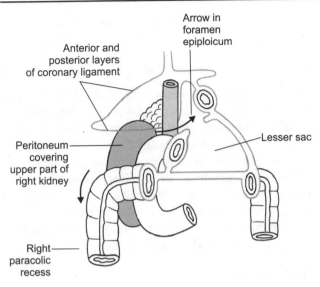

Fig. 4.20: The relations of the hepatorenal recess (Pouch of Morison)

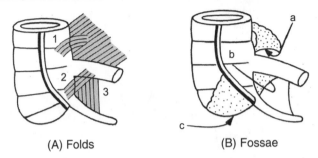

(A) Folds   (B) Fossae

Fig. 4.22: The peritoneal folds and fossae in the region of ileocaecal junction: (A) Folds: Superior (1), inferior (2), ileocaecal folds and mesoappendix (3). (B) Fossae superior (a), inferior (b), retrocaecal (c)

- **Apex** at the ileocaecal junction.
- **Base**—Attachment of transverse mesocolon between the hepatic flexure and duodenojejunal flexure.
- **Right side**—ascending colon.
- **Left side**—attachment of mesentery of small intestine.

This compartment has no free passage into the pelvic cavity.

Left Infracolic Compartment

It is quadrilateral in shape and is larger than the right infracolic compartment. It has the following boundaries:
- **Upper border**—attachment of transverse mesocolon between the duodenojejunal flexure and splenic flexure.

- **Right border**—attachment of the mesentery of small intestine.
- **Left border**—descending colon.

This compartment widens below to pass in a smooth sweep across the pelvic brim into the cavity of the pelvis.

Right Paracolic Recess (Gutter) (Figs. 4.19 and 4.20)

It is the space on the lateral side of the ascending colon. It commences in the supracolic compartment in the recess known as **hepatorenal pouch (of Morison)** and leads directly downward lateral to the ascending colon and caecum, crosses the pelvic brim to reach the cavity of pelvis.

The **hepatorenal pouch** has following boundaries:

Superiorly

- Reflection of the posterior layer of coronary ligament onto the upper pole of right kidney.

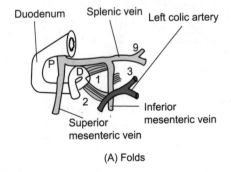

(A) Folds

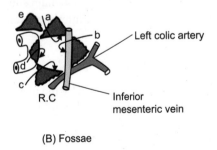

(B) Fossae

Fig. 4.21: The peritoneal folds and fossae in the region of duodenojejunal flexure: (A) Folds: Superior (1), Inferior (2) and paraduodenal (3). (B) Fossae: Superior (a), paraduodenal (b), Inferior (c), retroduodenal (d) and duodenojejunal (e)

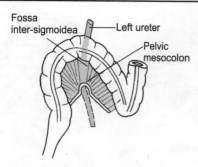

Fig. 4.23: The fossa intersigmoidea

Anteriorly

• Forwardly sloping visceral surface of liver.

Posteriorly

• Peritoneum covering the upper part of right kidney and diaphragm.

Inferiorly

• Leads directly into right paracolic recess.

Medially

• Leads into the lesser sac through the foramen epiploicum.

Left Paracolic Gutter

It lies wholly in the infracolic compartment lateral to the descending colon. It leads into the pelvis across the lateral limb of sigmoid mesocolon which is attached along the pelvic brim.

Peritoneal Fossae

(a) The Paraduodenal Fossae (Fig. 4.21)

The superior, inferior, left and right paraduodenal fossae occur in association with the terminal duodenum superior and inferior, and paraduodenal folds, the inferior mesenteric vein and the left colic artery.

(b) Fossae of the Caecal Region (Fig. 4.22)

The superior ileocaecal fossa is bounded by the mesentery proper and the superior ileocaecal (vascular) fold. It is open to the left.

The inferior ileocaecal fossa is bounded by the mesoappendix and the inferior ileocaecal or bloodless **fold of Treves.**

The retrocaecal fossa lies posterior to the caecum, is variable in extent and frequently contains the appendix.

(c) Fossa Intersigmoidea (Fig. 4.23)

The **pelvic mesocolon** has a parietal attachment shaped like an inverted V. The apex of this is at the bifurcation of the left common iliac artery. The lateral limb is attached to the left side of the pelvic brim and the medial limb diverges from the apex to the third piece of sacrum. At the apex is the **fossa intersigmoidea** which is always present in infancy but may disappear or be represented merely by a dimple in adults. The left ureter can be rolled on the underlying common iliac artery by a finger in this fossa and therefore, it is the surgeon's guide to the left ureter.

LESSER SAC

It is a diverticulum from the greater sac and since it provides a slippery surface for the posterior surface of stomach so it is also known as **omental bursa**.

Development (Fig. 4.5)

It appears as a pouch evaginating the dorsal mesogastrium from the right side. The pouch forms an irregular space which communicates in front with greater sac by a narrow opening. The cavity enlarges when the stomach rotates to bring its left surface to the anterior and the right surface to the posterior. The lesser sac thus comes to lie behind the stomach separating it from structures forming the stomach bed.

Opening into the Lesser Sac (Fig. 4.24)

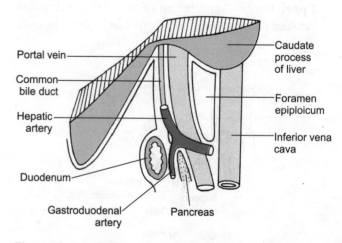

Fig. 4.24: Boundaries of foramen epiploicum with peritoneal reflection in its region

It is the communication with the greater sac and is known as **epiploic foramen (of Winslow)**. It is slit-like and can admit two fingers. The boundaries of the foramen are:

Anteriorly

- Free edge of lesser omentum containing within its layers, the **bile duct** in front and to the right, the **hepatic artery** in front and to the left and the **portal vein** behind.

Posteriorly

- The **inferior vena cava** covered by peritoneum.

Superiorly

- The **caudate process of the liver.**

Inferiorly

- The **first part of duodenum.**

SUBDIVISION OF LESSER SAC

The outline of the lesser sac looks like that of a hot water bag. It has the following subdivisions (Fig. 4.25):
- Vestibule
- Superior recess
- Inferior recess
- Splenic recess

Vestibule

It is a constricted area which lies behind the lesser omentum immediately to the left of the **foramen of Winslow** and separates the superior and inferior recesses. The constriction is produced on the left side by the **left gastropancreatic fold** raised by left gastric artery as it passes from the front of the aorta behind the posterior peritoneum upto the oesophageal opening to enter the lesser omentum. On the right side is the **right gastropancreatic fold** raised by the common hepatic artery as it curves down to the right, behind the peritoneum and then curves up behind the first inch of duodenum to enter the lesser omentum.

Superior Recess (Fig. 4.26)

It is the part lying behind the caudate lobe of the liver. It has following boundaries:
- **Roof-diaphragm**—Superiorly the recess is sealed by the reflection of peritoneum of the posterior wall of the lesser sac from the diaphragm onto the upper part of the caudate lobe of liver.
- **Anterior wall**—Caudate lobe of liver.
- **Posterior wall**—Diaphragm.
- **Right side**—The peritoneal lining over the diaphragm in the recess is continuous in front and on the right with

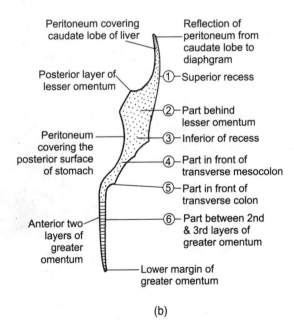

(a)   (b)

Fig. 4.25: Shape and subdivisions of the lesser sac as seen in a front view of a solid cast of its cavity: (a) Outline of lesser sac front view. (b) Sagittal section of the cast of the lesser sac showing its various parts and boundaries

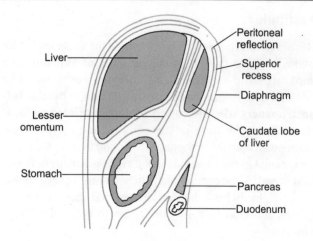

Fig. 4.26 (a): Superior recess: Anterior wall as seen in a sagittal section

the inferior layer of coronary ligament which limits the recess above and to the right of the caudate lobe. As the inferior vena cava passes through the diaphragm, the line of peritoneal reflection turns to the left, along the upper margin of the caudate lobe.

- **Left side**—It is closed by hepatogastric portion of the lesser omentum. The inferior layer of the coronary ligament terminates by becoming the posterior layer of lesser omentum.

Inferior Recess

It is below the right gastropancreatic fold and extends behind the stomach into the greater omentum. It has the following boundaries:

WALL

Anterior Wall (Fig. 4.27)

- Posterior layer of lesser omentum.
- Visceral layer of peritoneum covering the posterior surface of the stomach and the first 2.5 cm of dudoenum.
- Descending sheet of greater omentum.

Posterior Wall (Fig. 4.28)

- Ascending layer of transverse mesocolon covering the structures of stomach bed.
- Transverse mesocolon.
- Transverse colon.
- Posterior two layers of greater omentum.

BORDERS (FIG. 4.28)

Superiorly

- The vestibule opens it into the superior recess.

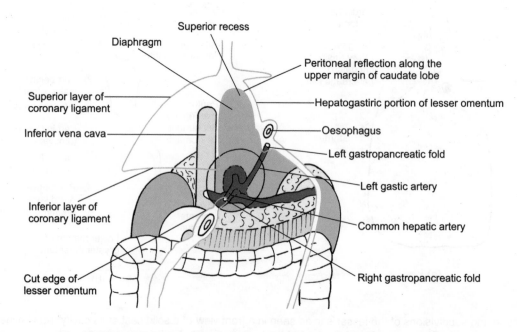

Fig. 4.26 (b): The boundaries of the superior recess of lesser sac in a frontal view

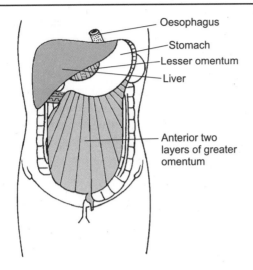

Fig. 4.27: Anterior wall of lesser sac as seen after the removal of the anterior abdominal wall

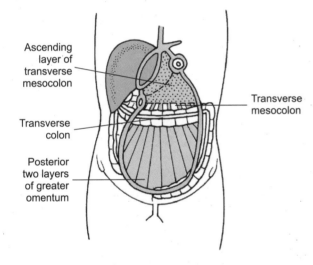

Fig. 4.28: Posterior wall of lesser sac after the removal of its anterior wall

Inferior Border

- Descending sheet of greater omentum becoming continuous with the ascending sheet.

Right Border from Below upward

- Anterior sheet of greater omentum becoming continuous with the posterior sheet on right side.
- The visceral peritoneum from the posterior surface of 2.5 cm of the first part of duodenum getting reflected to the anterior surface of head of pancreas.

- Above the first part of duodenum the border is absent as here lies the opening into the lesser sac.

Left Border from Below Upward

- Anterior layer of greater omentum becoming continuous with the posterior sheet by curving round the left border.
- By the converging gastrosplenic ligament and the lienorenal ligament to the hilum of spleen.
- By the attachment of the gastrophrenic ligament to the diaphragm.

Splenic Recess

- It is to the left of the gastropancreatic fold. Its relations are:

Anteriorly

- Stomach.
- Gastrolienal ligament.

Posteriorly

- Lienorenal ligament.
- Lying retroperitoneally are the left suprarenal gland, the upper pole of the left kidney and the diaphragm. The splenic artery running along the upper border of the pancreas demarcates the splenic and inferior recesses from one another.

CLINICAL APPLICATION

- The **epiploic foramen** is a potential site for intra-abdominal herniation. If a loop of bowel passes through the foramen, none of the boundaries can be incised because of the vessels and the bile duct associated with them. The bowel has to be deflated to withdraw the loop.
- The peritoneal recesses, spaces and fossae are potential sites of infection. The **pouch of Morison** is probably the most frequently infected abdominal space.
- Loops of bowel may get caught and strangulated in peritoneal fossae.
- The lesser sac may get filled with fluid as a result of perforation in the posterior wall of stomach or from an inflamed pancreas to form a pseudocyst of the pancreas.

- The greater omentum limits infection by forming a protective barrier around the site of infection.
- An increase in the fluid inside the peritoneal cavity is known as **ascites**.
- Considerable pain is experienced when the parietal peritoneum is inflamed because it is supplied by segmental nerves supplying the anterior abdominal wall. Reflex rigidity known as **'guarding'** results due to spasm of the overlying muscles.

- Pain arising from the viscera is diffuse and poorly localised and is usually referred to the abdominal wall receiving the same segmental nerve supply as the affected viscus. This is known as **referred pain**. A good example is the referred pain of **appendicitis,** where pain is felt in the umbilical region which is supplied by T_{10} segment and which also supplies the appendix.

Abdominal Viscera: Kidneys, Ureters and Suprarenals

5

THE KIDNEYS, URETERS AND SUPRARENAL GLANDS

Abdominal viscera are located in reference to the surface of the body with the help of the planes that intersect the surface of the body. These planes determine regions which help in learning the position of various viscera and form basis for the examination of the abdomen.

Planes of Abdomen (Fig. 5.1)

These are sagittal and horizontal planes.

Sagittal Planes

- **Median plane,** coincided with linea alba and passes through the umbilicus.

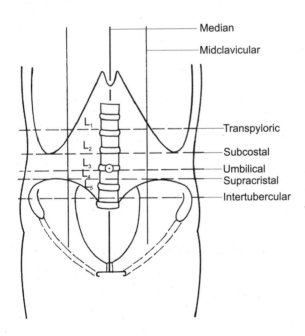

Fig. 5.1: Planes of abdomen

- **Midclavicular planes,** pass through the midclavicular point and intersect the costal arch close to the tip of the ninth costal cartilage.

Horizontal Planes

- **Transpyloric plane,** bisects the body between the jugular notch and the symphysis pubis. It passes through the lower border of the first lumbar vertebra and can also be drawn through a point midway between the xiphisternum and the umbilicus, or about a hand's breadth below the xiphisternal joint. It cuts each costal margin at the tip of the ninth costal cartilage, which is the lateral border of the rectus abdominis muscle defined by the linea semilunaris. It is so called because it usually passes through the pylorus of stomach. It marks the lower end of the spinal cord.
- **Subcostal plane,** connects the lowest points of the two costal arches and lies across the upper border of L_3 vertebra.
- **Supracristal plane,** marking the highest point of the iliac crests, passes through the lower part of the body of L_4. It is a landmark for the performance of lumbar puncture. The aorta bifurcates in this plane.
- **Umbilical plane,** passes through the umbilicus at the level of lower border of L_3 vertebra. The umbilicus is too variable to be a reliable landmark.
- **Intertubercular plane,** connects the tubercles of right and left iliac crests and passes through L_3 vertebra. The inferior vena cava begins in this plane.

Regions of Abdomen (Fig. 5.2)

For clinical purposes the abdomen is divided into nine regions by the two midclavicular planes, the subcostal and the intertubercular planes. The lateral six areas are from above downwards **right** and **left hypochondriac, right** and **left lumbar** and **right** and **left iliac.**

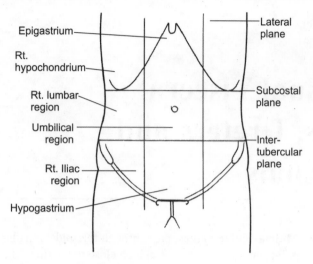

Fig. 5.2: Regions of abdomen

The middle three regions are from above downwards, the **epigastric, umbilical and hypogastric**. These regions are useful landmarks for ensuring a complete and systemic examination of the abdomen.

THE KIDNEYS

Shape and Size

Kidneys are large brown retroperitoneal viscera each about 11 cm in length, 5 cm in breadth and 3 cm in thickness.

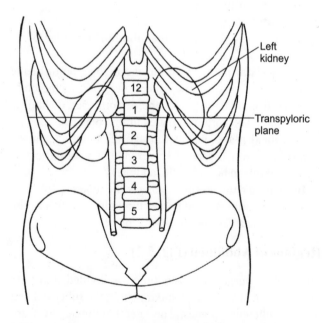

Fig. 5.3: The skeletal relationship of the kidney and ureters as seen from the anterior aspect of the body

They are bean-shaped and have an upper pole and a lower pole, anterior and posterior surfaces, a convex lateral border and a concave medial border. The vertical cleft on the medial border is the **hilum** which leads into a recess known as the **renal sinus**.

Position

The kidneys lie opposite the twelfth thoracic and upper three lumbar vertebrae (Fig. 5.3), with the right kidney lying at a lower level because of the large size of the right lobe of liver. The long axis of the kidney is parallel to, but not coincident with, the long axis of the twelfth rib. The right kidney reaches the upper border of the twelfth rib, the left reaches the lower border of the eleventh rib (Fig. 5.4). They are placed in such a way that their upper poles

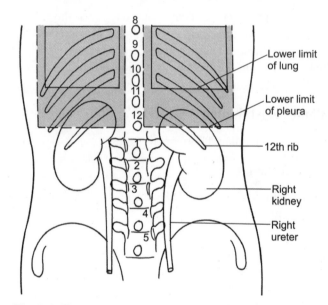

Fig. 5.4: The skeletal relationship of the kidney and ureters as seen from the posterior aspect of the body

are nearer the midline than the lower poles. They are slightly tilted in their transverse planes so that the hila are more anterior than their lateral borders (Fig. 5.5). The pelvis of the kidney lies opposite the first and second lumbar transverse processes.

Coverings of the Kidney (Fig. 5.6)

The kidney has three connective tissue coverings:
- **Renal capsule:** It is the fibrous capsule of the kidney. It strips easily from the organ.
- **Perirenal fat:** It is a substantial layer of fat lying outside the true capsule and is of more solid consistency than the

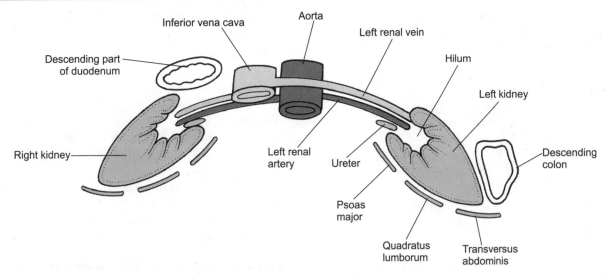

Fig. 5.5: Lie of the kidney and renal vessels in transverse section showing that the hila are more anteriorly placed than the lateral border of the kidney

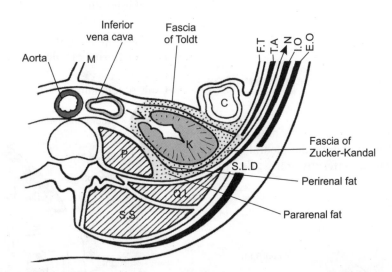

Fig. 5.6: Coverings of the kidney as seen in a transverse section of the body at the level of kidney (C = Colon, FT = Fascia transversalis, IO = Internal oblique, K = Kidney, M = Mesentery, P = Psoas major, QL = Quadratus lumborum, SS = Sacrospinalis, TA = Transversus abdominis)

general body fat. It retains the kidney in position as it is the only fat in the body which is solid at body temperature.

- **Renal fascia (Fascia of Gerota):** It is formed by the condensation of the perinephric fat at its periphery. It separates the kidney from the suprarenal gland as it ascends as a dome between the upper pole of the kidney and the suprarenal.

It is arranged as follows:

Laterally: At the outer border of the kidney it splits to enclose the organ. Lateral to this it is fused with fascia transversalis.

Medially: The anterior layer is thin and ill developed. The posterior layer is thicker and well-defined and fuses with the psoas sheath. Medially both layers merge with the tunica adventitia of the renal vessels and the connective tissue round the aorta and inferior vena cava.

Superiorly: The two layers join and fuse with fascia on the under aspect of the diaphragm (Fig. 5.7).

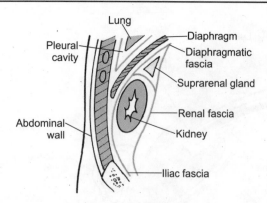

Fig. 5.7: Coverings of the kidney as seen in a vertical section going through the kidney

Inferiorly: The two layers are not fused and are open along each ureter (Fig. 5.7).

There is variable amount of fat behind the kidney outside the renal fascia **(the pararenal fat)** which is most abundant posterolaterally.

Relations (Fig. 5.8)

Posterior

These are same on both sides and form the **'bed'** of the kidney. They are:

- *Four muscles:*
  - Diaphragm behind the upper pole, separating it from the costovertebral reflection of the pleural cavity. Lower down lying **mediolaterally** are:
  - Psoas major.

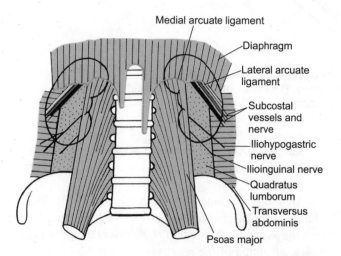

Fig. 5.8: The posterior relations of the kidneys, which are same on both side. Only the outline of the kidneys are given

- Quadratus lumborum.
- Transversus abdominis.
- **Three nerves:**
  - Subcostal.
  - Ilioinguinal.
  - Iliohypogastric.
- **Two ribs:**
  - The eleventh and twelfth on left side.
  - The twelfth only on the right side.
- **Two ligaments:**
  - Medial arcuate ligament.
  - Lateral arcuate ligament.
- **Subcostal artery and vein.**
  Anterior relations differ on the two sides:

Anterior Relations of the Right Kidney (Fig. 5.9)

- Suprarenal gland related to upper pole along a narrow strip.
- Inferior surface of right lobe of liver related to upper two-thirds of the surface leaving an area near the hilum.
- Descending (second) part of duodenum related to a narrow strip along the curved medial border.
- Hepatic flexure of colon is related just above the inferior pole.
- Coils of jejunum are related to inferior pole.

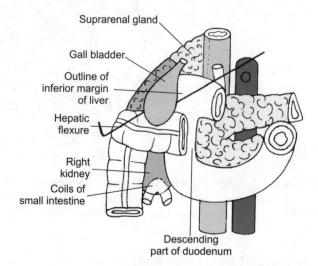

Fig. 5.9: Anterior relations of right kidney

The two areas related to the liver and small intestine are covered by peritoneum.

Anterior Relations of the Left Kidney (Fig. 5.10)

- Suprarenal gland to a small area along the upper medial border.

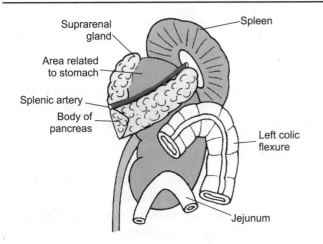

Fig. 5.10: Anterior relations of left kidney

- Spleen to the upper lateral half of the anterior surface.
- Stomach to the triangular area bounded by the upper two areas.
- Body of pancreas lies across the middle on a rectangular area below the area for stomach.
- Left colic flexure and commencement of descending colon laterally to the lower part.
- Upper coils of jejunum medially to the lower part.

The areas related to stomach, spleen and jejunum are covered by peritoneum.

Hilum of the Kidney (Fig. 5.11)

This is a vertical fissure in the middle of the medial border of the kidney. Between its two lips are situated from before backwards:
- Renal vein.
- Anterior division of renal artery.
- Pelvis of ureter.
- Posterior division of renal artery.

Renal Sinus

This is the recess into which the hilum of kidney leads. It is occupied by the pelvis of the ureter and renal vessels. There is a variable amount of fat between the various structures within the renal sinus.

Blood Supply

Renal Arteries (Fig. 5.5)

They are lateral branches of abdominal aorta, usually between L_1 and L_2, below the origin of the superior mesenteric arteries. The blood supply to the kidney through these arteries is profuse as the kidneys receive approximately one-fifth of the cardiac output. Each renal artery gives rise to:
- Inferior suprarenal artery to the suprarenal gland.
- Numerous twigs to the ureter.

Renal Segments (Fig. 5.12)

Each renal artery divides into five segmental branches within the renal sinus each with its own territory of distribution. On this basis the kidney can be divided into five renal segments. These are:
- **Superior:** Apical
- **Anterior superior:** Upper
- **Anterior inferior:** Middle
- **Inferior:** Lower
- **Posterior**

In the region of the hilum the renal artery typically divides into an anterior and a posterior division. The posterior division supplies the posterior segment, while the anterior division supplies all the other segments. There is no collateral circulation between the segments. The line along which the upper and middle segments meet, the posterior segment constitutes the **avascular line (Brodel's white line)**. An incision along this line produces minimal damage to the blood supply.

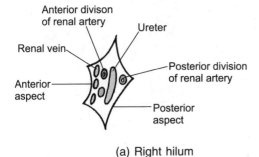

(a) Right hilum

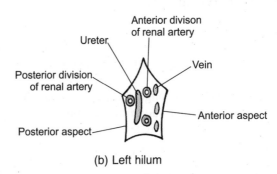

(b) Left hilum

Fig. 5.11: Arrangement of structures in the hilum of kidneys as seen from the medial aspect

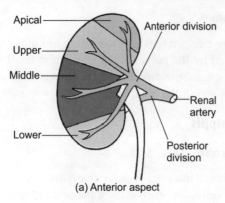

(a) Anterior aspect

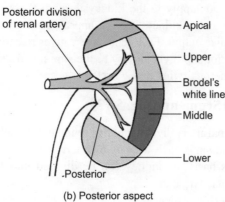

(b) Posterior aspect

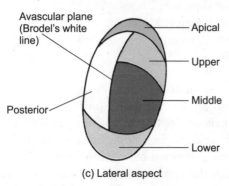

(c) Lateral aspect

Fig. 5.12: Segments of kidney and arteries depicted on various aspects of right kidney

Renal Veins (Fig. 5.5)

These are two:

- **Right renal vein** drains into the inferior vena cava at a lower level than the left renal vein, usually it has no significant tributaries.
- **Left renal vein** is longer than the right renal vein. As it crosses anterior to aorta in the middle, the superior mesenteric artery crosses in front of it. Its terminal portion is behind the head of the pancreas and in front of the right renal artery. It receives the following tributaries:

– Left gonadal vein
– Left suprarenal vein
– Left inferior phrenic vein

Veins from the renal segments communicate with one another profusely unlike the arteries. The five segmental veins unite at the hilum to form the single renal vein.

Lymph Drainage

The lymphatics follow both arteries and veins and drain into para-aortic nodes at the level of L_2.

The upper pole may drain into the nodes of posterior mediastinum through the diaphragm.

Nerve Supply

- Sympathetic preganglionic cells lie from T_{12} to L_1 and run in the least splanchnic nerve and lumbar splanchnic nerves. Postganglionic cells lie in aorticorenal ganglia and course within the renal plexus to the kidneys. Sympathetic fibres principally supply the renal vasculature.
- Some are sensory and convey painful sensation from the renal pelvis and upper part of ureter.
- Parasympathetic supply from vagus of uncertain function is also present. Some afferents may run with the vagal fibres.

Structure of Kidney (Fig. 5.13)

When the kidney is split into two halves the following features become visible:

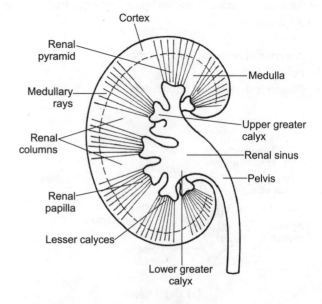

Fig. 5.13: Maexoscopic structure of the kidney

- **Renal sinus:** The space into which the hilum leads and in which there are the renal vessels, lymphatics, nerves and the renal pelvis.
- **Renal pelvis:** The expanded upper end of the ureter. Renal pelvis is formed by the union of three to four tubes, the upper, intermediate and lower major calyces. Each major calyx is formed by the union of three to four minor calyces. Each minor calyx is cup-shaped and fits over one to three renal papillae which are apices of renal pyramids.
- **Medulla:** It is the part internal to the bases of renal

pyramids which appear dark in the section of the kidney and are separated from each other by **renal columns** which are extensions of the cortical tissue.

- **Cortex:** It is the part of the kidney external to the bases of the renal pyramids. It is streaked, granular and paler in appearance.

Development (Fig. 5.14)

The intermediate cell mass is segmented in the cervical region, but in the thoracic and lumbosacral region, it is unsegmented and forms the nephrogenic cord. The cervical

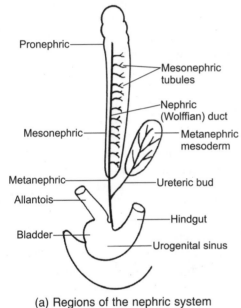

(a) Regions of the nephric system

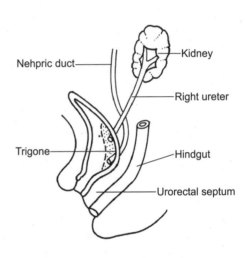

(c) Caudal ends of the nephric ducts expand and are taken up into the wall of the urinary bladder to form its trigone and so have separate openings

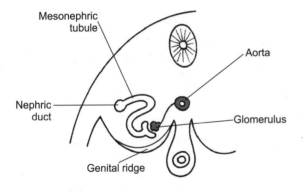

(b) Mesonephric tubules open successively into the nephric duct

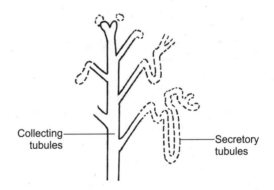

(d) Metanephric mesoderm forms secretory tubules while the collecting tubules, calyces, pelvis and ureter are formed by the ureteric bud

Fig. 5.14: Successive stages in the development of kidney

part is called the **pronephros,** the thoracic and upper lumbar part, the **mesonephros** and the lower lumbar and sacral part, the **metanephros**.

Pronephros is the first to form. It appears in early third week and disappears by fourth week. Its tubules lead into the pronephric duct which extends caudally to open into the cloaca.

Mesonephros appears as the pronephros fades. As it grows, it projects into the coelom lateral to the dorsal mesentery. On its medial aspect is a linear ridge, called the genital ridge. Mesonephros is a solid mass to begin with but later on in each segment of the embryo, the mass gives rise to the mesonephric tubules which end in the mesonephric duct. By about second month, mesonephros and the upper mesonephric tubules disappear. Those few which persist are found later near the testes. The lower mesonephric tubules connected to the testes become the **vasa efferentia** and the mesonephric duct becomes the **vas deferens** and terminates on the dorsal wall of the cloaca.

Metanephros the third kidney system, appears during the regression of mesonephros. It forms a solid mass of tissue called the metanephric blastema.

The kidney has double origin (Fig. 5.14 d).

- The collecting system of the kidney viz., distal part of the tubule, pelvis and ureter develops from the ureteric bud which arises from the mesonephric **(Wolffian)** duct near its cloacal end. It grows dorsally and cranially into the sacral region of the nephrogenic cord, where it induces the formation of a metanephric cap. The dilated tip of the ureteric bud then divides and gives rise to two or three major calyces. These, in turn, give rise to minor calyces. The division goes on till thirteen generations of division present. The tubules of the third and fourth generations are absorbed into the minor calyces. The tubules of the fifth and succeeding generations form the definitive collecting tubules.

- The secreting system viz., the glomerulus and proximal part of the tubule are formed from metanephros. The metanephric tissue proliferates and divides with the ureteric bud so that each branch tubule has its own cap. The metanephric cap on the end of each tubule becomes vesicular and then S-shaped, with one extremity tapping the collecting tubule and the other being invaginated by the glomerular tuft. Secretory and collecting tubules are thus developmentally and functionally distinct.

During development the kidney ascends from the pelvic region to the loin. This apparent migration is due to growth of the lumbar and sacral regions of the body and to straightening of its curvature. It is accompanied by growth and elongation of the ureter.

CLINICAL APPLICATION

- The twelfth rib is oblique and the lower border of the pleura is horizontal and the two cross like an X. The incision for operation on kidney begins in the renal angle which is between the twelfth rib and the outer border of the sacrospinalis muscle. In cases where the twelfth rib is very short, the eleventh rib might be mistaken for the twelfth rib and the pleura may be opened up on exposing the kidney.

- The nerve supply of the large bowel and kidney is same. A renal calculus may cause reflex interference with peristalsis, such cases may stimulate acute obstruction of the large bowel.

- The kidney is retained in place mainly by intra-abdominal pressure, the perirenal and pararenal fat assists. Diminution of this fat gives rise to a **floating kidney** which mostly moves downward because of respiratory movements and gravity.

- **Renal abscess** may be limited by the renal fascia and may track between the layers of this fascia into the pelvis.

- Pain originating from the kidney is referred to the T_{12} to L_2 dermatomal distribution (lumbar and inguinal regions as well as the antero-superior thigh), since the visceral afferent nerves from the kidneys reach the spinal cord via the least splanchnic nerve (T_{12}) and the lumbar splanchnic nerves (L_1 and L_2).

- A longitudinal incision on the kidney along the avascular line (Brodel's white line) produces minimal damage to the blood supply. This approach is utilized for removal of renal stones.

- Ligation of a segmental artery results in necrosis of the entire segment as there is no anastomosis between the segmental arteries.

- **Aberrant or supernumerary renal arteries,** seen arising from the renal artery or aorta are segmental arteries. They are derived from foetal lobation pattern, with failure of the renal arterial segments to fuse.

- Failure of union between secretory and collecting tubules may result in formation of cysts which may be single or multiple **(congenital polycystic kidney)**.

- As the renal rudiments are ascending from the pelvic region to the loin, they normally remain entirely separate. They may, however, come in contact and adhere resulting in a horseshoe kidney usually connected at the lower poles. The ureters descend in front of the connecting isthmus.
- Failure of the kidney to ascend results in pelvic kidney (ectopic kidney).

THE URETERS

The ureters are excretory ducts between the kidneys and the urinary bladder.

Extent

The renal pelvis, lying in the renal sinus, narrows at the ureteropelvic junction to form the ureter. The length form the ureteropelvic junction to the vesical orifice is about 25 cm. It is described in two parts, the abdominal and the pelvic parts which are almost equal in length. From the hilum of the kidney, it runs downwards and medially, retroperitoneally within the periureteral sheath which is an extension of renal fascia, to cross the pelvic brim to enter the pelvic cavity where it ends by opening into the lateral angles of the urinary bladder.

Relations of Abdominal Part

Posterior Relations (Common to both sides)
- Psoas major whose medial edge separates it from the tips of lumbar transverse processes.
- Genitofemoral nerve.
- The beginning of the external iliac artery and the adjacent vein.

Anterior Relation of Right Ureter (Fig. 5.15)
- Descending part of duodenum.
- Right colic, gonadal and ileocolic, vessels cross lower down.
- Root of mesentery of small intestine, with superior mesenteric vessels, crosses before it reaches pelvic brim.
- Terminal ileum.

Anterior Relations of Left Ureter (Fig. 5.16)
- Upper left colic and sigmoidal vessels cross it.
- Gonadal vessels.
- Pelvic mesocolon and pelvic colon overlap it near the pelvic brim.

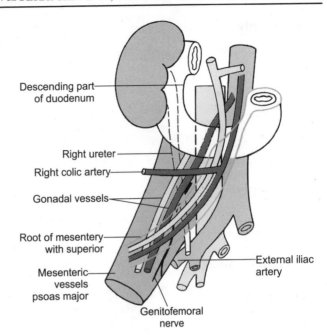

Fig. 5.15: Right ureter: Relations

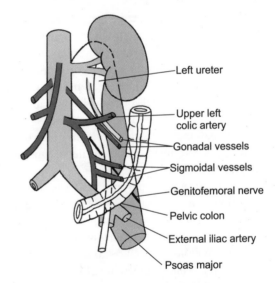

Fig. 5.16: Left ureter: Relations

Constrictions

There are three constrictions in the ureter:
- At pelviureteric junction below the hilum.
- At pelvic brim where it crosses in front of the external iliac artery.
- Just before it enters into the urinary bladder.

Blood Supply

Arterial supply is derived from the following:
- Renal artery
- Abdominal aorta
- Gonadal artery
- Common iliac artery

Venous drainage is from the corresponding veins.

Nerve Supply

It is from T_{11} to L_2 segments of the spinal cord via renal, hypogastric and pelvic plexuses.

Lymphatic Drainage

The lymph vessels of the abdominal part pass along the blood vessels to drain into para-aortic and common iliac nodes.

CLINICAL APPLICATION

- A stone may lodge or pass slowly through the three constrictions in the ureter. There is ureteral distension (hydroureter and hydronephrosis) proximal to stone. The distension causes excruciating pain (renal colic), which is among the most intense pains experienced by humans.
- Pain originating from specific regions of the ureter is referred according to splanchnic nerve supplying the region.
- Renal pelvis and upper ureteral obstruction distension pain is referred to the lumbar region (lesser splanchnic nerve: T_{12} segment).
- Middle ureteral obstruction pain is referred to inguinal and pubic regions, as well as to anterior scrotum and mons pubis and to superoanterior thigh (lumbar splanchnic nerves: L_1 and L_2 segments).
- Lower ureteral obstruction and distension pain is referred to the perineum (pelvic splanchnic nerves: S_2 to S_4).

THE SUPRARENAL GLANDS

Position

The suprarenal glands are paired retroperitoneal endocrine glands. They are yellowish pink in colour and are situated on the superomedial aspect of the kidneys.

Shape, Size and Weight

The right gland is pyramidal and the left semilunar in shape. It is about 5 cm vertically, 3 cm transversely and 1 cm anteroposteriorly. It is about 5 g in weight.

At birth it is about one-quarter of the size of the kidney but in the adult it is about one-thirtieth of the size of the kidney as shortly after birth it decreases in size and then increases again.

Covering (Fig. 5.7)

The suprarenal gland is enclosed with the kidney in a common envelop formed by the renal fascia but is separated from it by a plane of cleavage containing considerable amount of fat so that there is no danger of injuring the suprarenal gland during the removal of the kidney.

Relations

Each gland has an anterior and a posterior surface. Each of these surfaces has two relations (Figs. 5.17 and 5.18).

Relations of Right Suprarenal

Anterior (Figs. 5.17 and 5.18)

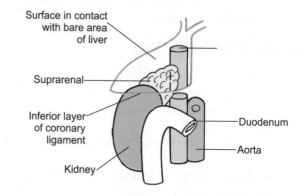

Fig. 5.17: Right suprarenal *in situ* showing its anterior relations

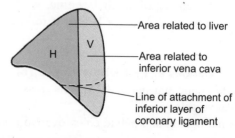

Fig. 5.18: Right suprarenal: Shape and relations of anterior surface

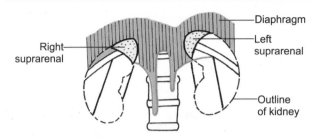

Fig. 5.19: Both suprarenals posteriorly lie on the diaphragm and the kidney

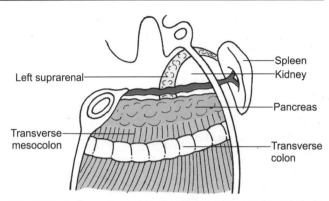

Fig. 5.21: Left suprarenal *in situ* showing its anterior relations

- Inferior vena cava medially.
- Bare area of liver laterally. The anterior surface is not covered by peritoneum except a tiny area below.

Posterior (Figs. 5.19 and 5.20)

- Kidney inferiorly.
- Diaphragm superiorly.

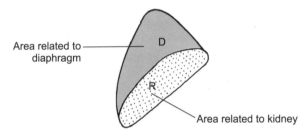

Fig. 5.20: Right suprarenal: Relations of posterior surface

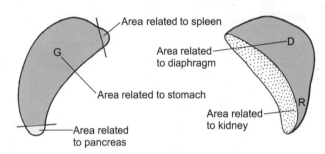

Fig. 5.22: Left suprarenal: Shape and (a) Anterior (b) Posterior surfaces and relations

Medial

- Right coeliac ganglion.
- Right inferior phrenic artery.

Relations of Left Suprarenal

Anterior (Figs. 5.21 and 5.22 a)

- Stomach with the lesser sac in between.
- Body of pancreas and splenic vessels. This area is devoid of peritoneum.

Posterior (Figs. 5.19 and 5.22 b)

- Crus of diaphragm medially.
- Kidney laterally.

Medial

- Left coeliac ganglion.
- Left inferior phrenic artery.

Blood Supply (Fig. 5.23)

Arteries

It is very vascular organ and each has three arteries supplying it.
- **Superior suprarenal** from the inferior phrenic artery.
- **Middle suprarenal** from the aorta.
- **Inferior suprarenal** from the renal artery.

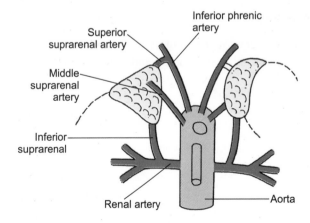

Fig. 5.23: The arterial supply of suprarenals

Veins (Fig. 5.24)

Each gland has only one vein emerging from the hilum. Hilum of the right gland is near the upper and while that of the lower is near the lower end.

- **Right suprarenal vein** drains into the inferior vena cava.
- **Left suprarenal vein** drains into the left renal vein.

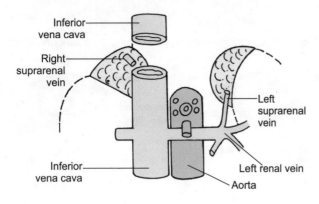

Fig. 5.24: The venous drainage of suprarenals

Nerve Supply

Preganglionic sympathetic fibres pass from T_8 to T_{11} segments via the greater and lesser splanchnic nerves and end directly on the cells of medulla.

There is no parasympathetic supply.

Lymphatics

Lymph vessels drain into the para-aortic nodes.

Structure

The gland consists of an outer cortex and inner medulla. Developmentally, structurally and functionally the cortex

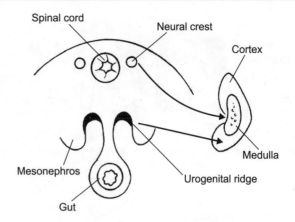

Fig. 5.25: Development of suprarenal

and medulla are different. Cortex produces three classes of steroid hormones. Medulla secretes epinephrine.

Development (Fig. 3.25)

The suprarenal gland develops from two sources:
- Cortex is derived from the mesoderm of the embryonic urogenital ridge.
- Medulla is derived from embryonic neural crest ectoderm.

CLINICAL APPLICATION

- The right suprarenal gland is more difficult to approach surgically than the left, because it is in part posterior to inferior vena cava.
- Pheochromocytoma is a tumour of adrenal medulla which causes paroxysms of hypertension due to excessive bursts of epinephrine and norepinephrine.
- Right suprarenal vein is very short and the inferior vena cava may be torn during its ligation.
- The gland is handled as little as possible before venous ligation, which is done before the arteries, to prevent hormone release.

6

Gastrointestinal Tract

INTRODUCTION

The general arrangement of the gastrointestinal tract is as follows (Fig. 6.1):

- The **oesophagus** and **stomach** lie in the upper left part of the abdominal cavity below the diaphragm. The stomach ends just to the right of the midline at about the level of first lumbar vertebra.
- The **small intestine:** It follows the stomach. It has three parts:
- **Duodenum** is the first part. It curves around the second lumbar vertebra like a letter C.
- **Jejunum** is the second part.
- **Ileum** is the third part. These second and third parts lie in coils in the middle of the abdomen.
- **The large intestine:** The end of ileum passes upwards and to the right into the large intestine known as **colon,** which more or less frames the intestine.
- Caecum is the beginning of large intestine.
- Ascending colon ascends upwards on the right side.
- Transverse colon lying horizontally loops downward from above.
- Descending colon descends on the left side.

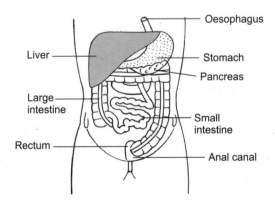

Fig. 6.1: The gastrointestinal tract

- Rectum and anal canal, the end of the large intestine, pass towards the right to be in the midline, to end in the posterior part of pelvis.
- In addition to the glands in the walls of the stomach and intestine which produce digestive juices, there have also developed glandular organs known as the **liver** and **pancreas,** which arise by specialization of the glands in the walls of the gut. They are connected by special ducts with the interior of the intestine.
- **Liver** lies in the upper right part of the abdomen below the diaphragm. It is the largest glandular organ of the body.
- **Pancreas** passes from the right to the left behind the stomach and lies against the posterior abdominal wall behind the peritoneum.

PERITONEUM

The peritoneum is the serous membrane lining the abdominal and pelvic cavities. Its arrangement is complex due to the way the organs develop within the abdomen. All organs lie outside the peritoneum. Some of them which are invaginated in it are almost wholly covered by peritoneum and then are connected by a double fold of peritoneum to the lining of the body wall. The double folds of peritoneum are called **mesenteries** and **ligaments.** Certain structures are partly covered by peritoneum viz., the diaphragm, commencement of abdominal aorta, left suprarenal gland, upper pole of left kidney and pancreas.

THE ABDOMINAL OESOPHAGUS

The oesophagus enters the abdominal cavity through the oesophageal opening in the right crus of the diaphragm situated to the left of the midline at the level of T_{10} vertebra. The abdominal part of the oesophagus is 1.5 cm long and enters the stomach at its cardiac orifice. It lies in a groove on the upper part of the posterior aspect of the liver and is covered by peritoneum anteriorly and to the left.

THE STOMACH

Stomach is the most dilated part of the alimentary tract.

Position (Fig. 6.2)

It lies in the upper left quadrant of the abdominal cavity.

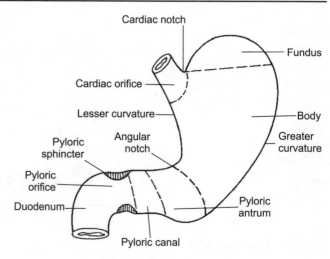

Fig. 6.3: Parts of stomach

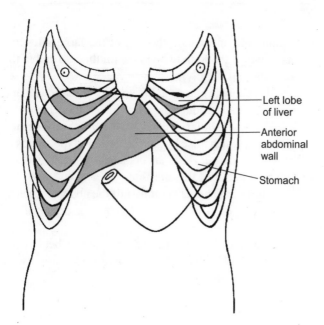

Fig. 6.2: Position and anterior relations of stomach

Shape (Fig. 6.3)

It is shaped like the letter J. Its upper part is broader than the lower part. It has anterior and posterior surfaces and a right border known as **lesser curvature** and a left border called the **greater curvature**. There is a **cardiac orifice** where the oesophagus enters the stomach and a **pyloric orifice** through which it opens into the duodenum.

Parts (Fig. 6.3)

Stomach is divided into the following parts:
• **Fundus** is the part which lies above the cardiac orifices.
• **Body** is below the fundus.
• **Pyloric part** is the part marked off from the body by the **angular notch** at the lower end of the lesser

curvature. It consists of two subdivisions, the **pyloric antrum,** a dilated part next to the body and the **pyloric canal** which is a canal of uniform size. The pyloric canal is thickened along its circumference by an aggregation of circular muscle constituting the **pyloric sphincter**.

Relations

The anterior surface is related to (Fig. 6.2):
• Inferior surface of the left lobe and the quadrate lobe of liver.
• Left half of the diaphragm.
• Anterior abdominal wall.

The posterior surface is related to structures which are referred to as **stomach bed**. These are (Fig. 6.4):
• Diaphragm
• Gastric surface of spleen
• Left suprarenal gland
• Left kidney
• Pancreas
• Transverse mesocolon
• Transverse colon

Arterial Supply (Fig. 6.5)

The stomach receives its arterial supply from the coeliac artery or its branches which run along its curvatures. The coeliac artery should be considered to fully understand the arterial supply of stomach.

The **coeliac artery** supplies the abdominal part of the foregut whose derivatives are:
• Lower end of oesophagus.

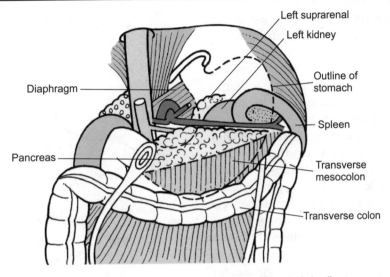

Fig. 6.4: Stomach: Posterior relations (Stomach bed)

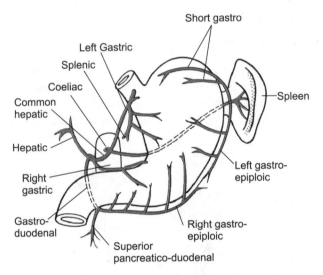

Fig. 6.5: Arterial supply of stomach

- Stomach.
- Duodenum, upto immediately distal to the opening of the hepatopancreatic duct.
- Pancreas.

The biliary apparatus and the spleen which develop in the ventral and dorsal mesogastria respectively are also supplied by the branches of the coeliac artery. Owing to the leftward intrusion of the lesser sac, the three branches of the coeliac trunk cannot pass directly to the part of the gut which they supply. Each makes a U-turn. The proximal limb of the U is retroperitoneal, on the posterior abdominal

wall. The distal limb is in a fold of peritoneum viz., lesser or greater omentum.

Origin

From front of aorta, just below the aortic opening of the diaphragm (T_{12}).

Course and Relations

The coeliac artery is short. It passes forwards and has following relations:

Above: Caudate lobe of liver.
Below: Pancreas.
In front: Lesser sac.
To the right: Caudate process of liver.
On either side: The coeliac ganglion and coeliac plexus and crurae of diaphragm.

Branches

- Common hepatic.
- Splenic.
- Left gastric.
- The **common hepatic artery** runs downwards and to the right below the epiploic foramen to reach the upper border of first part of duodenum. It then turns upwards to reach the free edge of lesser omentum. Here, it divides into **hepatic artery proper** and the **gastroduodenal artery**. The hepatic artery proper makes a U-turn upto the liver. The common hepatic artery gives a **right gastric branch** which runs along the lesser curvature of stomach. The gastroduodenal gives a **right**

gastroepiploic branch which runs along the greater curvature of stomach and a superior pancreaticoduodenal branch. In the free margin of lesser omentum the bile duct is on its right side and the portal vein is behind it. The opening in the lesser sac separates the free margin of lesser omentum from peritoneum covering the inferior vena cava (Fig. 4.24). At the porta hepatics the hepatic artery divides into its terminal **right** and **left branches**. The right branch gives the **cystic artery** to gall bladder.

- **Splenic artery** is a large artery. It runs sinuously retroperitoneally to the left along the upper border of the pancreas. Its omental part turns forwards between the layers of the lienorenal ligament to the spleen (Fig. 7.29). **Short gastric** and **left gastroepiploic branches** of the splenic continue between the layers of the gastrosplenic ligament and then between the anterior two layers of the greater omentum.

- Left **gastric artery** has its proximal part running up on the diaphragm to reach its oesophageal opening. It sends **oesophageal branches** through the opening, then makes a U-turn into the lesser omentum.

To summarise the arterial supply of stomach:

- Along the lesser curvature lying within the lesser omentum are the **left gastric artery** (a direct branch from the coeliac) and **right gastric artery** (a branch of the common hepatic which is a branch of the coeliac).

- Along the greater curvature lying within the greater omentum are the **left gastroepiploic** (a branch of the splenic artery which arises from the coeliac) and the **right gastroepiploic** (a branch of the gastroduodenal which is a branch of the common hepatic arising from the coeliac).

- **Short gastric branches** from the splenic artery supply the fundus of stomach.

Venous Drainage (Fig. 6.6)

The veins draining the stomach pass to the **portal vein** which goes to the liver. The portal vein is formed behind the neck of pancreas by the union of the **splenic vein** with the **superior mesenteric vein**. The veins draining the stomach are:

- **Right** and **left gastric veins** running along the lesser curvature drain directly into the portal vein which also receives some pancreaticoduodenal veins.

- The **right gastroepiploic vein** on the greater curvature drains into the superior mesenteric vein which also receives some pancreaticoduodenal veins. It is connected to the right gastric vein by a **prepyloric vein (of Mayo)** which lies on the anterior surface of the pylorus.

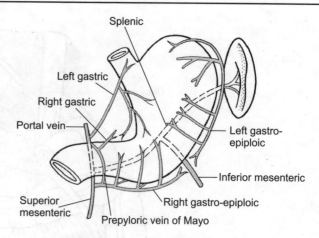

Fig. 6.6: Venous drainage of stomach

- The **left gastroepiploic** and **short gastric veins** on the greater curvature drain into the splenic vein which also receives pancreatic veins.

Nerve Supply (Fig. 6.7)

- Parasympathetic nerve supply is by the **anterior gastric** (mainly formed by left vagus) and **posterior gastric** (mainly formed by right vagus) nerves.

- Sympathetic nerves come from the **coeliac plexus**.

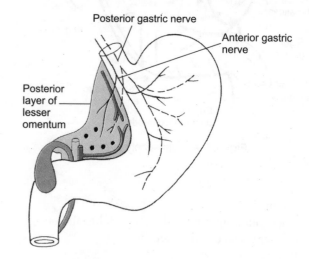

Fig. 6.7: Nerve supply of stomach

Lymphatic Drainage (Fig. 6.8)

The stomach can be divided into four lymphatic areas which correspond fairly closely to the arterial territories.

The division is done by drawing a curved line in its long axis, so that two-thirds of the stomach is to

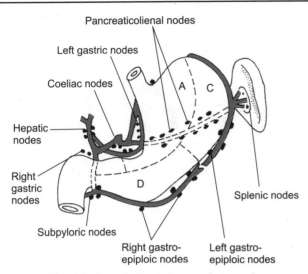

Fig. 6.8: Lymphatic drainage of stomach

the right of this line and one-third to the left. The right two-thirds is divided into a larger upper area (A) and a smaller area (B). The left third is again divided into two by a line at the junction of its upper third (C) and lower two-thirds (D).

- The lymphatics from the right two-thirds drain as follows:
(i) (A) the largest area along the lesser curvature, including the cardia, fundus and oesophagus drains to the **left gastric nodes**.
(ii) (B) which is pyloric antrum along the lesser curvature, is drained by the **right gastric** and **hepatic nodes**.
- The lymphatics from the left one-third drain as follows:
(iii) (C) area along the left part of the greater curvature is drained by the **left gastroepiploic, pancreaticolienal nodes** and **splenic nodes**.
(iv) (D) area which includes the pyloric antrum and pyloric canal along the greater curvature is drained by the **right gastroepiploic** and **subpyloric** nodes.

The efferent lymphatics from all these nodes pass through the coelic nodes before they enter the cisterna chyli through an intestinal lymph trunk.

CLINICAL APPLICATION

- A posterior wall gastric ulcer may perforate into the lesser sac or erode into the pancreas causing pancreatitis or into the splenic artery resulting in massive hemorrhage as these structures lie in the stomach bed.

- The blood supply of stomach is so profuse that any artery supplying it is sufficient to maintain its vitality providing the marginal anastomotic vessels are patent.
- Section of the gastric branches of the anterior and posterior vagal trunks (selective vagotomy) reduces peptic secretion.
- In the surgical treatment of cancer of stomach, it becomes necessary to remove the stomach along with lower third of the oesophagus and the superior part of duodenum as they share a common lymphatic drainage.

THE SMALL INTESTINE

The small intestine consists of three parts, duodenum, jejunum and ileum.

THE DUODENUM

The duodenum is the first part of the small intestine and is the shortest, widest, thickest and the most fixed part of the small intestine. Its name refers to its length, which is twelve fingers breadth (Duodenum = Duodenum digitorum = Space of 12 fingers breadth, Latin).

Situation (Fig. 6.9)

- It is situated on the posterior abdominal wall opposite the bodies of L_1 to L_3.

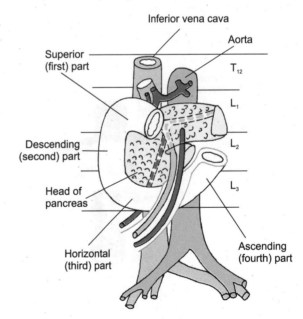

Fig. 6.9: Situation, shape and subdivisions of duodenum

Shape

- It is curved like the letter "C" around the head of the pancreas.

Subdivisions

- It is divided into four parts which were previously called first, second, third and fourth. The first part is now named the superior, the second the descending, the third the horizontal or inferior and the fourth the ascending.

Relations

SUPERIOR (FIRST) PART

Superior part is 5 cm (2 inch) in length and starts at the pylorus of the stomach and therefore, is in the transpyloric plane, 2.5 cm to the right of the midline. It runs upwards to the right side and also posteriorly.

Its first 2.5 cm are completely covered by peritoneum so that its upper and lower borders give attachment to the right extensions of the lesser and greater omentum respectively. Its posterior surface is, therefore, related to the lesser sac.

The second 2.5 cm of the superior part is covered with peritoneum only on the anterior surface. The relations of the superior part are (Figs. 6.10 and 6.11):

Anteriorly

- Quadrate lobe of liver.
- Gall bladder.

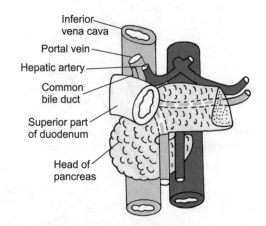

Fig. 6.10: Relations of the superior part of duodenum from the anterior aspect

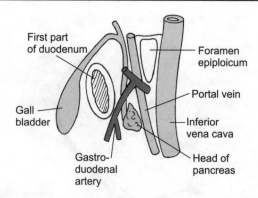

Fig. 6.11: Relations of the superior part of duodenum in sectional view

Posteriorly

- Lesser sac.
- Gastroduodenal branch of hepatic artery.
- Common bile duct.
- Portal vein behind the upper two structures.
- Inferior vena cava further back behind the peritoneum.

Superiorly

- Foramen epiploicum.

Inferiorly

- Head of pancreas.

This part of duodenum is visualised in radiographs as the **duodenal cap**.

DESCENDING (SECOND) PART

It is 7.5 cm (3 inch) in length and descends from the neck of the gall bladder to the right side of the bodies of L_2 and L_3. Its relations are:

Anteriorly (Fig. 6.12)

- Transverse colon crosses in the middle and this is the only part not covered by peritoneum.
- Right lobe of liver above the colon.
- Coils of small intestine below the transverse colon.

Posteriorly (Fig. 6.13)

- Hilum and adjoining anterior surface of the right kidney.
- Right renal vessels and pelvis of right ureter.

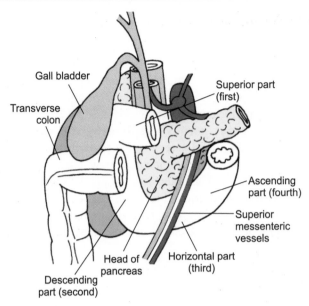

Fig. 6.12: Anterior relations of descending part of duodenum

Medially

- Head of pancreas.

Laterally

- Right kidney.
- Right colic flexure.

HORIZONTAL (THIRD) PART

It is 10 cm (4 inch) in length and cross the midline transversely from the right side of the third lumbar vertebra to its left side. It has following relations:

Anteriorly (Fig. 6.9)

- Root of the mesentery.
- Coils of small intestine.
- Trunk of superior mesenteric artery.
- Super mesenteric vein.
- This part is nipped between the two great vessels lying posteriorly (IVC and aorta) and the superior mesenteric vessels lying anteriorly.

Posteriorly from Right to Left (Fig. 6.13)

- Right ureter.
- Psoas major.
- Inferior vena cava.
- Right gonadal vessels.
- Aorta with the origin of inferior mesenteric artery.

Superiorly

- Head and uncinate process of pancreas.

Inferiorly

- Coils of jejunum.

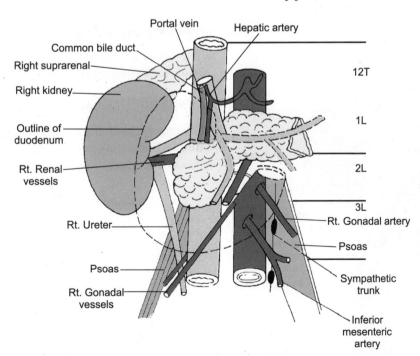

Fig 6.13: Posterior relations of all the four parts of duodenum only outline of duodenum is shown

ASCENDING (FOURTH) PART

It is 2.5 cm (1 inch) long, passes upwards to the left of the L$_2$ vertebra and bends forward to become the jejunum at the duodenojejunal flexure.

Anteriorly

• Coils of jejunum.

Posteriorly (Figs. 6.13 and 6.14)

• Left margin of abdominal aorta.
• Left psoas major.
• Left sympathetic trunk.
• Left gonadal artery.

Laterally (Fig. 6.14)

• Left kidney.
• Left ureter.
• Inferior mesenteric vein.

The first and fourth parts of duodenum have peritoneum on their anterior and posterior surfaces where they are adjacent to the stomach and jejunum, and this gives considerable mobility to these parts. The rest of the duodenum is covered by peritoneum only on its anterior surface.

The **suspensory ligament of Treitz** is a fibromuscular structure which arises from the right crus of diaphragm and descends deep to the pancreas to get inserted into the muscular coat of the duodenojejunal flexure. It may exaggerate the duodenojejunal kink.

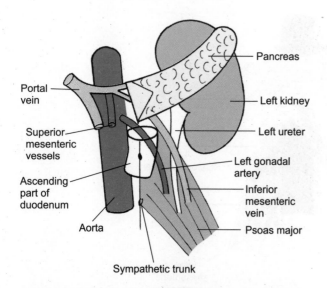

Fig. 6.14: Posterior and lateral relations of ascending part of duodenum

Arterial Supply (Fig. 6.15)

Since, the duodenum is derived from both the foregut and midgut, which meet just distal to the common opening of the bile and pancreatic ducts, its blood supply comes from the artery of foregut viz., the coelic and the artery of midgut viz., the superior mesenteric.

The foregut part is supplied by the **superior pancreaticoduodenal artery,** a branch of gastroduodenal which is given off by common hepatic which comes from the coeliac artery. The midgut part is supplied by **inferior pancreaticoduodenal** which is a branch of superior mesenteric. Ascending part is also supplied by the first jejunal branch from the superior mesenteric artery.

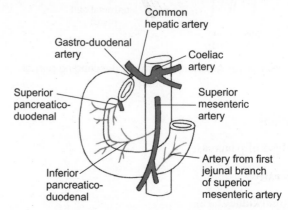

Fig. 6.15: Arterial supply of duodenum

Venous Drainage (Fig. 6.16)

The veins of the duodenum, **superior and inferior pancreaticoduodenal,** drain into the portal vein.

Lymphatic Drainage

The lymphatics drain into the **pancreaticoduodenal lymph nodes** lying between the head of pancreas and the duodenum. These nodes drain into the **preaortic nodes**.

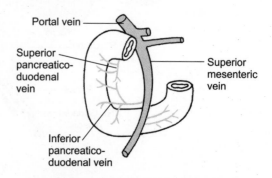

Fig. 6.16: Venous drainage of duodenum

Interior of Duodenum (Fig. 6.17)

The descending part of duodenum has a common opening on the middle of its posteromedial wall for the main pancreatic duct and the bile duct.

The opening is on a **major duodenal papilla**. Within the wall, the common opening is dilated and forms the **hepatopancreatic ampulla (of Vater)** which is surrounded by the **ampullary sphincter (of Oddi)**. The opening is guarded by a fold of mucous membrane. The accessory pancreatic duct, if present, opens on top of a **minor duodenal papilla** above the main one.

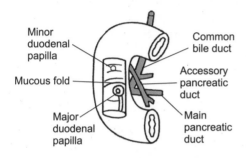

Fig. 6.17: Mucous surface of the descending part of duodenum showing the aperture of the ducts. The accessory pancreatic duct if present opens on top of a minor duodenal papilla above the main one

CLINICAL APPLICATION

- Perforation of an ulcer situated on the postero-medial wall of proximal part of the superior part of duodenum causes infection of the lesser sac.
- A gallstone may ulcerate from the fundus of the gall bladder into the duodenum as it is overlapped by it.
- Since duodenum is fixed to the posterior abdominal wall it is ruptured following a very heavy blow, as the aorta and L_3 vertebra is posterior relation of the horizontal part of duodenum.
- The blood supply to the proximal part of the superior part of duodenum by the superior pancreati-coduodenal artery is poor. In 70% cases a **supraduodenal artery (of Wilkie)** from the common hepatic or gastroduodenal artery vascularises this part. Its terminal twigs are end arteries and so its thrombosis or obstruction leads to duodenal ulcer.
- The superior mesenteric vascular bundle may

compress the horizontal part of the duodenum against the aorta and the vertebral column producing duodenal obstruction (superior mesenteric artery syndrome). It is more likely to occur with wasting or after severe dieting.
- The junction of pylorus of stomach with duodenum is marked by a constriction externally and also by a constant **vein (of Mayo)** which crosses it at this level.
- The duodenojejunal junction is identified by the presence of the **suspensory ligament of Treitz**, which is a well marked peritoneal fold descending from the left crus of the diaphragm of the duodenal termination.

THE JEJUNUM AND ILUEM

Position

The jejunum and ileum lie in coils in the middle of the abdominal cavity framed by the large intestine. The coils lie more or less in the middle of the abdominal cavity and also hang down into the pelvis (Fig. 6.18).

Extent

The length of the small intestine varies from 3–10 metres (10 to 33 feet) in different subjects. The jejunum starts at the **duodenojejunal flexure** on the left side of the second lumbar vertebra. The upper two-fifths are designated as jejunum and lower three-fifths as ileum. This is arbitrary as there is no clear-cut demarcation between the two. The

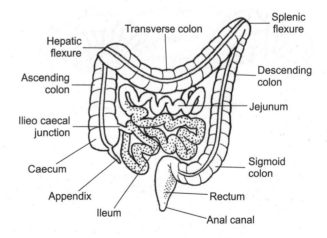

Fig. 6.18: General position of small intestine and colon and their various parts

ileum ends at the **ileocaecal junction** in the right iliac fossa. The calibre of the small intestine becomes wider from the duodenal to the caecal end.

Relations

Anteriorly (Fig. 4.18)

- Anterior abdominal wall.
- Greater omentum.

Posteriorly

- Retroperitoneal structures of posterior abdominal wall.

Superiorly (Fig. 4.19)

- Transverse mesocolon.
- Transverse colon.

Differences between Jejunum and Ileum (Fig. 6.19)

The chief differences are:
- Mucous surface of jejunum presents numerous transverse folds while ileum has fewer transverse folds.
- Jejunum has a thick wall, the ileum is thin walled due to fewer mucous transverse folds.
- The mesentery of jejunum has fewer arterial arcades and that of the ileum has more arterial arcades.
- Jejunum has longer vasa recta while ileum has shorter vasa recta.
- Jejunum has less fat in its mesentery and so the visibility of the vessels is good accounting for **"peritoneal windows"**. The reverse is the case in ileum.
- Mucous surface of ileum has solitary and aggregated lymph nodes.

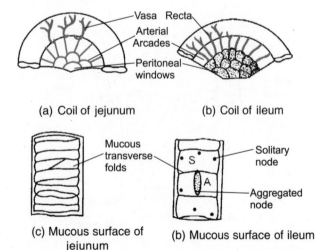

(a) Coil of jejunum   (b) Coil of ileum

(c) Mucous surface of jejunum   (b) Mucous surface of ileum

Fig. 6.19: Differences between jejunum and ileum

Mesentery (Fig. 6.20)

The mesentery is a peritoneal fold suspending the jejunum and ileum from the posterior abdominal wall. It has two layers (right or upper and left or lower) and two borders (anterior and posterior). The posterior border is known as the **root of the mesentery**.

The root of mesentery is 15 cm in length and its line of attachment runs obliquely downward and to the right from duodenojejunal flexure to the right iliac fossa. The root is much shorter than the anterior or intestinal border which is about 5.5 metres or more long. This difference results in marked folding, so that the mesentery resembles a partly opened fan. The width from root to intestine may be 15 cm to 20 cm, being widest opposite the middle part.

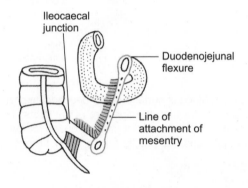

Fig. 6.20: Mesentery of small intestine extending from the doudenojejunal flexure to ileocaecal junction

The obliquely of the mesentery divides the infracolic compartment of peritoneal cavity into right and left parts.

The mesentery contains the superior mesenteric vessels, nerve plexuses, lymphatics and lymph nodes.

Along its line of attachment, it crosses successively the following structures (Fig. 6.21):
- Horizontal part of the duodenum.
- Aorta.
- Inferior vena cava.
- Right ureter.
- Right genitofemoral nerve.
- Right gonadal vessels.
- Psoas major muscle.

Blood Supply

The arterial supply is by the superior mesenteric artery and the venous drainage is into the superior mesenteric vein.

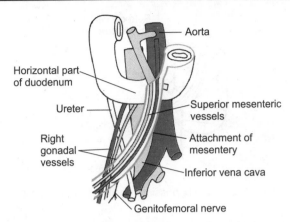

Fig. 6.21: Line of attachment of mesentery on the posterior abdominal wall and the structures crossed by it

CLINICAL APPLICATION

- The 1.5 m (5 ft.) of the small intestine at a point 1.8 m (6 ft.) from the duodenojejunal flexure to a point 3.3 m (11 ft.) from the flexure lie in the pelvis due to the fact that the mesentery to this part is longer than the other parts. These are the parts of small intestine which are likely to be affected in pelvic peritonitis.
- During abdominal operations the jejunum and ileum are differentiated by the number of arterial arcades and the length of parallel vessels in its mesentery. Jejunum has one or two arterial arcades with 3.75 cm (1.5 inch) long parallel vessels and the ileum has two or three arterial arcades with 1.25 cm (0.5 inch) long parallel vessels. This is the only distinction of use to the operating surgeon.
- A short **diverticulum (Meckel's)** may be found on the antimesenteric border of the ileum in cases where the vitellointestinal duct persists. It is 5 cm (2 inch) in length, 50 cm (2 ft.) proximal to the ileocaecal junction and is found in 2% of individuals. It may give rise to following conditions:
- Non-closure of the vitellointestinal duct results in small intestinal contents discharging at the umbilicus **(umbilical fistula)**.
- A long diverticulum predisposes to obstruction; a short one with a broad base to **intussusception**.
- Mucosa of diverticulum may present accessory pancreatic tissue (because at one time of its development it is very near the developing pancreas) or gastric mucosa, the secretions of

which may lead to ulcer formations, perforations or diverticulitis.
- Often a fibrous band may connect the diverticulum with the umbilicus and this may give rise to **volvulus** and intestinal obstruction.
- If the vitellointestinal duct closes at both ends but remains patent in the middle, it causes a cyst behind the navel **(enteromata)**.

THE LARGE INTESTINE

The large intestine consists of caecum, vermiform appendix, colon, rectum and anal canal (Fig. 6.18). Except for the appendix, rectum and anal canal, the large intestine has the following features which distinguish it from the small intestine.

- **Taenia coli** which are three thickened bands formed by the aggregation of the longitudinal muscle coat.
- **Haustrations** which are sacculations of the wall, produced since the taenia coli are shorter than the length of the colon.
- **Appendices epiploicae** which are fatty projections of the serous coat on the antimesenteric border of the different parts of the colon.

CAECUM

The caecum is the blind (Caecum = Blind in *Latin*) commencement of the large intestine inferior to the entry of the ileum. It is situated in the right iliac fossa above the lateral end of the inguinal ligament lateral to the right lateral plane (Fig. 6.22). It is fully covered with peritoneum.

Relations

Anteriorly

- Anterior abdominal wall.

Posteriorly (Fig. 6.23)

- Retrocaecal recess (Fig. 4.22 b).

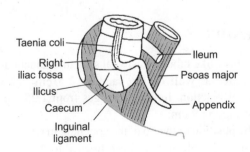

Fig. 6.22: Caecum in the iliac fossa

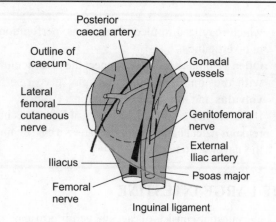

Fig. 6.23: Posterior relations of caecum. Outline of caecum is shown by dotted lines

- Iliacus and psoas muscles.
- Lateral femoral cutaneous nerve.
- Femoral nerve.
- Genitofemoral nerve.
- External iliac artery.
- Posterior caecal artery.

Interior (Fig. 6.24)

- **Ileocaecal opening** is transverse and is on the postero-medial wall of the caecum. It is bounded by two horizontal folds which project inwards.
- Appendicular opening is 2.5 cm below the ileocaecal orifice and is slit-like.

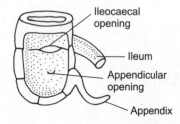

Fig. 6.24: The orifices within the caecum

APPENDIX

It is a worm-like tubular vestigeal structure attached to the posteromedial wall of the caecum 2.5 cm below the ileocaecal junction. Its length ranges from 1.25 cm to 22 cm, average is 9 cm.

The position of the tip of the appendix in relation to the caecum is variable and has been likened to the hands of a clock (Fig. 6.25).

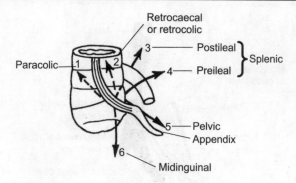

Fig. 6.25: The six possible positions of appendix

- 10 o'clock (right paracolic).
- 12 o'clock position (retrocaecal or retrocolic) in 65% of cases.
- 2 o'clock position (left paracaecal). In this position it may be preileal or postileal (1.5% of cases).
- 5 o'clock position (pelvic) when it crosses the pelvic brim. It is so in 20% of cases.
- 6 o'clock position (midinguinal).

The three taenia of the caecum always converge on to the appendix irrespective of its site of attachment. It is usually connected to the ileum by a triangular extension of the posterior leaf of the mesentery forming a **mesoappendix** along which the appendicular artery runs to supply it (Fig. 4.22 a).

The appendix is characterized by a large accumulation of lymphoid tissue. Its overwhelming importance is because it is a common site of infection (appendicitis) necessitating its surgical removal.

The appendix is characterised by a large accumulation of lymphoid tissue. Its overwhelming importance is because it is a common site of infection (appendicitis) necessitating its surgical removal.

Arterial Supply (Fig. 6.26)

The appendicular artery, a branch of the ileocolic artery reaches the appendix through its mesentery (meso-appendix). This may arise from the posterior caecal artery.

Lymphatic Drainage

The lymph vessels terminate in the **ileocaecal nodes** situated close to the ileocaecal artery and **appendicular nodes** at the base of mesoappendix.

Nerve Supply

The sympathetic fibres are derived from T_{10} and T_{11}

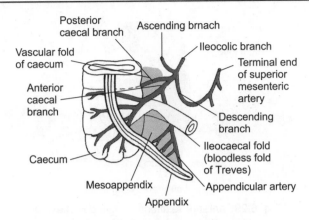

Fig. 6.26: Arterial supply of appendix

segments of the spinal cord and the parasympathetic fibres are derived from the vagi.

Development

At an early embryonic stage it has the same calibre as the caecum and is in line with it. It is formed by the excessive growth of the right wall of caecum which pushes the appendix to the inner side.

CLINICAL APPLICATION

- When the appendix occupies preileal or postileal position then its inflammation may affect the terminal ileum and cause much vomiting (an unusual thing in appendicitis) and even obstruction of the small gut.
- A retrocaecal appendix gives rise to symptoms very late. The infection from it may go upwards and reach **Morison's pouch** causing a subphrenic abscess.
- Inflammation of a pelvic appendix may be confused with inflammation of a pelvic organ e.g., fallopian tube or ovary.
- Because appendix is innervated by the lesser splanchnic nerve, initial **colicky pain** is referred to the T_{10} and T_{11} dermatomes, which include the periumbilical region. As the adjacent parietal peritoneum becomes inflamed, pain becomes localised to the lower right quadrant and the overlying muscle exhibits the reflex spasm characteristic of acute abdomen (guarding).
- The appendicular artery is the sole arterial supply of appendix. It is an end artery with a relatively narrow lumen. Acute appendicitis may result in thrombosis of

this artery with rapid development of gangrene and subsequent perforation, if appendectomy is delayed.
- The teniae coli, all of which converge into the appendix, are useful landmarks in locating the appendix at operation.

COLON

The colon extends from the caecum in the right iliac fossa to its junction with the rectum which is in front of the middle piece of sacrum.

Subdivisions

It is divided into:
- Ascending colon
- Transverse colon
- Descending colon
- Sigmoid or pelvic colon

ASCENDING COLON

It is about 20 cm long and ascends up from the caecum to the inferior surface of the right lobe of liver, where it makes a sharp bend at the level of second lumbar vertebra called the right colic or hepatic flexure to become the transverse colon (Fig. 6.27).

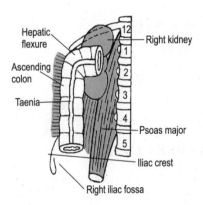

Fig. 6.27: Ascending colon and its position

Relations

Anteriorly

- Anterior abdominal wall.
- Coils of small intestine.
- Right edge of greater omentum (Fig. 4.18).

Posteriorly (Fig. 6.28)

- Iliacus, quadratus lumborum and transverses abdominis.
- Right kidney.
- Subcostal nerve and vessels.
- Iliohypogastric and ilioinguinal nerves.

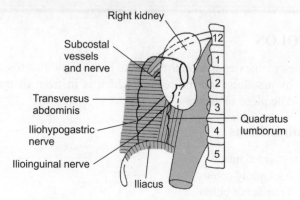

Fig. 6.28: Posterior relations of ascending colon

RIGHT COLIC OR HEPATIC FLEXURE

This is formed by the terminal part of the ascending colon which turns downward, forward and to the left to become continuous with the transverse colon. It lies below the level of transpyloric plane.

Relations

Anteriorly (Fig. 6.29)

- Inferior surface of the right lobe of liver.

Posteriorly (Fig. 6.30)

- Anterior surface of the lower pole of right kidney.
- Transversus abdominis muscle.

TRANSVERSE COLON

Transverse colon lies in upper abdomen from the hepatic flexure to the splenic flexure which is situated below the lateral end of the spleen. It is suspended from the anterior margin of the pancreas by the transverse mesocolon with its longest part in the middle and shortest parts at the hepatic and splenic flexures which are consequently relatively fixed. Greater part of transverse colon hangs down to a variable extent, sometimes into the pelvis.

Relations

When the transverse mesocolon is short the transverse colon has the following relations:

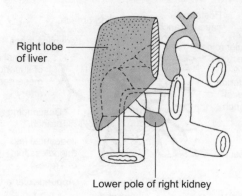

Fig. 6.29: Anterior relations of right colic flexure

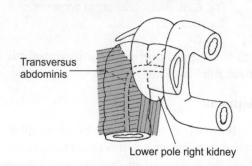

Fig. 6.30: Posterior relations of right colic flexure

Anteriorly (Fig. 6.31)

- Descending sheet of greater omentum.

Posteriorly (Fig. 6.32)

- Right kidney
- Descending (second) part of duodenum
- Head of pancreas
- Duodenojejunal flexure.
- Left kidney.

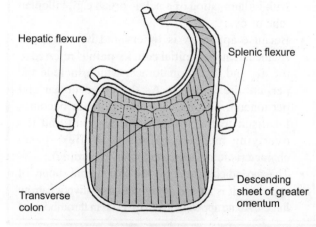

Fig. 6.31: Transverse colon: Anterior relations

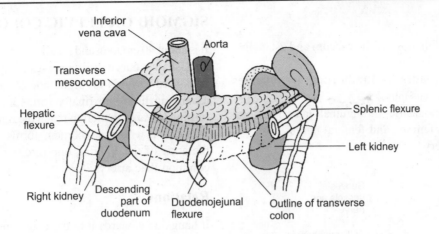

Fig. 6.32: Transverse colon: Posterior relations

LEFT COLIC OR SPLENIC FLEXURE

It is more acute than the hepatic flexure and is also at a higher level.

Relations (Fig. 6.33)

Anteriorly

- Stomach.
- Left costal margin.

Posteriorly

- Left kidney
- Colic surface of the spleen.

The flexure is anchored to the diaphragm opposite the eleventh rib in the midaxillary line by a peritoneal fold, the **phrenicocolic ligament**.

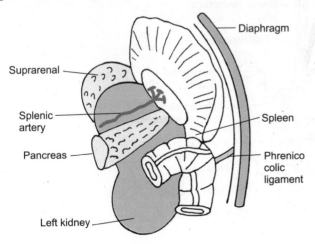

Fig. 6.33: Relations of left colic flexure

DESCENDING COLON

It is about 20–25 cm in length and extends from the splenic flexure to the pelvic brim. First, it passes down along the lateral margin of the left kidney to its lower end, then it runs vertically to the iliac crest and to the medial side of the left anterior superior iliac spine. It then turns medially to the pelvic brim where it becomes the sigmoid colon (Fig. 6.34).

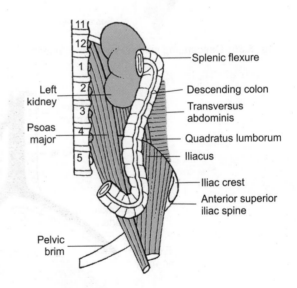

Fig. 6.34: Descending colon position

Relations

Anteriorly

- Coils of small intestine.

Posteriorly

These correspond with those of the caecum and ascending colon on the right side (Fig. 6.35).

- Psoas major, quadratus lumborum, transverses abdominis and iliacus muscles.
- Subcostal, iliohypogastric, ilioinguinal, lateral femoral cutaneous, genitofemoral and femoral nerves.
- External iliac artery.

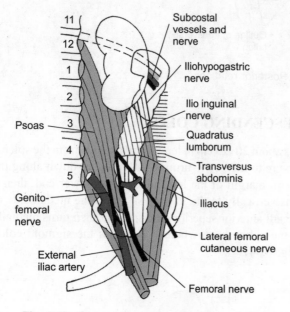

Fig. 6.35: Descending colon: Posterior relations

SIGMOID OR PELVIC COLON (FIG. 6.36)

It is about 40 cm long and is called sigmoid since it describes an S-shaped curve. It first passes from the left pelvic brim backward towards the right side of the pelvis to form an ascending limb and finally forms a descending limb by turning towards the left to reach the midline. It has a pelvic mesocolon whose attachment forms an inverted V with the apex of the V lying opposite the division of the left common iliac artery.

Relations

It hangs downwards into the pelvis in front of the rectum and behind the bladder or uterus.

ARTERIAL SUPPLY OF COLON

The colon is supplied by the superior and inferior mesenteric arteries.

SUPERIOR MESENTERIC ARTERY

The superior mesenteric artery is the artery of midgut and therefore supplies its derivatives which are:

- Duodenum distal to the opening of the bile duct
- Jejunum and ileum
- Appendix
- Caecum
- Ascending colon
- Right two-thirds of transverse colon

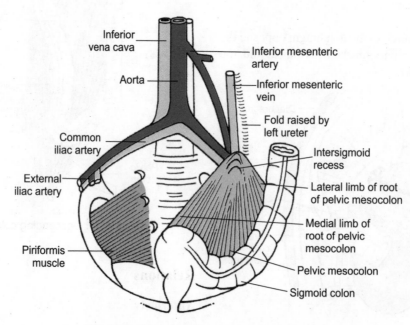

Fig. 6.36: Sigmoid colon and pelvic mesocolon

Origin

It is the second ventral branch of abdominal aorta and arises at the level of L_1 vertebra (Fig. 6.37).

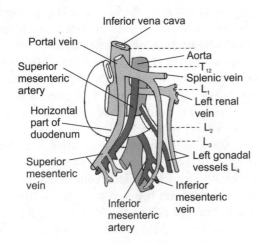

Fig. 6.37: Superior and inferior mesenteric arteries and their relation to duodenum and the big vessels and their vertebral levels of origin (Note the formation of portal vein at the level of L_1)

Course and relations (Figs. 6.13 and 6.21): At its origin it lies behind the pancreas and is crossed by the splenic vein. Just below its origin, it crosses the left renal vein which separates it from the aorta. It appears at the lower border of pancreas and crosses its uncinate process and the horizontal part of duodenum and enters the mesentery. In the mesentery, it is accompanied on its right side by the **superior mesenteric vein** and with it runs downward and to the right to reach the right iliac fossa. With inferior vena cava, right psoas major, right ureter and genitofemoral nerve lying posterior to it (Fig. 6.21). Throughout its course, it is surrounded by a plexus of sympathetic nerves. It ends by anastomoses with one of its own branches.

It presents a curved course with the convexity facing downwards and to the left.

Branches (Fig. 6.38)

These are:
- **Inferior pancreaticoduodenal branch** which runs upwards to anastomose with the superior pancreatic-coduodenal artery.
- **Jejunal** and **ileal branches** about 12 to 15 in number arising from the left convex side of the artery. They pass between the layers of the mesentery and form a series of arterial arcades before reaching the jejunum and ileum.

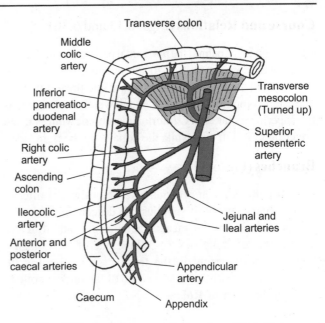

Fig. 6.38: Superior mesenteric artery: Branches

- **Ileocolic branch** is the lowest branch arising from the right side of the artery. It divides into an ascending and a descending branch. The descending branch anastomoses with the terminal end of the superior mesenteric artery.

Ileocolic branch also gives rise to:
- Ileal branches supplying the terminal ileum.
- Anterior and posterior caecal branches to the caecum.
- Appendicular artery to appendix.
- Colic branch to supply lower one-third of ascending colon.
- **Middle colic branch** is the first to arise, it passes downwards between the layers of transverse mesocolon and divides into left and right branches. It supplies the right two-thirds of transverse mesocolon.
- **Right colic branch** is the second branch, it divides into an ascending and a descending branch. It supplies upper two-thirds of the ascending colon and right colic flexure.

INFERIOR MESENTERIC ARTERY

The inferior mesenteric artery is the artery of the hindgut and therefore supplies its derivatives which are:
- Left one-third of transverse colon.
- Descending colon.
- Sigmoid colon.

Origin

It is the third ventral branch of the abdominal aorta and arises at the level of L_3 vertebra (Fig. 6.37).

Course and Relations (Figs. 6.13 and 6.36)

At its origin it lies behind the horizontal part of the duodenum. It descends downwards and to the left to cross the aorta, left sympathetic trunk, left psoas major and the termination of the left common iliac artery beyond which it continues as the superior rectal artery. Inferior mesenteric vein and left ureter lie to its left side while the aorta is on the right side.

Branches (Fig. 6.39)

- **Left colic** is given off soon after the origin of inferior mesenteric artery. It supplies the descending colon. It passes up and to the left at an acute angle and bifurcates near the left colic flexure. Where one of the branches passes to the right in the transverse mesocolon, to anastomose with a similar branch of the middle coilc to form the **arch of Rolan**.

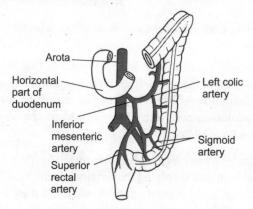

Fig. 6.39: Inferior mesenteric artery: Branches

- **Sigmoidal arteries** supply the sigmoid colon and anastomoses with the descending branch of the left colic artery.

Along the concavity of the three sided square made by the large bowel, there courses an artery made up by anastomotic vessels from the different main vessels going to the large intestine. It is known as **marginal artery (Drummond's)** and from it arise the terminal arteries to the colon **(vasa recta)** (Fig. 6.40). It extends from the ascending colon to the end of pelvic colon. This artery can maintain the vitality of the left colon even after the inferior mesenteric artery has been ligated at its origin. The **Rolan's arch,** formed by the anastomosis of one of the branches of left colic with a branch of middle colic, provides a strong anastomotic connection between the inferior mesenteric artery and the middle colic artery thereby supplementing the marginal artery which is sometimes poor near the flexure.

Anastomotic connection between the lowest sigmoid branch and the upper rectal branch of the superior rectal artery is sometimes by a very small vessel incapable of providing adequate collateral circulation in the vicinity.

CLINICAL APPLICATION

- In resection of caecum with removal of ileocolic artery, the terminal ileum is also removed as it shares the same blood supply. This avoids the possibility of ischemic necrosis.

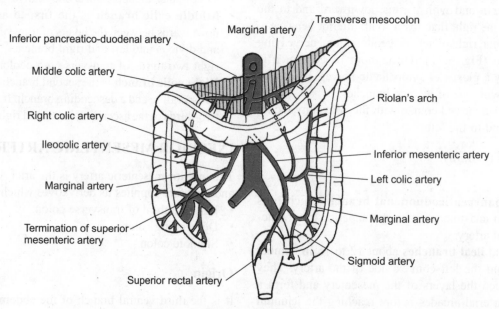

Fig. 6.40: Marginal artery of Drummond

- **The marginal artery (of Drummond),** made up of anastomotic vessels from the main arteries going to the large intestine, is capable of supplying the gut even though one of the large feeding trunks be severed. It can maintain the vitality of the left colon even after the inferior mesenteric artery has been ligated at its origin.
- The **arch of Rolan,** formed by the anastomosis of one of the branches of left colic with a branch of middle colic, plays an important part in supplementing the marginal artery which is in 5% cases poor near the splenic flexure.
- The weakest point of anastomosis in the marginal artery is in the region of left colic flexure, between the middle colic and left colic branches and not between the left colic and sigmoid arteries as suggested by **Sudeck.**

Venous Drainage of Large Intestine

The large intestine drains into the hepatic portal system.

The **hepatic portal system** begins as the venous capillaries of the gastrointestinal tract and ends as the venous sinusoids of liver. It has no valves.

Formation: It is formed by the union of the splenic vein and superior mesenteric vein behind the neck of pancreas at the level of L_1 (Fig. 6.37).

Course: It ascends up to reach the right edge of porta hepatic where it divides into a right and a left branch.

Relations (Fig. 6.41)

- **Below the superior part of duodenum,** it is related anteriorly to the neck of pancreas, posteriorly to the inferior vena cava and on the right side to the common bile duct and the pancreaticoduodenal vessels.
- **Behind the superior part of duodenum,** the gastroduodenal artery and common bile duct lie anterior to it. The artery being medial to the duct. The inferior vena cava lies posterior to it.

- **Above the superior part of duodenum,** anteriorly lies the common bile duct and the hepatic artery. The artery is medial to the duct. The duct, artery and the portal vein lie enclosed in the free margin of lesser omentum **(hepatoduodenal ligament).** Posteriorly the foramen epiploicum intervenes between the portal vein and the inferior vena cava.
- **Within the right of porta hepatic,** the terminal part divides into a right and a left branch. The right branch enters the right lobe of the liver while the left branch enters the left lobe. The left is joined in front by the ligamentum teres (obliterated left umbilical vein) and behind by ligamentum venosum (obliterated ductus venosus) (Fig. 6.41a).

Tributaries (Fig. 6.42)

The portal vein receives three major veins and numerous smaller veins to drain the alimentary tract, spleen, pancreas and gall bladder.

- **Superior mesenteric vein** parallels and receives tributaries from the regions supplied by the superior mesenteric artery. It also receives the **right gastroepiploic vein.** It is the largest tributary of the portal vein.
- **Splenic vein** drains the spleen, as well as portions of the stomach and pancreas. It generally parallels the splenic artery and may be embedded in the pancreatic

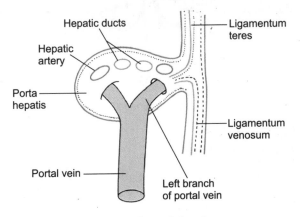

(a) In the region of duodenum.

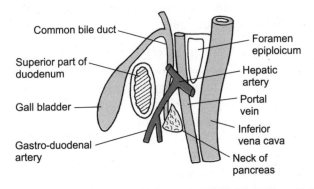

(b) In the region of porta hepatis. Relations of portal vein at the porta hepatis.

Fig. 6.41(a and b): Relations of the portal vein

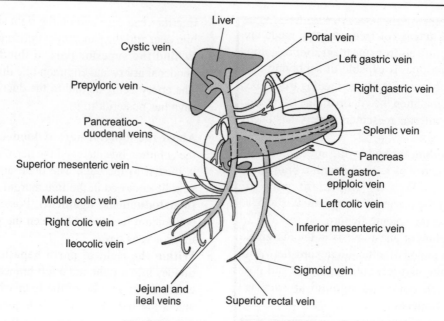

Fig. 6.42: Tributaries of the portal vein

parenchyma. Its tributaries correspond to the branches of the splenic artery. In addition, it receives the inferior mesenteric vein.

- **Inferior mesenteric vein** drains the regions supplied by the inferior mesenteric artery. It usually enters the splenic vein but may enter the superior mesenteric vein.
- Smaller tributaries are:
  - **Left gastric vein** runs upwards along the lesser curvature of stomach and joins the retro-duodenal part of the portal vein.
  - **Right gastric vein** runs downwards along the lesser curvature of stomach and joins the portal vein as it enters the free margin of lesser omentum. It receives the **prepyloric vein of Mayo**.
  - **Cystic vein,** when present, drains into the right branch of portal vein.

CLINICAL APPLICATION

- Obstruction of the portal circulation may give rise to portal hypertension which may cause varicosity of the veins (varices) at the regions where the portal and systemic veins communicate e.g., **oesophageal varices** at the lower end of oesophagus, **piles** at the lower end of rectum and **caput medusae** in the region of umbilicus.

LYMPHATIC DRAINAGE

In general, the lymphatic drainage follows the arteries.

The glands are arranged on a plan common to all parts of the large and small intestines. They are very numerous and are arranged in three groups (Fig. 6.43):

- Proximal.
- Intermediate.
- Distal.

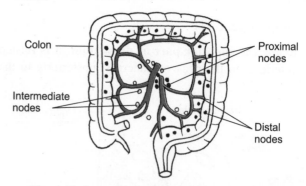

Fig. 6.43: Lymphatic drainage of large intestine

The Proximal Nodes

These are situated on the main blood vessels to the gut and are named accordingly as:

- Superior mesenteric

- Ileocolic
- Right colic
- Left colic
- Middle colic
- Inferior mesenteric
- Superior rectal
- Sigmoid

The Intermediate Nodes

These are situated on the larger branches of the above named vessels.

The Distal Nodes

These are situated near the gut between the numerous small vessels entering the gut. Some of these nodes lie on the gut.

The lymph goes for the most part from the gut to the distal nodes and then to the intermediate and proximal set. This plan is the same throughout the large and small intestines. The lymphatics from the territory of any one of the arteries converge on the main trunk of the vessel so that the lymph drainage is divided fairly accurately into areas corresponding to the main arteries.

CLINICAL APPLICATION

- The lymphatic drainage field of each segment of the bowel corresponds fairly accurately to its blood supply. This fact governs the operative treatment of cancer of the large intestine. If cancer occurs in caecum or ascending colon, the whole of the gut supplied by branches of superior mesenteric and the related peritoneum, is removed to ensure the removal of the whole lymph territory which converges on these vessels.
- Since, the afferent nerves from the descending colon reach the spinal cord via lumbar splanchnic nerves (L_1 and L_2), so the pain originating within the descending colon is referred to the inguinal region and thigh.
- The afferent nerves from the sigmoid colon reach the spinal cord via pelvic splanchnic nerves (S_2 to S_4), so the pain originating within the sigmoid colon is referred to the perineum and legs.
- Congenital absence of autonomic plexus in areas of large bowel results in stasis, obstinate constipation and enormous dilatation of large bowel (**megacolon** or **Hirschsprung's disease**).

Nerve Supply

The transverse colon is the most caudal part of the gastrointestinal tract to be supplied with parasympathetic innervation from the vagus nerve.

The innervation of the descending colon is by two pathways. It receives parasympathetic innervation from the pelvic splanchnic nerves (S_2 to S_4) and sympathetic innervation from the lumbar splanchnic nerves (L_1 and L_2).

7

Liver, Extrahepatic Biliary Apparatus, Pancreas and Spleen

INTRODUCTION

The liver is the largest gland in the body weighing about 1500 gm. It is soft in consistency. It develops from the foregut and remains attached to it through the bile duct through which it drains bile into the second part of duodenum.

Position (Fig. 7.1)

It is surrounded by a thin fibrous **capsule (Glisson's)** that lies just beneath the visceral peritoneum. The liver is mostly well protected by the rib cage, except the part within the infrasternal angle. It almost fully occupies the right hypochondrium and extends across the epigastrium to reach the left hypochondrium as far as the left lateral line. It extends upwards under the rib cage as far as the fifth rib anteriorly on the right side and fifth intercostal space on the left. The sharp inferior border crosses the median plane at the level of L_1 vertebra. The liver is relatively very large at birth and occupies much of the abdominal cavity, this is normal finding until the child is 2 to 3 years old.

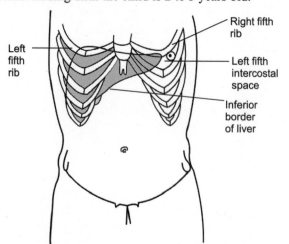

Fig. 7.1: Position of the liver in relation to the anterior abdominothoracic wall

Left fifth rib

Right fifth rib

Left fifth intercostal space

Inferior border of liver

Shape

It is a wedge-shaped organ, its base faces to the right and its apex to the left (Fig. 7.2). Out of the five surfaces and various borders of this wedge, only two surfaces and one margin are described as three surfaces smoothly run into each other.

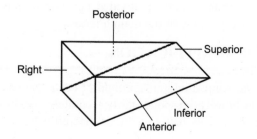

Posterior

Superior

Right

Inferior

Anterior

Fig. 7.2: Liver is wedge-shaped. Schematic five surfaces of liver

LOBES

The liver is divided into anatomical right and left lobes by the following ligaments and fissures (Figs. 7.3 and 7.4):

- **Falciform ligament,** which attaches the anterior and superior surfaces of the liver to the diaphragm and the anterior abdominal wall. Below the two layers, of the ligament are continuous and its free margin encloses the **ligamentum teres.**
- **Ligamentum teres,** a solid fibrous cord formed by the obliteration of the **left umbilical vein** soon after birth, runs forward across the inferior surface and border of the liver in a fissure to the left end of the porta hepatis which is a depressed oval area on the inferior surface of the liver. From the liver the ligamentum teres runs downward to reach the umbilicus.

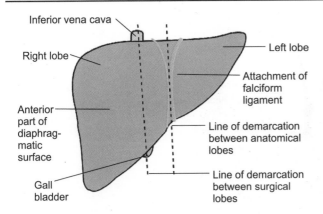

Fig. 7.3: Lobes of liver: Anatomical and surgical subdivisions as seen on the anterior part of diaphragmatic surface of liver

- **Ligamentum venosum,** a second fibrous cord formed by the obliteration, of the **ductus venosus,** runs upward across the posterior surface of the liver, in a deep fissures, first forwards and then to the right. It diverges from the left end of porta hepatic.

The **surgical subdivision into right and left lobes** is defined by the following landmarks:
- **Fossa for the gall bladder** lying on the inferior surface of the liver. The narrow neck of the gall bladder passes into the right end of porta hepatis.
- **Groove for inferior vena cava,** a deep vertical groove on the posterior surface of the liver, containing the upper part of inferior vena cava.

The fissures for the ligamentum teres and venosum, the fossa for the gall bladder, the groove for the inferior vena cava along with the porta hepatis form an H-shaped pattern on the posteroinferior aspect of the liver. The portion of liver behind the porta hepatis and between the sulcus

for the inferior vena cava and the fissure for ligamentum venosum is the **caudate lobe,** so called because it is attached to the right lobe by the tail-like **caudate process,** which is between the sulcus for inferior vena cava and the porta hepatis. The caudate process forms the upper boundary for the opening into the lesser sac (foramen epiploicum). The rectangular portion of the liver between the fossa for gall bladder and the fissure for ligamentum venosum is the **quadrate lobe**.

The caudate and quadrate lobes belong to the left lobe in clinical practice although anatomists include them in the right lobe.

Porta Hepatis (Figs. 7.5(a) and (b))

The porta hepatis is a transverse fissure separating the quadrate lobe from the caudate lobe. Its lips give attachment to the lesser omentum. The right and left branches of the hepatic artery and the portal vein enter it, and the right and left hepatic ducts come out of it. Hepatic lymph nodes and a pad of fat are situated near it.

Peritoneal Fold of Liver (Fig. 7.6)

Falciform Ligament

It is a sickle-shaped double fold of peritoneum which stretches from the liver to the diaphragm and the anterior abdominal wall. It has a convex and concave margin and a right and left layer. The convex margin is attached to the inferior surface of the diaphragm and the anterior abdominal wall upto the umbilicus. The concave margin contains the **obliterated left umbilical vein** which is represented by the ligamentum teres. The right layer is continuous with the upper layer of **coronary ligament**.

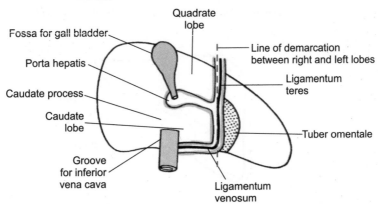

Fig. 7.4: Lobes of liver: As seen on the posterior part of diaphragmatic surface and inferior surface of liver

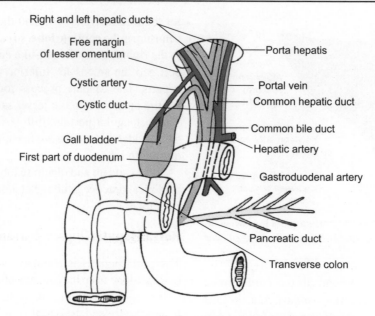

Fig. 7.5 (a): Porta hepatis: Structures entering and leaving it

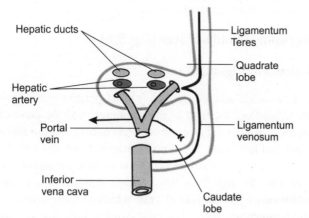

Fig. 7.5 (b): Porta hepatis: Structures entering and leaving it

Left Triangular Ligament

The left layer of coronary ligament is continued onto the left on the upper surface of left lobe and folds upon itself to form the left triangular ligament.

Coronary Ligament

It is on the posterior surface of the right lobe of liver and has a superior and an inferior layer.

- Superior layer stretches between the posterosuperior aspect of right lobe of liver and the diaphragm along upper part of bare area. It is continuous with the right layer of **falciform ligament**.

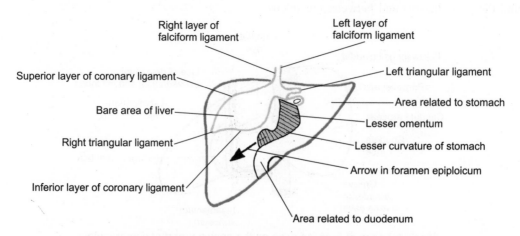

Fig. 7.6: Peritoneal folds of liver as related to the inferior and posterior surfaces of liver

- Inferior layer stretches between the posteroinferior aspect of the right lobe of liver and the diaphragm along lower part of bare area.

Right Triangular Ligament

The two layers of coronary ligament fuse on the right to form the **right triangular ligament** and between them is the bare area of liver.

Lesser Omentum

It is derived from ventral mesogastrium and is a two layered fold of peritoneum:
- **Attachments:** Superiorly to the fissure for ligamentum venosum and the lips of porta hepatic along an L-shaped line. Inferiorly to the lesser curvature of stomach and to the first inch of the superior part of duodenum.
- **Relation:** Its free margin forms the anterior boundary of foramen epiploicum. Posterior to it is the lesser sac. Anterior to it is the left intraperitoneal subdiaphragmatic space.
- **Contents:** The free margin contains the portal vein hepatic artery and the common bile duct (Fig. 6.7). The other contents are left and right gastric vessels, lymphatics from stomach, lymph nodes and nerve plexuses (Fig. 6.7).

Surfaces and their Relations (Fig. 7.7)

The liver has two surfaces:

Diaphragmatic Surface

It is related to the diaphragm and has four parts which are smoothly continuous with each other.

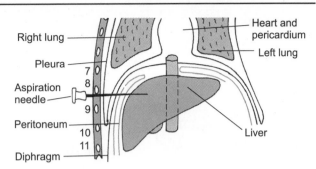

Fig. 7.7: Relations of the right part and superior part of the diaphragmatic surface of liver. The needle for liver puncture transverse both pleural and peritoneal cavities. Numbers indicate the rib number

- **Right part** is the base of the wedge and lies against the 7th to 11th ribs. The diaphragm separates the upper one-third of this surface from the right pleura and lung, the middle one-third from the right pleura only and lower one-third from the thoracic wall (Fig. 7.7).
- **Superior part** is in contact with the diaphragm and is related to the heart and pericardium in the middle and to the bases of the lungs and pleural cavities on either side (Fig. 7.7).
- **Anterior part** apart from being related to the diaphragm, it is also related to the anterior abdominal wall in the infrasternal angle. On either side of the midline the respective lungs and pleural sacs overlap it.

The falciform ligament, a sagittal fold of peritoneum, is attached to this surface (Fig. 7.3).
- **Posterior part** is small and triangular in outline and presents the following features from left to right (Fig. 7.8):

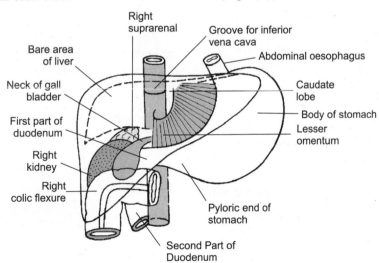

Fig. 7.8: Relations of the posterior part of the diaphragmatic surface of liver

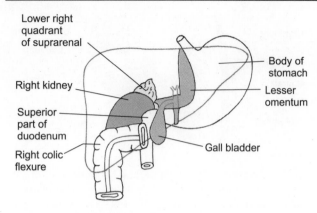

Fig. 7.9: Relations of inferior or visceral surface of liver

- A groove which is related to the abdominal part of oesophagus.
- Fissure for ligamentum venosum.
- Caudate lobe which is related to the superior recess of lesser sac.
- Groove for inferior vena cava.
- Bare area of liver which is a rough triangular area not covered by peritoneum and bearing the suprarenal impression for the right gland.

Visceral Surface or Inferior Surface

It is the only surface not related to the diaphragm. It sits upon the upper abdominal viscera which form the **"liver bed"** and from the left to right side these are:
- Part of the body of stomach and its pyloric end.
- Superior and descending part of duodenum which cross the neck of gall bladder.
- Gall bladder in the fossa for gall bladder which is non-peritoneal.
- Lesser omentum related to a prominence on the left lobe called the tuberomentale.
- Right colic flexure.
- Upper part of right kidney.
- Lower right quadrant of right suprarenal.

Blood Supply

The liver receives its blood supply from the **hepatic artery,** a continuation of common hepatic which is a branch of coeliac.

The liver also receives blood from the **portal vein** which receives the venous blood from the alimentary tract. It is formed behind the neck of pancreas by the union of superior mesenteric and splenic veins at the level of L_1 vertebra. It ascends behind the superior part of duodenum where the bile duct and the gastroduodenal artery are

anterior to it and the inferior vena cava is posteriorly situated. In the lesser omentum it is behind the hepatic artery and bile duct. At the porta hepatis it divides into right and left branches. The right branch supplies the right lobe while the left branch supplies the caudate and quadrate lobes and left lobe of liver.

Liver Segments

On the basis of the subdivision of the portal vein and hepatic artery, each lobe of liver is divided into two segments. The segments of left lobe are (Figs. 7.3 and 7.4):
- **Left lateral** which is equivalent to the left anatomic lobe.
- **Left medial** which includes the quadrate and part of caudate lobe. The line of the fissure for ligamentum venosum and ligamentum teres demarcate the above two segments.

The two segments of right lobe are:
- **Right anterior.**
- **Right posterior:** The line of division runs obliquely and medially from the middle of the front of the right lobe towards the vena caval groove.

Lymphatic Drainage (Fig. 7.10)

- **Portal nodes** at the hilum drain the inferior aspect of liver and end in hepatic nodes.
- **Vena caval nodes** at the vena caval orifice of the diaphragm drain the posterior parts of liver and end in middle diaphragmatic nodes.
- **Retrosternal nodes** drain the anterior and upper parts. The lymphatics pass out between the two layers of falciform ligament.

There are, therefore, two main lymph streams from the liver, one via the coeliac nodes to the cisterna chyli and the other via thorax to the mediastinal trunks of both sides.

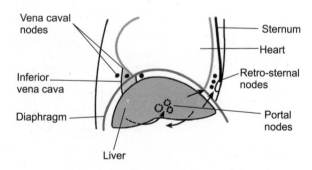

Fig. 7.10: The lymphatic drainage of liver

Development

The liver appears by the third week as the hepatic diverticulum of the foregut. It develops within the septum transversum and the ventral mesogastrium, dividing the ventral mesogastrium into the lesser omentum and the falciform ligament (Fig. 4.3).

CLINICAL APPLICATION

- Fracture of right lower ribs or penetrating wounds of upper abdomen or thorax can injure the liver as it is closely related to them.
- The liver is punctured for abscesses in its interior. The needle is inserted in the 10th, 9th or 8th space on the right side. Above this it will injure the lung. The needle passes successively through intercostal muscle, parietal pleura, costodiaphragmatic recess of pleura, diaphragmatic pleura, diaphragm, peritoneum over the undersurface of diaphragm, peritoneal recess between the liver and the diaphragm, peritoneum covering the diaphragm and finally the liver (Fig. 7.7).

- Liver abscesses usually lie in the upper part of the right lobe and produce irritation of the overlying diaphragm which causes referred pain over the shoulder. This is because the nerve impulses ascend through the phrenic nerves (C_3 to C_5) and the supraclavicular nerves (C_3 and C_4) which supply the skin over the shoulder share the same spinal segments.
- Because of its great vascularity secondaries from cancers of almost any part of body can spread to liver.
- If the portal vein is obstructed (e.g., cirrhosis of liver) the portal blood find its way to the heart by the vena cavae via communication between the portal and systemic circulations. The sites of portal-systemic anastomosis are (Fig. 7.11):
- At the lower end of oesophagus. The oesophageal branches of left gastric vein (draining to the portal vein) communicate with oesophageal veins (draining into the inferior hemiazygos vein which ends in azygos vein which joins the superior vena cava of systemic circulation). In portal obstruction these veins may become varicose and burst into

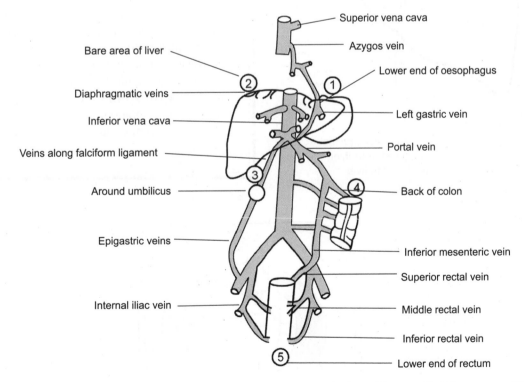

Fig. 7.11: Sites of portal systemic communication: (1) At lower end of oesophagus; (2) At bare area of liver; (3) Around the umbilicus; (4) At the back of colon; (5) At the lower end of rectum

the oesophagus causing vomiting of blood **(haematemesis)**.

- At the umbilicus veins pass along the falciform ligament to the umbilicus, connect the veins of the liver (portal) with the superficial and deep epigastric veins (systemic) around the umbilicus. Enlargement of these veins results in distended veins radiating from the umbilicus which is known as **"Caput medusae"**.
- At the lower end of the rectum, at the **Hilton's line** in the anal canal, the submucous venous plexuses is drained above by the superior rectal vein which continues as the inferior mesenteric vein to end in the splenic vein which joins the portal vein. The plexuses are drained below by the inferior and middle rectal veins which drain into systemic veins. In portal obstruction the veins in the rectum become varicose and form **haemorrhoids** or **piles**.
- At the back of colon the colic and splenic veins

(portal) in the extraperitoneal fat, anastomose with twigs of renal vein and veins of body wall (systemic).

- At base area of liver, small vessels unite the diaphragmatic veins (systemic) with the liver veins (portal).
- In relation to the periphery of liver there are potential spaces known as **"subphrenic"** because they are all related to the diaphragm. They are of great clinical importance as they may become filled with pus. The ligaments of the liver delimit them to a large extent. Three spaces are on the right side and three on the left side (Fig. 7.12).
- **Right and left subphrenic spaces** (right and left anterior intraperitoneal). They are intraperitoneal compartments lying between the diaphragm and the liver and separated from each other by the falciform ligament.
- **Right and left subhepatic spaces** (right and left posterior intraperitoneal) lie below the liver. They are intraperitoneal compartments.

The right is the **hepatorenal pouch of Morison**. It communicates anteriorly with the right subphrenic space around the anterior margin of the right lobe of liver and below both open into the general peritoneal cavity from which infection may track, for example, from a perforated appendix or a perforated peptic ulcer (Fig. 4.20).

The left subhepatic space is the **lesser sac** which communicates with the Morison's pouch through the foramen of **Winslow**. It may fill with fluid as a result of a perforation in the posterior wall of the stomach or from an inflamed pancreas to form a pseudocyst.

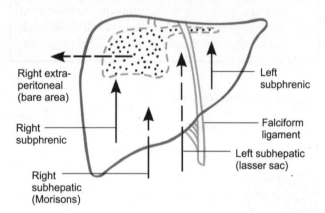

Fig. 7.12 (a): Anatomy of subphrenic spaces. Subphrenic spaces in relationship to liver. Dotted arrows are posterior to liver

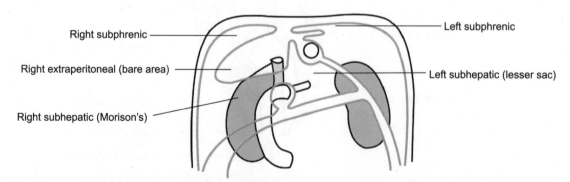

Fig. 7.12 (b): Subphrenic spaces in relation to the peritoneal reflection with viscera removed

- **Right extraperitoneal space (bare area of liver)** lies between the bare area of the liver and the diaphragm. It is entirely shut in and if it be distended with fluid, the liver tends to be pushed down.
- **Left extraperiotoneal space** is merely the connective tissue around the upper pole of the left kidney. It is seldom infected and is the least important of the six spaces.
- Because of its peritoneal attachments the liver moves with the diaphragm during respiration.
- Liver abscesses can erode through the diaphragm into the pleural cavity while lung abscesses can erode through the diaphragm into the subphrenic space and involve liver.
- Acute enlargement of liver and venous congestion is associated with pain as the result of sudden stretching of Glisson's capsule.
- Liver bleeds profusely when ruptured as it is an extremely vascular organ.
- Because of direct drainage of blood from the intestines to the liver via the portal vein, the liver is a common site of secondary involvement of both infection and cancer of the bowels.
- Sometimes due to abnormal lobulation of the liver a tongue-shaped projection extends from the inferior margin of the liver usually from the right lobe. It is known as **Riedel's lobe**. It may be mistaken for an abnormal abdominal mass.

THE EXTRAHEPATIC BILIARY APPARATUS

The extrahepatic biliary apparatus comprises (Fig. 7.13):
- Right and left hepatic ducts.
- Common hepatic duct formed by the union of the two hepatic ducts.
- Cystic duct which joins the common hepatic duct to form the common bile duct.
- Gall bladder which is drained by the cystic duct.
- Common bile duct which opens into the duodenum.

HEPATIC DUCTS

Right and left hepatic ducts emerge from the porta hepatic and unite to form the common hepatic duct. In the porta hepatic the relations from before backwards are (Fig. 7.5):
- Hepatic ducts.
- Right and left branches of hepatic artery.
- Right and left branches of the portal vein.

Common Hepatic Duct

Common hepatic duct is 3 cm long and is formed at the right edge of porta hepatis.

Cystic Duct

The cystic duct runs inferomedially in the lesser omentum to join the common hepatic duct to form the bile duct. It is 1.5 cm long. A spiral fold known as the **valve of Heister** maintains its patency.

GALL BLADDER

The gall bladder is a fibromuscular sac which stores and concentrates bile. It holds about 1½ oz of bile.

Situation

It is located in a fossa on the visceral surface of the liver between the right lobe and the quadrate lobe (Fig. 7.4). In terms of vertebral level, the commonest position is the angle between the twelfth rib and first lumbar vertebra (Fig. 7.14).

Shape and Subdivisions

Gall bladder is piriform in shape and is 6 to 10 cm long with a capacity of about 50 mL.

It is divided into three parts (Fig. 7.13):
- **Fundus** which is the bulbous end that projects beyond the inferior border of the liver. It is related to the anterior abdominal wall behind the tip of the ninth costal cartilage

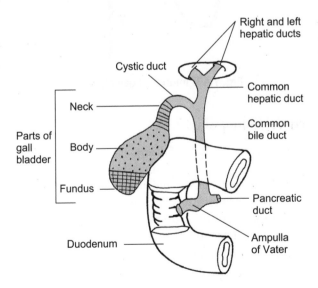

Fig. 7.13: The extrahepatic biliary apparatus

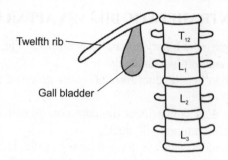

Fig. 7.14: Situation of gall bladder in terms of vertebral level is vertically in the angle between the 12th rib and L₁ vertebra

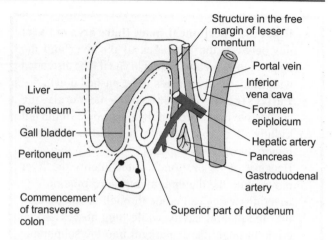

Fig. 7.16: Anterior and posterior relations of the gall bladder in a sectional view

opposite the lateral border of the rectus abdominis. Posteriorly it lies on the commencement of the transverse colon, just to the left of hepatic flexure (Fig. 7.15). It is completely covered by peritoneum.

- **Body** is the dilated part following the fundus and passes backwards and upwards towards the left to join the neck. It has upper and lower surfaces. The upper surface is in direct contact with fossa for gall bladder and is not covered by peritoneum (Fig. 7.16). The lower surface is covered by peritoneum and is related to the superior part of duodenum and the right end of transverse colon.
- **Neck** is formed by tapering of the body and curves medially to be continuous with the cystic duct. The part between the body and the neck may sag down as a pendulous pouch **(Hartmann's)** in a diseased gall bladder.

Interior of Gall Bladder (Fig. 7.17)

The circular muscle in the gall bladder throws the mucous membrane into spiral folds **(the valve of Heister)**. This spiral value is place in the S-shaped bend formed by the neck and the cystic duct. It prevents any obstruction to inflow or egress resulting from kinking of the neck of gall bladder.

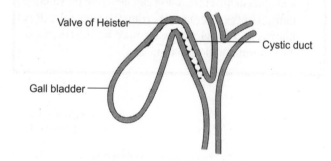

Fig. 7.17: Interior of gall bladder

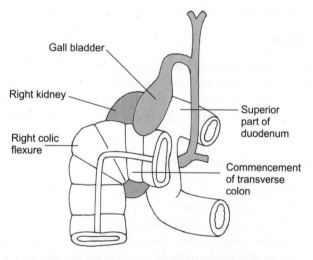

Fig. 7.15: Posterior relations of gall bladder

Arterial Supply (Fig. 7.18)

Cystic artery is a branch of the right hepatic artery supplies the gall bladder. It passes behind the cystic duct to reach the neck of the gall bladder and then divides into an anterior and a posterior branch to supply the gall bladder.

The cystic artery crosses the cystohepatic triangle (Calot's) which has following boundaries:
- Cystic duct on right side.
- Common hepatic duct on left side.
- Hilum of liver above.

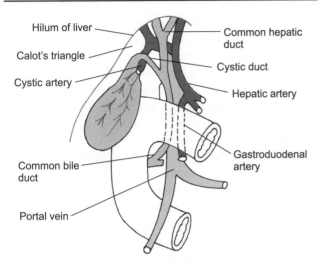

Fig. 7.18: Blood supply of gall bladder and relations of the common bile duct

Venous Drainage

The cystic artery has no accompanying vein. Venous drainage of the gall bladder is by a number of small vessels which run directly from its upper surface into the liver. The rest of the gall bladder is drained by vessels which join to form one or two cystic veins which join the portal vein.

Lymphatic Drainage

The gall bladder drains into:
- Nodes in porta hepatis
- Cystic node in Calot's triangle.
- A node at the anterior border of epiploic foramen.

COMMON BILE DUCT

The common hepatic duct and cystic duct converge to form the common bile duct, which empties into the duodenum. It is 10 cm long and 1 cm in diameter. It lies above, behind and below the first part of duodenum. It joins with the pancreatic duct to open into the middle of the second part of duodenum in its posteromedial part.

Relations

- **Supraduodenal part** runs in the free margin of lesser omentum with the following relations (Fig. 7.18):
- Hepatic artery on the left.
- Portal vein posteriorly.
- **Retroduodenal part** passes downward behind the superior part of duodenum with (Fig. 7.16):
- Gastroduodenal branch of hepatic artery to the left.
- Portal vein and inferior vena cava posteriorly.

- **Infraduodenal part** enters the second part of duodenum about 3 to 8 cm beyond the pyloric sphincter. It is the narrowest part of the common bile duct. The hepatopancreatic ampulla or duodenal papilla **(Vater's)** is formed by the confluence of the common bile duct and pancreatic duct. It is surrounded by the sphincter of Oddi. This part has following relations:
  - Head of pancreas anteriorly.
  - Superior pancreaticoduodenal artery medially.
  - Inferior vena cava posteriorly.

CLINICAL APPLICATION

- The phrenic nerve (C_3 to C_5) takes no part in the innervation of the peritoneum overlying the gall bladder or bile ducts. Shoulder tip pain can only occur if the peritoneum on the under surface of the diaphragm is irritated by inflammatory exudate. The skin over the acromion process is supplied by the supraclavicular nerve (C_3 and C_4).
- An enlarged gall bladder may be palpated in the right hypochondrium at the junction of the linea semilunaris and the costal margin corresponding to the tip of ninth costal cartilage.
- The numerous variations in the biliary tree and in branches of and relations of the hepatic artery in the Calot's triangle and in hepatoduodenal ligament constitute a major hazard in surgery. Calot's triangle is the most important area in billiary surgery.
- Biliary obstruction is painful. Pain associated with the inflammation of gall bladder (cholecystitis) reaches the spinal cord, levels T_5 and T_6 via the greater splanchnic nerves and is referred to T_5 and T_6 dermatomes, which include the right upper quadrant of the abdomen and epigastrium, as well as the region of the right scapula.

PANCREAS

The pancreas is a combined exocrine and endocrine gland. The exocrine part sends digestive secretions through its ducts into the second part of duodenum. The endocrine or ductless part secretes insulin directly into the blood stream to control blood sugar level. It is soft lobulated yellow gland.

Shape and Situation

The whole organ is about 15 cm long.

It has roughly the shape of an inverted tobacco pipe, and lies almost horizontally across the upper part of the posterior abdominal wall in the epigastric and left

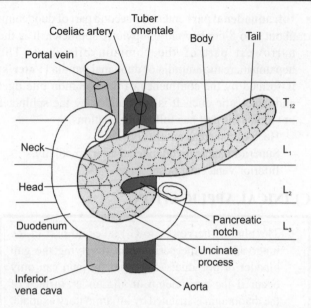

Fig. 7.19: General position of pancreas and its various parts

hypochondriac regions. Because of its deep position, it cannot be palpated.

Subdivisions

The adult pancreas consists of:
- Head
- Neck
- Body
- Tail

- The **head** forms an irregularly shaped disc and lies within the concavity of C-shaped duodenal loop in front of the second lumbar vertebra. It is flattened from before backwards and has anterior and posterior surfaces. From its lower part the hook-like **uncinate process** extends up and to the left forming the **pancreatic notch** above it.
- The **neck** is a constricted portion which connects the head and body of pancreas.
- The **body** inclines upwards in front of the first lumbar vertebra. It is first flattened but soon becomes somewhat prismatic in shape, with superior, inferior and posterior surfaces and superior, anterior and inferior borders.
- The **tail** is the continuation of the body and lies at the level of the twelfth thoracic vertebra. Along with the splenic vessels, it runs in the lienorenal ligament.

Relations

Anteriorly (Fig. 7.20)

- Head:
  - Pylorus of stomach to the upper part
  - Transverse colon and root of transverse mesocolon also to upper part. Aorta
  - Coils of small intestine to the lower part.
  - Superior mesenteric vessels are anterior to uncinate process.

- Neck:
  - Pylorus of stomach.

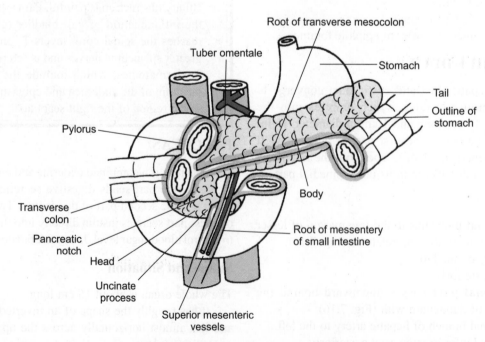

Fig. 7.20: Anterior relations of pancreas

– Gastroduodenal artery (Fig. 6.41b).
– Transverse mesocolon is attached anteriorly towards the lower border of the neck.
– **Tuberomentale,** an elevation at the junction of the head and neck, is related to the lesser omentum. The coeliac artery arises just above it.

• Body:
– The root of the transverse mesocolon is attached to the anterior border.
– The superior surface of the body is covered by the peritoneum of the posterior wall of lesser sac and is related to stomach.
– The inferior surface is covered by peritoneum reflected from the posterior wall of the greater sac and is related to the duodenojejunal flexure and coils of small intestine.

• Tail:
– It along with the splenic vessels runs in the lienorenal ligament and lies on the gastric surface of the spleen between the hilus and the colic flexure. The tip of the tail is the only part of the pancreas which is completely surrounded by peritoneum (Fig. 7.30).

Posteriorly (Fig. 7.21)

Posteriorly from right to left the various parts of pancreas are related as follows:

• Head:
– Inferior vena cava and right crus of diaphragm.
– Terminal part of left renal veins.
– Aorta is posterior to uncinate process.

• Neck:
– Beginning of the portal vein formed by the union of superior mesenteric and splenic veins.

• Body:
– Abdominal aorta.
– Origin of superior mesenteric artery.
– Left crus of diaphragm.
– Left sympathetic trunk.
– Left suprarenal gland.
– Hilum of the left kidney and middle of its anterior surface.
– Left renal vein which runs transversely from left to right side.
  Splenic vein is embedded in the posterior surface and runs transversely above the origin of the superior mesenteric artery. Inferior mesenteric vein crosses the left renal vein to join the splenic vein.

• Tail, together with the splenic vessels, lies between the two layers of lienorenal ligament and is related to:
  A limited area of spleen behind its gastric surface.

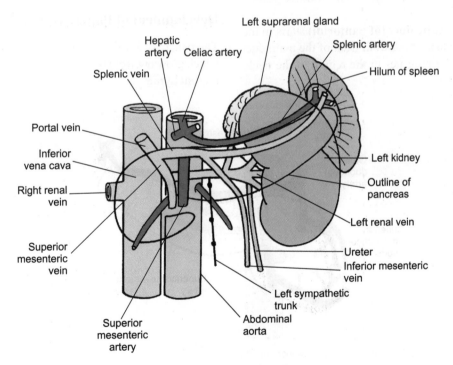

Fig. 7.21: Posterior relations of pancreas

Ducts of Pancreas

There are two ducts which communicate with each other (Fig. 7.22):

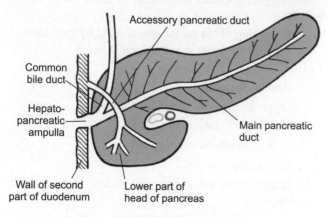

Fig. 7.22: The ducts of pancreas

- **Main pancreatic duct (of Wirsung)** begins in the tail and runs through the body to the neck, receiving tributaries from above and below in a **Herring** bone pattern. It bends down into the head and joins the end of the bile duct to form the **hepatopancreatic ampulla** which opens into the posteromedial aspect of the descending part of duodenum. A sphincter guards the end of the bile duct and another guards the ampulla.
- **Accessory pancreatic duct (of Santorini)** starts in the lower part of the head, crosses in front of the main duct with which it communicates in the region of the neck,

and enters the second part of duodenum 2.5 cm above the main duct.

Arterial Supply (Fig. 7.23)

- Head and neck are supplied by:
  - **Superior pancreaticoduodenal** branch from the gastroduodenal artery.
  - **Inferior pancreaticoduodenal** branch of the superior mesenteric artery.
- Body and tail are supplied by:
  - Branches of **splenic artery** and a large branch from it called the **arteria pancreatica magna**.

Venous Drainage

- **Portal vein** through the tributaries of the splenic and superior mesenteric veins.

Lymphatic Drainage

- **Pancreaticosplenic nodes** on the superior border, which drain into coeliac nodes.
- **Superior mesenteric nodes** in the root of mesentery.

Nerve Supply

The sympathetic nerve supply is from the splanchnic nerves and the parasympathetic supply is from the vagus.

Development of Pancreas (Fig. 7.25)

The pancreas develops from two buds, ventral and dorsal, which grow out from the duodenal wall into the surrounding mesenchyme.

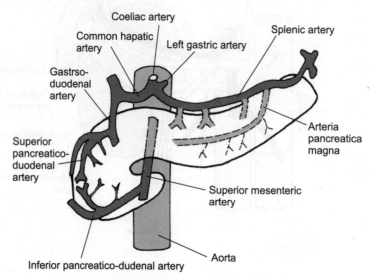

Fig. 7.23: Arterial supply of pancreas

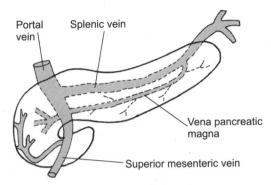

Fig. 7.24: Venous drainage of pancreas

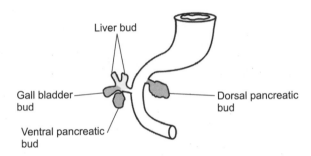

Fig. 7.25 (a): Ventral and dorsal buds of pancreas grow into ventral and dorsal mesogastrium, respectively

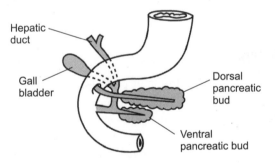

Fig. 7.25 (b): Due to rotation of stomach and duodenum, the ventral bud is brought dorsal and caudal to the dorsal bud

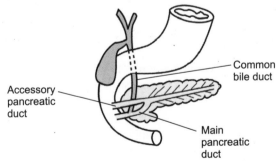

Fig. 7.25 (c): Fusion of dorsal and ventral pancreatic buds with the communication of their duct systems

- **Ventral bud** arises in common with the hepatic diverticulum and so grows into the ventral mesogastrium.
- **Dorsal bud** arises a little cranial to the level of hepatic diverticulum and extends into the dorsal mesogastrium.

As the stomach and duodenum rotate, growth changes in the duodenal wall cause the ventral pancreas and the common hepatopancreatic orifice to migrate around the dorsal (originally right) wall of the duodenum until the concavity of the duodenal loop is reached. The ventral bud is thus brought dorsal and caudal to the dorsal bud. Fusion between the dorsal and ventral pancreas occurs. The ventral bud contributes to the lower part of the head and the uncinate process while the dorsal bud forms the upper part of the head, neck, body and tail of pancreas. Their duct systems communicate. One major anastomosis connects the distal part of the duct of the dorsal bud with that of the ventral bud to form the main pancreatic duct which opens at the duodenal papilla. The proximal part of the duct of the dorsal bud usually disappears but in 10% of cases it persists as the accessory pancreatic duct.

CLINICAL APPLICATION

- Because of its deep position the pancreas is difficult to palpate. Its retroperitoneal position contributes to severe epigastric pain radiating to the back in cases of acute pancreatitis.
- The tail of pancreas contains the majority of the islets of **Langerhans** and this is to be kept in mind in pancreatic resection.
- Because the pancreatic duct and common bile duct join and enter the duodenum via a common opening, spasm of sphincter of Oddi or blockage of the duct and the duodenal papilla results in reflux of bile into the pancreatic duct causing acute pancreatitis.
- 80% of carcinoma of pancreas are located in its head. It may press upon the following structure which lie in close relationship to it and cause following signs and symptoms:
  - Jaundice due to obstruction of common bile duct.
  - Ascites due to portal hypertension caused by pressure on the portal vein.
  - Pyloric obstruction due to pressure on pylorus of stomach.
- Sometimes the two developing buds of the pancreas may completely surround the descending part of

> duodenum giving rise to **"annular pancreas"**. This may produce duodenal obstruction.
> - The lesser sac lies anterior to the pancreas and so it may get distended with fluid in acute pancreatitis causing a **"pseudocyst of the pancreas"**.

SPLEEN

The spleen is the largest lymphoid organ, red brown in colour, soft and pulpy in consistency. It is haemopoietic in the fetus and later functions in blood destruction. It has the capacity for blood and lymphocyte storage and also participates in immunologic activity.

Shape and Size

It is ovoid in shape and is flattened anteroposteriorly. It has two ends, anterior and posterior, two borders superior and inferior and two surfaces, diaphragmatic and visceral.

The size of the normal spleen varies within wide limits but is usually 12 cm × 7 cm × 3 cm and weighs 150 to 200 g.

Situation

It occupies the left hypochondrium anterior to the 9th, 10th and 11th ribs behind the midaxillary line. Its long axis is parallel to the tenth rib. Lower pole generally lies between L_1 and L_2 (Figs. 7.26 and 7.27).

The spleen is an intraperitoneal viscus.

- **Anterior end** lies against the lateral margin of the left kidney, in the transpyloric plane and at the midaxillary line, opposite the eleventh rib.

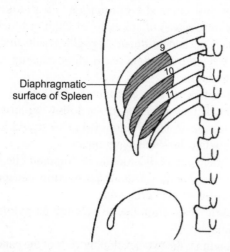

Fig. 7.26: Position of spleen from the posterior aspect under cover of 9th, 10th and 11th ribs

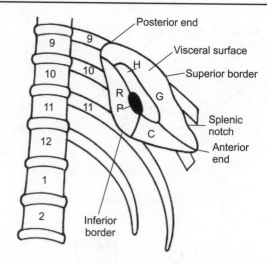

Fig. 7.27: Position of spleen from within showing the various impressions on its visceral surface (C = Colic, G = Gastric, H = Hilum, P = Pancreatic, R = Renal).

- **Posterior** end lies on the upper end of the left kidney, in the scapular line, opposite the ninth rib.
- **Superior border** is convex upward, is sharp and shows one or more notches near the anterior end. There is one prominent and constant notch on the anterior end of the upper border called the **splenic notch** which is helpful in identifying a palpably enlarged spleen.
- **Inferior border** is rounded and blunt.

Relations

- Visceral surface (Fig. 7.27) presents four impressions produced by the related viscera:
  - **Renal impression** for the superolateral part of the anterior surface of the left kidney. It faces medially, backwards and downwards.
  - **Gastric impression** is the uppermost. It faces forward and medially and forms part of the stomach bed. Near its medial edge is the elongated hilum for the splenic vessels.
  - **Colic impression** is a small area below the gastric impression meant for the left colic flexure. It rests on the phrenicocolic ligament.
  - **Pancreatic impression** is in contact with the tail of pancreas and is a narrow strip posterior to the hilum just below its lateral end.
- Diaphragmatic surface (Fig. 7.28) is convex, completely covered by peritoneum and is related to the diaphragm, left costomediastinal recess of the pleura, with its contained thin basal margin of the left lung, which separates it from the 9th, 10th and eleventh ribs.

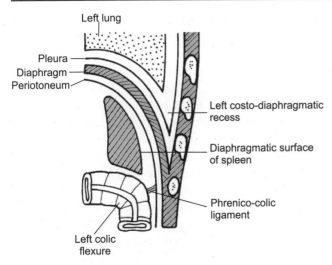

Fig. 7.28: Relations of the diaphragmatic surface of spleen shown in a coronal section

Peritoneal Folds

The spleen is completely surrounded by peritoneum which passes from its hilum as two peritoneal folds which form the lateral limit of the lesser sac (Fig. 7.29).

- **Lienorenal ligament** stretches from the front of the left kidney to the hilum of spleen and carries the splenic vessels and tail of pancreas within it.
- **Gastrosplenic ligament** stretches from the hilum of spleen to the greater curvature of stomach and carries the short gastric arteries (branches of the splenic or the left gastroepiploic artery) which supply the left half of greater curvature and fundic area of stomach.

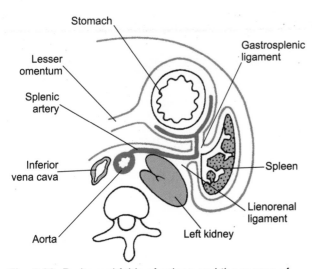

Fig. 7.29: Peritoneal folds of spleen and the course of splenic vessels

Blood Supply (Fig. 7.30)

- **Splenic artery**, a branch of the coeliac axis, supplies spleen. It splits into five or six branches at the hilum to enter it.

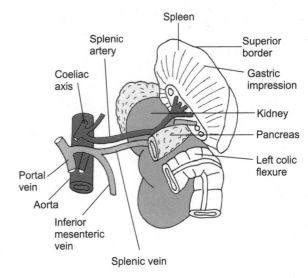

Fig. 7.30: Blood supply of spleen

- **Splenic vein** emerges from the hilum to join the portal vein after being joined by the inferior mesenteric vein behind the neck of pancreas.

Segments of Spleen (Fig. 7.31)

The intrasplenic branches of the superior and inferior terminal branches of splenic artery do not usually anastomose. Each supplies its own segment and so there is a **superior** and **inferior vascular segment** of spleen separated by a relatively avascular plane perpendicular to the long axis of the organ.

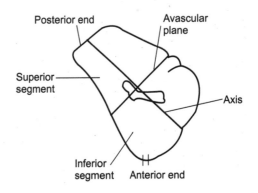

Fig. 7.31: Segments of spleen

Lymphatic Drainage

- **Pancreaticolienal nodes** which drain into the coeliac nodes.

Development (Fig. 4.4)

Spleen develops as lobules of mesenchymal condensation in the dorsal mesogastrium. These lobules soon fuse and project into the left layer of the mesogastrium. When the lesser sac forms and the dorsal mesogastrium shifts to the left, the spleen also shifts to the left (Fig. 4.5 a).

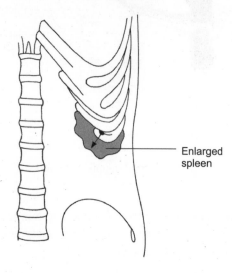

Enlarged spleen

Fig. 7.32: Enlarged spleen is felt below the subcostal margin

CLINICAL APPLICATION

- The spleen is palpable only when splenomegaly occurs. When it enlarges in diseased condition it can be felt below the left subcostal margin (Fig. 7.32). It must be enlarged to twice its normal size before its lower pole can be felt on inspiration.
- Due to its vascularity and its close proximity to the lower ribs, the spleen is the commonest intra-abdominal organ to be ruptured by blunt injury such as by a broken eleventh rib.
- The close relation of the pancreatic tail to the hilum of the spleen and the vessels there has to be kept in mind during splenectomy as the tail of pancreas is easily wounded.
- **Accessory spleens** in the dorsal mesogastrium are common. When splenectomy is done all accessory splenic tissue is located and excised, if left behind, the symptoms of the disease for which the operation was performed will persist. Accessory splenic tissue may lie in the tail of pancreas, the mesentery of spleen, the omentum, mesentery of small intestine, ovary and even testis (since spleen develops in close relationship with the genital ridge).
- Blood from a ruptured spleen irritates the peritoneum under the diaphragm (phrenic nerves C_3 and C_4) causing referred pain in the left shoulder (supraclavicular nerves C_3 and C_4) —Kehr's sign.
- Presence of vascular segments in spleen makes a segmental surgical resection possible which is important where preservation of splenic tissue is necessary.

8

The Pelvis: Walls, Nerves, Vessels and Floor

INTRODUCTION

The **pelvis** is divided in the greater **(false)** pelvis and the lesser **(true)** pelvis by a circular opening known as **inlet**. The **inlet** is formed by the promontory of sacrum, the ala of sacrum, the arcuate line of ilium, the iliopubic eminence, the pectineal line, the pubic crest and the upper border of pubic symphysis. The **greater pelvis,** formed largely of the ala of ilium and the ala of sacrum on each side, actually forms the lower lateral wall of the abdominal cavity. The **lesser pelvis,** therefore, is usually referred to as the pelvis. The plane of the inlet of pelvis lies at an angle of 60° with the horizontal and the pelvic cavity is directed backwards in relationship with the abdominal cavity (Fig. 8.1).

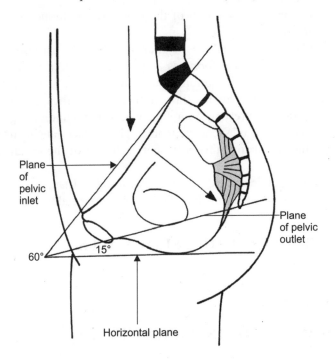

Fig. 8.1: Abdominopelvic cavity: The pelvic cavity is directed backwards

PELVIC WALLS

Arrangement of structures in the pelvic walls

The arrangement from outside to inside is as follows (Fig. 8.2):
- Pelvic bones, joints and ligaments.
- Muscles.
- Nerves.
- Pelvic fascia (parietal).
- Blood vessels.
- Peritoneum.

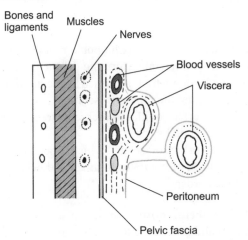

Fig. 8.2: Arrangement of structures in the pelvic walls

The viscera project into the pelvic cavity so that they have a peritoneal covering or lie outside the peritoneum.

BONY PELVIS

Internal aspect of the side wall

The bony side wall of the true pelvis is formed by (Fig. 8.3):

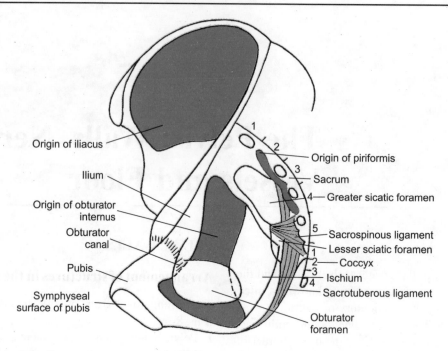

Fig. 8.3: Osteoligamentous pelvis cut in the median plane to show the side wall of the pelvic cavity

- The posterior surface of the body of pubis.
- The pelvic surface of the superior ramus of pubis which is directed backwards and upwards to meet the ilium and ischium.
- The internal surface of ischiopubic ramus which runs backwards and laterally (forming the medial boundary of obturator foramen). It is formed by the inferior ramus of pubis joining the ramus of ischium.
- The pelvic surface of ilium which is lower and posterior part of the medial surface.
- The pelvic surface of ischium which is bounded in front by the margin of obturator foramen and behind by the posterior border.

The posterior border of ilium and ischium go downwards and backwards to form the **greater** and **lesser sciatic notches** separated by the ischial spine.

The **sacrotuberous** and **sacrospinous ligaments** convert these notches into **greater** and **lesser sciatic foramina**.

The **obturator foramen,** a gap in the hip bone, is bounded above and in front by the superior ramus and body of pubis, medially and below by the ischiopubic ramus, behind by the body of ischium and above by the inferior margin of acetabulum. It is occupied by the **obturator membrane** which is attached to the margins of the foramen except superiorly where there is a gap which is known as the **obturator canal**.

Internal aspect of the posterior wall

The bony posterior wall of the true pelvis is formed by (Fig. 8.4):
- The pelvic surface of sacrum which is directed downwards and forwards and is concave from above downwards. It exhibits four pairs of anterior sacral foramina. The median area between the sacral foramina presents four transverse ridges indicating the fusion of sacral vertebrae. The surface lateral to the sacral foramina represents a fusion of the costal elements.
- The pelvic surface of the coccyx which is triangular in shape and is formed by the fusion of four rudimentary vertebrae.

MUSCLES OF THE PELVIC WALLS

These comprise:
- Obturator internus.
- Piriformis.

OBTURATOR INTERNUS (FIG. 8.5)

Clothes most of the side wall of pelvis.

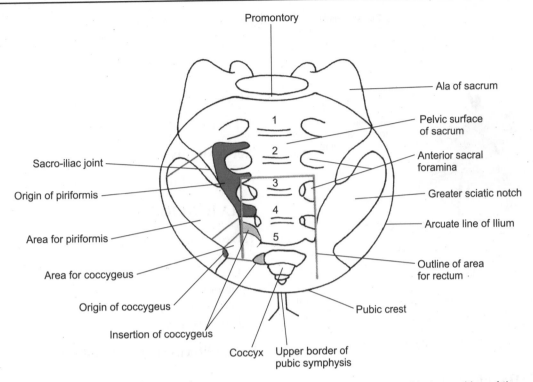

Fig. 8.4: The bony posterior wall of pelvis as seen through the pelvic inlet with the position of the piriformis, coccygeus and the rectum

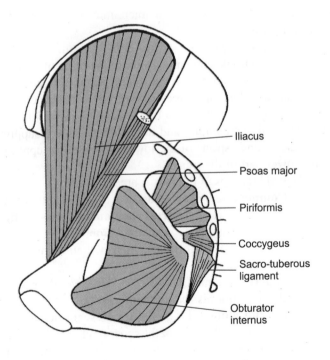

Fig. 8.5: Obturator internus muscle

Origin (Fig. 8.3)

- Inner surface of the margins of the obturator foramen except near the obturator canal.
- Inner aspect of the obturator membrane.
- Pelvic surface of the hip bone above and behind the obturator foramen.

Insertion (Fig. 8.6)

- The fibres converge and form a strong tendon which almost fills the lesser sciatic foramen as it turns at about a right angle to leave the pelvis to get inserted into the medial surface of greater trochanter of femur in front of the trochanteric fossa.

Nerve supply

- Nerve to obturator internus (L_5, S_1 and S_2) which enters the perineal surface of the muscle.

Action

- Lateral rotator of the thigh.

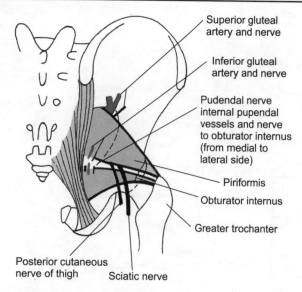

Fig. 8.6: The osseoligamentous foramina in the lateral pelvic wall seen from behind and the site of exit of some structures of the lateral pelvic wall and the insertions of obturator internus and piriformis

PIRIFORMIS (Fig. 8.7)

It is a muscle of the posterior wall of pelvis.

Origin (Fig. 8.4)

- Pelvic surface of the middle three pieces of sacrum.
- Upper margin of greater sciatic notch.
- Pelvic surface of the sacrotuberous ligament.

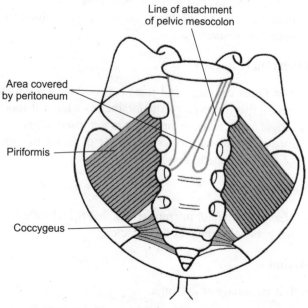

Fig. 8.7: Muscle of posterior pelvic wall: Piriformis

Insertion (Fig. 8.6)

- Top of the greater trochanter of femur after passing out of the greater sciatic foramen into the gluteal region.

Action

- Lateral rotator of the thigh.

Nerve supply

- Branches from S_1 and S_2 enter its pelvic surface.

PELVIC NERVES

These comprise the following:
- Sacral plexus.
- Coccygeal plexus.
- Obturator nerve.
- Pelvic part of sympathetic trunk.
- Hypogastric plexuses.

Sacral Plexus (Figs. 8.8 and 8.9)

The sacral plexus lies on the posterior wall of the pelvis, just lateral to the sacral foramina and most of it disappears into the buttocks as soon as it gives rise to its branches. The major part of the plexus lies on the anterior surface of the piriformis muscle and all the larger branches pass through the greater sciatic foramen, most of them below the piriformis.

    The sacral plexus is formed by the union of the lumbosacral trunk, containing some of the fibres of ventral ramus of L_4, all those from the ventral ramus of L_5 and the ventral rami of the first three sacral nerves. Like the general plan of other limb plexuses (branchial and lumbar) these roots divide into ventral and dorsal divisions and supply corresponding aspects of the lower limb. It also supplies the lower part of the trunk.
- Dorsal branches of the plexus are six in all:
  - **Common peroneal** (L_4 and L_5, S_1 and S_2): It is the smaller, lateral and **dorsal component of the sciatic nerve**. It may arise separately from the plexus, in front of the piriformis, which it then commonly pierces.
  - **Superior gluteal** (L_4 and L_5, S_1): It leaves the pelvis above piriformis (hence **"superior"**).
  - **Inferior gluteal** (L_5, S_1 and S_2): Its segmental origin is one lower than that of the superior gluteal. It leaves the pelvis below the piriformis, behind (superficial to) the sciatic nerve.
  - **Perforating cutaneous nerve** (S_2 and S_3): It is so

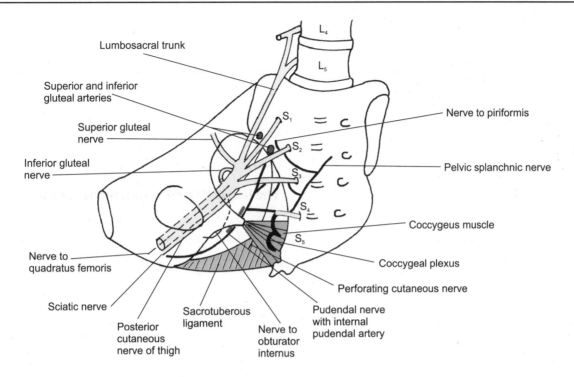

Fig. 8.8: The sacral plexus and its branches

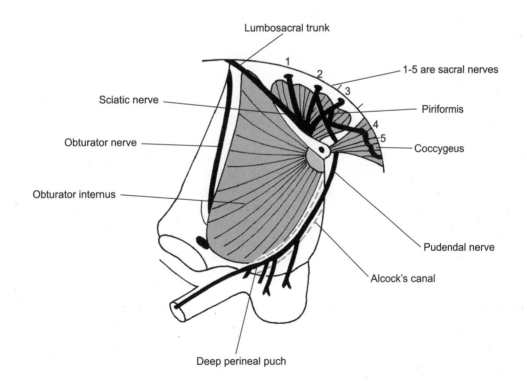

Fig. 8.9: Nerves of the lateral pelvic wall: The sciatic and pudendal nerves are the two main branches of sacral plexus. The obturator nerve comes from the lumbar plexus. The nerves lie on the muscles and are external to pelvic fascia

called as it perforates the sacrotuberous ligament and then winds around the lower border of gluteus maximus.

- **Posterior cutaneous nerve of thigh:** It has both dorsal (S_1 and S_2) and ventral (S_2 and S_3) components and its root value is (S_1 to S_3). It leaves the pelvis behind (superficial to) the sciatic nerve close to the inferior gluteal nerve.
- **Branches to piriformis** (S_1 and S_2): These sink into the pelvic surface of the muscle, on which the plexus lies.
- Ventral branches of the plexus are seven in all:
  - **Tibial nerve** (L_4 and L_5, S_1 to S_3): It is the larger, medial and **ventral component of the sciatic nerve**.
  - **Pudendal nerve** (S_2 to S_4): It leaves the pelvic cavity medial to all the other structures emerging below piriformis, including the accompanying internal pudendal vessels.
  - **Pelvic splanchnic nerves or nervi erigentes** (S_2 to S_4): These are parasympathetic nerves. They pierce the parietal pelvic fascia to reach the pelvic viscera, in the extraperitoneal plane, after joining the inferior hypogastric plexus.
  - **Nerve to quadratus femoris** (L_4 and L_5, S_1): It leaves the pelvic as an anterior (deep) relation of the sciatic nerve.
  - **Nerve to obturator internus** (L_5, S_1 and S_2): It leaves the pelvic cavity medial to the sciatic nerve but lateral to the internal pudendal vessels and pudendal nerve. It turns dorsally around the ischial spine and then lies on the side wall of the pelvis.
  - **Posterior cutaneous nerve of thigh**, already described as it has both dorsal (S_1 and S_2) and ventral (S_2 and S_3) components.
  - **Muscular branches** to the pelvic diaphragm and external anal sphincter. Fibres from S_3 and S_4 supply the pelvic diaphragm on its pelvic aspect. The perineal branch of S_4 pierces coccygeus and enters the ischiorectal fossa from under cover of the edge of coccyx. It supplies the superficial part of the sphincter which arises from the coccyx.

Coccygeal Plexus

The ventral rami of S_5 and Co 1 turn forward, between the sacrum and coccyx and below the transverse process of Co 1 respectively, pierce coccygeus to enter the pelvic cavity. They join to form a trunk which is joined by a twig from the ventral ramus of S_4 to form the coccygeal plexus, actually a nerve. This gives off the **anococcygeal nerves**

which pierce the sacrotuberous ligament below coccygeus and supply the skin over the coccyx.

The Obturator Nerve (Fig. 8.9)

The obturator nerve is a branch of the lumbar part of lumbosacral plexus. It crosses the ala of the sacrum near the sacroiliac joint, enters the pelvis by crossing the pelvic brim and leaves the pelvic cavity by passing through the obturator canal. It supplies the medial side of the thigh.

The Pelvic Part of Sympathetic Trunk

This part of the sympathetic trunk crosses the ala of sacrum close to the promontory and descends just medial to the sacral foramina to lie in the extraperitoneal tissue. It ends on the coccyx by joining its fellow of the opposite side in **ganglion impar**. There is a ganglion at each sacral foramen which communicates with each sacral ventral ramus and coccygeal nerve by a gray ramus communicans. There are normally 4 to 5 sacral ganglia. Medial branches join the inferior hypogastric plexus (Fig. 3.15).

The Hypogastric Plexuses

The **superior hypogastric plexus** or presacral plexus lies in front of the promontory. It is formed by strands from the aortic plexus, receiving branches from the sympathetic trunk on each side. The plexus divides into two nerves which run down on each side of the rectum to form the inferior hypogastric plexus.

The **inferior hypogastric plexus** lies on the side of the lower third of the rectum, below the peritoneal reflection. It receives numerous branches from the sacral sympathetic trunk, from the corresponding hypogastric nerves descending from the superior hypogastric plexus, and from the pelvic splanchnic nerves. Branches from the plexus accompany the visceral branches of the internal iliac artery and some parasympathetic fibres derived from the pelvic splanchnic nerves ascend either with the hypogastric nerve to join the inferior mesenteric plexus or independently in the extraperitoneal tissue, to supply the colon distal to the left colic flexure.

The sympathetic trunks and the hypogastric nerves lie in the extraperitoneal tissue internal to the fascia.

PELVIC FASCIA (FIG. 8.10)

The connective tissue within the pelvis is divided into parietal and visceral pelvic fascia.

Parietal pelvic fascia forms more or less dense membranes on the pelvic surface of the muscles (obturator

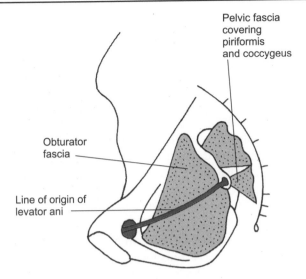

Fig. 8.10: Parietal layer of pelvic fascia

internus and piriformis) and blends with the periosteum at their margins. Particularly well defined is the **obturator fascia** over the obturator internus muscle. The anterior limit of this fascia is along a line extending from the pelvic brim to the back of the pubis. This line is not straight as it hooks downwards to allow the obturator nerve and vessels to get to the obturator foramen without having to pierce it.

Superiorly it blends with the psoas sheath at the pelvic brim. Posteriorly it extends back in front of the piriformis and sacral plexus and is bound down to the margins of sciatic foramina. Inferiorly it covers the obturator internus and is attached to the bony rim of the pelvic outlet. Much thinner layers cover the piriformis. Elsewhere the bone of the pelvis is devoid of fascia.

The sacral plexus lies external to the fascia and internal to the piriformis muscle and its branches to the lower limb do not pierce the fascia. The vessels, the sympathetic trunks and the hypogastric nerves lie internal to it. The blood vessels of the gluteal region have to pierce the fascia to reach the buttock.

Visceral pelvic fascia invests the pelvic viscera and is loose or dense depending upon the distensibility of the organ. It forms the vesical, genital and rectal parts of the visceral layer of endopelvic fascia.

PELVIC VESSELS (FIG. 8.11)

ARTERIES

These are:
- Internal iliac
- Median sacral
- Superior rectal

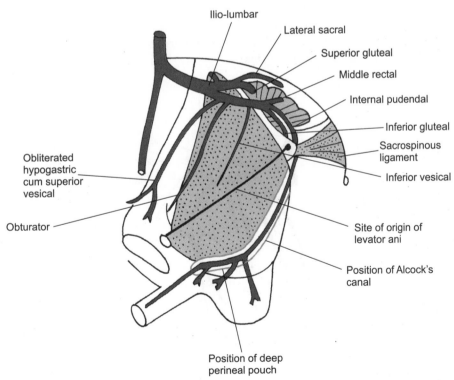

Fig. 8.11: The internal iliac artery and its branches are internal to pelvic fascia

The **INTERNAL ILIAC ARTERY,** the arterial stem of the pelvis, begins as one of the two terminal branches of the common iliac artery at the level of the lumbosacral disc. It crosses the brim with its vein immediately behind it and the ureter immediately in front. It ends near the greater sciatic notch into a larger anterior and a smaller posterior division.

The **ANTERIOR DIVISION** gives parietal and visceral branches.

The parietal branches are:
- **Obturator artery** runs forward along the side wall of the pelvis below the obturator nerve. It leaves the pelvis through the **obturator canal** to reach the thigh.
- **Inferior gluteal artery** is a terminal branch of the anterior division. It leaves the pelvis through the greater sciatic foramen below the piriformis between S_1 and S_2 roots (Figs. 8.8 and 8.12).
- **Internal pudendal artery** is one of the two terminal branches of the anterior division. It is the main artery of the perineum and accompanies the pudendal nerve after piercing the parietal pelvic fascia. It passes out of the pelvis through the greater sciatic foramen.

The visceral branches are:
- **Umbilical artery** is the first branch of the internal iliac artery. It runs forward crossing the medial aspect of the obturator nerve, it passes into the anterior abdominal wall where it continues as a fibrous cord known as the **medial umbilical ligament**. The **superior vesical** artery arises from the patent portion of the umbilical artery. It supplies the upper part of bladder, the lower part of ureter and ductus deferens.
- **Inferior vesical artery** runs anteriorly below the obturator artery to supply the base of the bladder, and in male the prostate and seminal vesicle and gives branches to the ureter and ductus deferens. It is represented in the female by the **vaginal artery**.
- **Uterine artery** descends on the pelvic wall in the female and turns medially along lateral cervical ligament. It passes above and in front of the ureter, just lateral to the cervix. The vaginal artery may arise from the uterine artery.
- **Middle rectal artery** arises from the lower end of the anterior division. It runs towards the lower rectal wall to supply its musculature, in male also the prostate and seminal vesicle. It is usually small.

The **POSTERIOR DIVISION** breaks up into three branches, all of which are parietal:
- **Iliolumbar artery** arises near the pelvic brim and passes upward between the obturator nerve and the lumbosacral trunk to run deep to the medial edge of psoas major. It divides into an iliac and a lumbar branch. The **lumbar branch** may replace the dorsal branch of the fifth lumbar artery and supply the psoas major and quadratus lumborum. The **iliac branch** supplies psoas and iliacus.
- **Lateral sacral arteries** are two viz., upper and lower. They run medially across the sacral ventral rami and

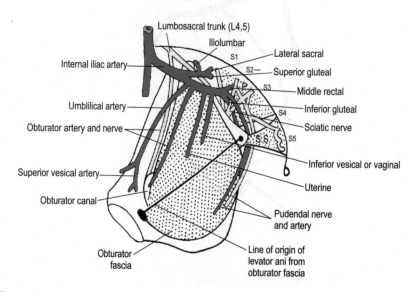

Fig. 8.12: The nerves and arteries of the lateral pelvic wall as related to each other

send branches into the sacral foramina to supply the contents of sacral canal and the muscles and skin behind the sacrum.

- **Superior gluteal artery** is the largest branch of the internal iliac. It leaves the pelvis above the piriformis, passing between the lumbosacral trunk and the ventral ramus of S_1, accompanied by the superior gluteal nerve (Figs. 8.8 and 8.12).
- The **Median sacral artery,** a branch of the aorta, descends in the midline, on the posterior wall formed by the sacrum, to end in the coccygeal body.

The Superior Rectal Artery is the terminal branch of inferior mesenteric. It crosses the common iliac artery and descends into the pelvis in the sigmoid mesocolon to supply the rectum.

VEINS – These are:
- Superior rectal.
- Internal iliac.
- Median sacral.
- **Superior rectal:** Upper part of rectum drains into the superior rectal vein and so by the inferior mesenteric vein into the portal system.
- **Internal iliac:** Internal iliac vein drains the rest of the pelvic viscera.
- **Median sacral:** Median sacral vein accompanies the median sacral artery on its right side. It ends in the left common iliac vein.

PELVIC FLOOR

The pelvic floor consists of the **pelvic diaphragm** formed by two muscles viz., the coccygeus and levator ani and the pelvic fascia covering it. It encloses the urethra and anal canal and in the female the vagina which lie in the midline.

Levator Ani (Figs. 8.13 and 8.14)

It is a wide flat muscle which slopes from the side wall of the pelvis towards the median plane in a downward and backward direction. It consists of two parts, pubococcygeus and iliococcygeus.

- *Pubococcygeus*
  It consists of three group of fibres:
- **Levator prostate (in males)** or **pubovaginalis (in females):** They are the most medial fibres which arise from the back of the body of pubis and form a U-shaped sling around the prostate gland in the male or vagina in the female. Fibres of the two sides are inserted into the perineal body.
- **Puborectalis:** It is formed by the fibre arising more laterally from the body of the pubis. It swings more medially and inferiorly to loop around the anorectal junction to join with the fibres of the opposite side and blend with the posterior fibres of the deep part of the external anal sphincter.
  The muscles of the two sides form a U-shaped sling which maintains the anorectal junction angled forwards.
- **Pubococcygeus proper:** It arises from the posterior surface of the body of pubis and from the anterior half of the white line (arcus tendineus). It is inserted into the anococcygeal body and coccyx. It is a flat muscle and its fibres are in different functional sets.
- *Iliococcygeus*
  It arises from the posterior half of the arcus tendineus

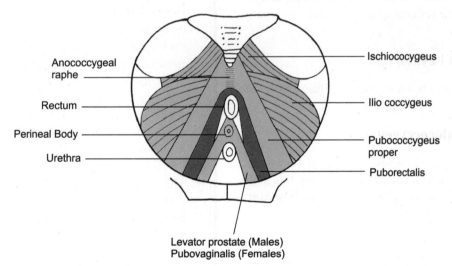

Fig. 8.13: The pelvic diaphragm seen through the pelvic inlet showing the three parts of pubococcygeus

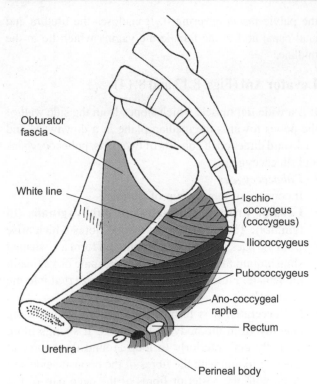

Fig. 8.14: The pelvic diaphragm : Side view.

and the pelvic surface of the ischial spine. It is inserted into the side of coccyx and the anococcygeal raphe, which extends from the tip of coccyx to the anorectal junction. The fibres of iliococcygeus are covered on their pelvic aspect by the backward running fibres of pubococcygeus. At the arcus tendineus, a diaphragmatic fascial layer splits to cover both superior and inferior surfaces of lavator ani as the **superior** and **inferior fascia of pelvic diaphragm**. The superior fascia reflects onto the pelvic viscera as visceral fascia.

Nerve Supply of Levator Ani

Ventral rami of S_3 and S_4 on its pelvic surface and by the pudendal nerve on its perineal surface.

Coccygeus (Ischiococcygeus)

It is a fan-shaped muscle whose superficial fibres have atrophied and remain as sacrospinous ligament. It is in the same plane as iliococcygeus. It is a rudimentary **"tailwagger"**.

Origin

• Pelvic surface of ischial spine.

Insertion

• Side of coccyx and last piece of sacrum.

Nerve supply

• Perineal branch of S_4.

Functions of the Pelvic Diaphragm

• It supports the pelvic viscera.
• It helps in maintaining increased intra-abdominal pressure by counteracting the actions of the diaphragm and anterior abdominal wall.
• The puboprostatic and pubovaginalis may help in expelling the urine during micturition.
• The puborectalis sling is drawn forwards so that the anorectal junction can maintain the continence of faeces. The sling relaxes during defaecation.

The puborectalis sling also directs the head of the foetus during the second stage of labour.

CLINICAL APPLICATION

• A process of peritoneum is rarely pushed out of the pelvis through the obturator foramen alongside the obturator vessels and nerve. It is known as **obturator hernia** and occurs only in elderly females.
• Rarely the gut and peritoneal sac escape from the pelvis at either the upper or lower border of piriformis. It is present in the buttock under cover of the gluteus maximus muscle and is known as **sciatic hernia**.
• At times the arcus tendineus which gives origin to the levator ani is attached only to the pubic bone in front and the ischial spine behind and not to the obturator fascia at all. Then there is a potential gap between the arcus tendineus sling and the obturator fascia, known as **hiatus of Schwalbe**. It is important as a process of pelvic peritoneum may be pushed through the hiatus causing a hernia into the ischiorectal fossa.
• The pubococcygeus part, although capable of considerable relaxation is often torn during childbirth. This causes defective support of the viscera, leading sometimes to prolapse of the uterus.

9

Pelvic Peritoneum and Pelvic Viscera

ARRANGEMENT OF PELVIC VISCERA

The pelvic viscera have the following arrangement (Figs. 9.1 and 9.2).
- Posteriorly is the termination of the gastrointestinal tract.
- Anteriorly is the urinary bladder and the termination of the urinary tract.
- Between the upper two are the internal female genitalia or parts of the male genitalia.

Pelvic Peritoneum

The pelvic peritoneum does not reach the bottom of the pelvic cavity, but is reflected over the pelvic viscera. The posterosuperior surface of the pelvis is covered with peritoneum down to the second piece of sacrum, except where the medial limb of the sigmoid mesocolon is attached.

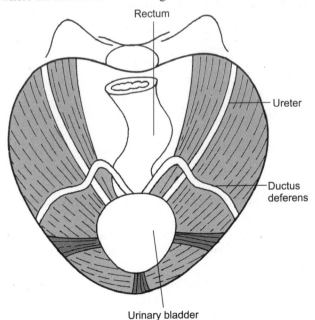

Fig. 9.1: Arrangement of pelvic viscera in the male

Inferior to this the rectum intervenes between the sacrum and peritoneum. Anteriorly and posteriorly the arrangement of peritoneum is identical in the male and female, but differs in the intermediate region.

In the male (Fig. 9.3): The peritoneum posteriorly covers the front and sides of the upper third of rectum and only the front of its middle third. The lowest third is below the level of the peritoneum. From below the middle third it passes forward on the upper edge of the back of the bladder. From there it covers the upper surface of the bladder and then runs upwards the anterior abdominal wall. The space between the rectum and the bladder is called the **rectovesical pouch** and usually contains loops of small intestine.

In the female (Fig. 9.4): The peritoneum has the same relationship with the rectum as in the male. It leaves the rectum and passes forward onto the posterior aspect of the upper third of vagina. From there it runs upwards over the entire posterior surface and fundus of the uterus. It passes downwards on the front of the upper two-thirds of the uterus and then bends forward over the superior surface of the bladder and then passes directly onto the posterior surface of the anterior abdominal wall. There is a deep **recto-uterine pouch (of Douglas)** between the rectum and the uterus, but the pouch is actually rectovaginal. A shallow **uterovesical pouch** is formed between the uterus and the bladder.

THE PELVIC VISCERA

THE RECTUM

The rectum is the part of the large intestine, about 13 cm long, between the sigmoid colon and the anal canal. It is a retroperitoneal structure located from the middle piece of sacrum to about 2.5 cm beyond the coccyx where it is continuous with the anal canal.

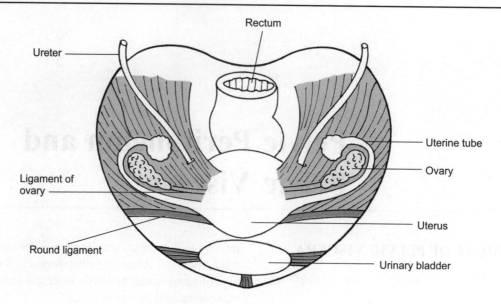

Fig. 9.2: Arrangement of pelvic viscera in the female

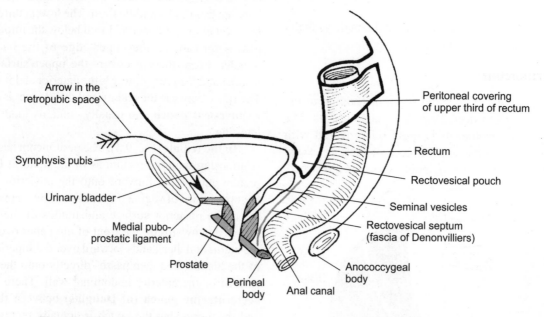

Fig. 9.3: Reflection of pelvic peritoneum in the male as seen in a sagittal section of pelvis

Shape (Fig. 9.5)

It is tubular organ not of uniform calibre. The ampulla which lies just above the pelvic floor, is the widest part of the rectum and is capable of considerable distension and is usually empty since the faeces are stored in the sigmoid colon. It presents curvature in both anteroposterior and lateral directions.

• There are two anteroposterior curvatures:

– An upper sacral curvature with concavity facing forward.
– A lower perineal curvature with the concavity facing backward and continuous with the anal canal.

• There are three lateral curvatures:
– Upper convex to the right.
– Middle convex to the left.
– Lower convex to the right.

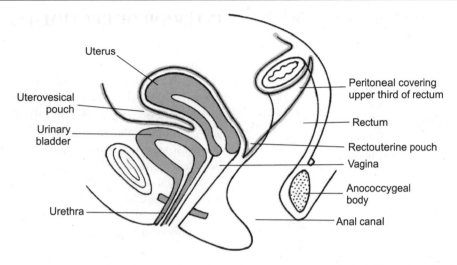

Fig. 9.4: Reflection of pelvic peritoneum in the female as seen in a sagittal section of pelvis

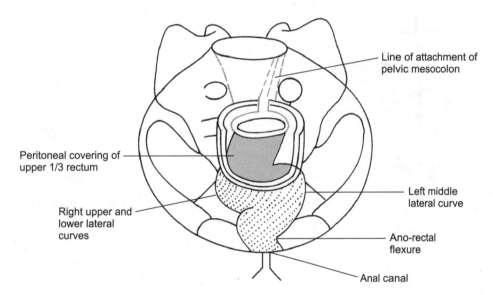

Fig. 9.5: Schematic rectum *in situ* : The peritoneal reflection and the lateral flexures, two on the left and one on the right

Peritoneal Reflection

The rectum has no mesentery (Figs. 9.3 and 9.4).

- Upper one-third is covered by the peritoneum on its anterior surface and sides (Fig. 9.5).
- Middle one-third is covered by the peritoneum only on the anterior surface.
- Lower one-third has no peritoneal covering as it is below the level of peritoneum which is reflected forward onto the superior surface of the urinary bladder in the male or the upper part of vagina in the female to form the **rectovesical pouch** or **rectouterine pouch** respectively.

Relations

Anteriorly

In Males (Fig. 9.3)
- Peritoneum and pelvic colon to the upper two-thirds.
- Urinary bladder, vas deferens, seminal vesicles and prostate to the lower third.
- Rectovesical fascia **(of Denonvilliers)** between the rectum behind and the urinary bladder and prostate in front.

In Females (Fig. 9.4)
- Pelvic colon and rectouterine pouch to the upper two-thirds. The pouch separates it from the uterus and vagina.

- Posterior fornix and middle part of posterior wall of vagina are related to the lower third.

Posteriorly (Figs. 9.6 and 9.7)

- Sacrum coccyx and anococcygeal rape.
- Coccygeus piriformis and levator ani.
- Median sacral and lateral sacral vessels.
- Sympathetic nerves and ganglion impar.
- S_3 to S_5 nerves and coccygeal nerves.

Lateral

- Lateral ligaments of rectum in both sexes.
- Uterosacral folds and ligaments in the female.

INTERIOR OF RECTUM (FIG. 9.8)

The interior of rectum usually presents three sickle-shaped transverse folds corresponding to the three curves seen externally, with the exception of the outer longitudinal muscular coat. All the coats of the rectum take part in their formation. Formerly they were called **valves of Houston**. They get obliterated during the distention of rectum. The middle fold, which is on the anterior and right walls is the best development and constant.

It is immediately above the ampulla. The upper and lower folds are less definite and are present 2.5 cm above and below the middle fold. They are supposed to give shelf-like support to faecal masses.

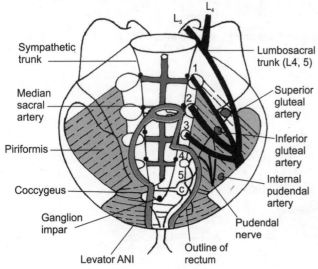

Fig. 9.6: Posterior relations of rectum (1-5 are sacral nerves C is coccygeal nerve)

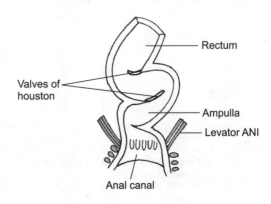

Fig. 9.8: Interior of rectum

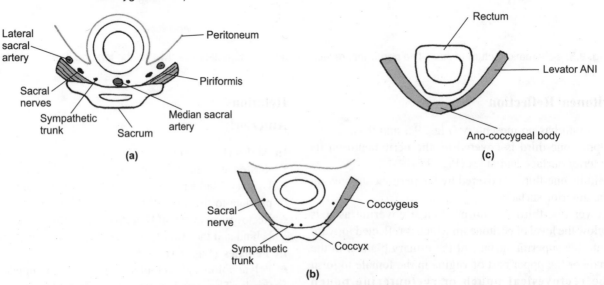

Fig. 9.7: Posterior relations of rectum: (a) Posterior relations of upper one-third. (b) Posterior relations of middle one-third. (c) Posterior relations of lower one-third

Arterial Supply (Fig. 9.9)

The rectum is supplied by the following arteries:
- **Superior rectal:** It is the continuation of inferior mesenteric artery and divides into a right and a left branches which descend on the sides of the rectum.
- **Middle rectal:** It is a branch of the anterior division of internal iliac.
- **Inferior rectal:** It is a branch from the internal pudendal.

Venous Drainage (Fig. 9.9)

The rectum is drained by the following veins:
- **Superior rectal** which continues up as inferior mesenteric vein and ends in the splenic vein. This drainage is into the portal system.
- **Middle rectal**.
- **Inferior rectal** end in the internal iliac vein. These two drain into the systemic system.

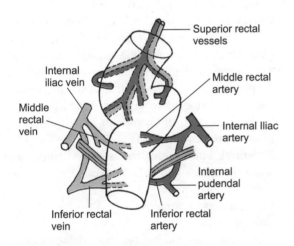

Fig. 9.9: Blood supply of rectum

Lymphatic Drainage (Fig. 9.10)

The rectum is divided into upper half and lower half for study of its lymphatic drainage.
- **Upper half:** The lymphatics of the upper half of rectum drains upward along the superior rectal vessels to finally reach the nodes at the origin of inferior mesenteric artery.
- **Lower half:** The lymphatics of the lower half of rectum and upper part of anal canal down to the mucocutaneous junction pass with the middle rectal vessels to the nodes along the internal iliac vessels. Some of the lymphatics reach the ischiorectal fossa and then accompany the internal pudendal vessels.

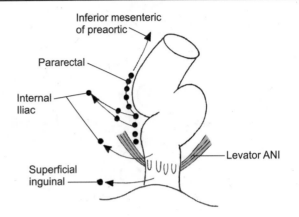

Fig. 9.10: Lymph nodes draining rectum and anal canal

Nerve Supply

Sympathetic Innervation

- The pelvic plexuses.
- The aortic plexus via inferior mesenteric and superior rectal arteries.

Parasympathetic Innervation

- The pelvic splanchnic nerves (S_2 to S_4) which stimulate contraction of the smooth muscle together with relaxation of the internal sphincter as in defaecation.
- Both sympathetic and parasympathetic fibres are associated with pain arising from the rectum and upper part of anal canal.

Fascia of the Rectum

It consists of loose areolar tissue surrounding the rectal venous plexus. The following condensations are noteworthy (Fig. 9.11):
- **Rectal stalks or lateral ligaments:** These are condensations of areolar tissue around the middle rectal vessels and are situated on each side of the back of rectum, 2 to 5 cm above the levator ani running from the third piece of sacrum to the rectal wall. It contains the pelvic splanchnic nerves also.
- **Fascia of Waldeyer** is a strong thick layer of parietal fascia which suspends the lower part of the ampulla to the hollow of the sacrum. It encloses the superior rectal vessels.
- **Fascia of Denonvilliers** is a layer of visceral pelvic fascia. It lies anterior to the lower extraperitoneal part of the rectum and is closely adherent to it. It extends from the anterior peritoneal reflection above to the

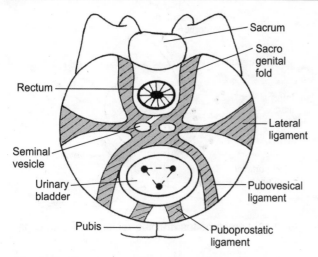

Fig. 9.11: The rectal stalks or lateral ligaments of rectum

superior layer of the urogenital diaphragm below. Laterally it becomes continuous with the lateral ligaments of rectum.

Supports of Rectum

The rectum is held in position by:
- The attachments of the levators ani between the internal and external sphincters (Fig. 10.5).
- The visceral layer of pelvic fascia.
- The **recto-urethralis muscle (of Roux)** which extends from the anterior surface of the lower end of rectum to apex of prostate and urethra in male and to the back of vagina in female (Fig. 9.16).
- The rectal stalk or lateral ligament (Fig. 9.11).
- The fatty tissue of the pelvis and ischiorectal fossae.
- The sacral curve.

Development (Fig. 9.20)

A coronal mesodermal septum, the wedge of tissue between the allantois and hindgut, called the **urorectal septum** extends caudally and divides the cloaca into a dorsal rectum and a ventral primitive urogenital sinus. It also divides the cloacal membrane into a ventral part, the urogenital membrane and a dorsal part, the anal membrane.

CLINICAL APPLICATION

- The close relation of the rectum to the lumbosacral plexus explains the sciatic and perineal distribution of pain noted at times as an early symptom of carcinoma of rectum.

- Pelvic abscesses form in the rectovesical or recto-uterine pouches because these are the most dependent portions of the peritoneal cavity, into which infected fluid or blood can drain by gravity.
- Lymphatics of the lower third of rectum course upwards, laterally as well as downwards so the resection for the cancer of this part is extensive.
- The veins draining the rectum constitute an important communication between the systemic and hepatic portal veins. Internal haemorrhoids (piles) are the enlarged, distended (varicose), submucosal veins in the anal columns and especially affect the left lateral and right anterior and posterior veins. They occur due to conditions associated with increased portal venous pressure or in pregnancy, in which there is increased pressure on the pelvic veins due to the fetal head. The lack of submucosal connective support may be an important factor in causing varicosity of veins.
- **Rectal examination:** The anal canal and lower part of the rectum are examined by means of a gloved finger. The tone of the sphincters is assessed. The sacrum and coccyx can be palpated through the posterior wall. Many structures situated outside but related to the anorectal canal can be identified. In the male, the following can be felt anteriorly from above downwards (Fig. 9.12):
- **Prostate:** The base of the urinary bladder and seminal vesicles which lie above the prostate are normally not palpable.
- Membranous urethra.
- Bulb of penis.
  In the female, anteriorly from above downwards are:
- The cervix of the uterus.
- The upper part of vagina.
- Fascia of Denonvilliers which separates the rectum from the anterior structures forms the plane of dissection in excision of the rectum.
- Prolapse of the rectum through the anus is often related to damage of the levator ani muscle usually the result of injury during childbirth.
- If the nervous pathways are intact, faecal continence depends on the integrity of the levator ani.

THE URINARY BLADDER

Situation

It is the most anterior organ in the pelvic cavity lying behind

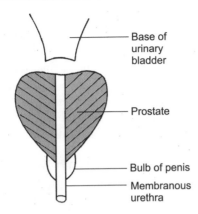

Fig. 9.12: Structures felt per rectum in the male

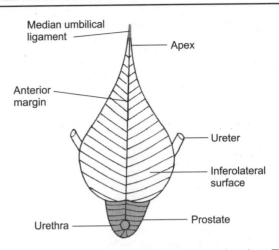

Fig. 9.14: Urinary bladder and prostate: anterior view. The rounded anterior border and the inferolateral surfaces of the bladder continue into those of prostate

the pubic symphysis and the superior pubic rami. Behind it is the rectum in the male and the uterus in the female. When it distends it rises above the symphysis pubis.

Form and Size (Figs. 9.13 and 9.14)

The distended bladder is globular in both sexes. In the empty state it is a three-sided pyramid with following features:

- Apex
- Base or posterior surface.
- Superior surface.
- Inferolateral surfaces.
- Neck.

The **apex** is directed anteriorly and is situated where the superior and inferolateral surfaces meet. It is continuous with the median umbilical ligament which is a remnant of the urachus and extends in the midline on the back of the anterior abdominal wall from the apex to the umbilicus.

The **base** or **posterior surface** is directed backwards and slightly downwards. It is somewhat triangular in shape. The ureters open into its superolateral angles.

The **superior surface** is also triangular in shape and bounded on each side by the lateral borders which extend from the ureteric orifices posterolaterally to the apex anteriorly. Its posterior border joins the ureteric orifices.

The **inferolateral surfaces** on either side are directed downwards and laterally. They along with the base slope inferiorly to meet at the neck of the bladder.

Relations

- **Posterior surface or base**

In the male its relations are:
- Peritoneum covering a small triangular area, in the uppermost part, related to rectum.

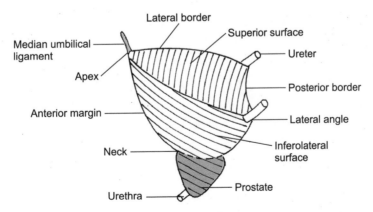

Fig. 9.13: Side view of urinary bladder and prostate. Both have identical surfaces and borders

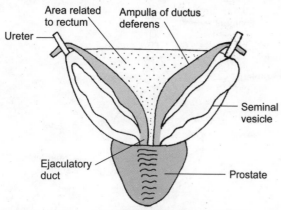

Fig. 9.15: Relations of the posterior surface of the urinary bladder in the male

- Ductus deferens and seminal vesicle on either side of midline diverge to leave the triangular area in direct relation to rectum.
- Rectovesical fascia, **(of Denonvilliers)** intervening between the above structures and the rectum (Fig. 9.16).

In the female it is related to (Fig. 9.17):
- Anterior wall of vagina and its anterior fornix.
- **Superior surface**

In the male is completely covered by peritoneum and is related to (Fig. 9.16):
- Pelvic colon.
- Coils of ileum.

In the female the peritoneum is reflected onto the under surface of the uterus to form the uterovesical pouch and does not reach as far back as the vaginal fornix. It is thus related to (Fig. 9.17):
- Supravaginal cervix.
- Body of the uterus.
- **Inferolateral surfaces** in both sexes are related anteriorly to:
- **Retropubic space (of Retzius)** (Fig. 9.18), containing loose fatty tissue and pubovesical and puboprostatic ligaments in the male and the pubovesical ligaments in the female.

The **boundaries of the cave of Retzius,** which is a prevesical space, are (Figs. 9.3 and 9.18):
- **Anteriorly:** Posterior surface of pubis and posterior sheath of rectus abdominis.
- **Posteriorly:** Inferolateral surfaces of the urinary bladder.
- **Superiorly:** Reflection of peritoneum from the superior surface to the back of anterior abdominal wall upto the umbilicus, here limited on each side by lateral umbilical ligament with the median umbilical ligament bisecting the space.
- **Inferiorly:** Puboprostatic or pubovesical ligaments.
- **Neck of the bladder**

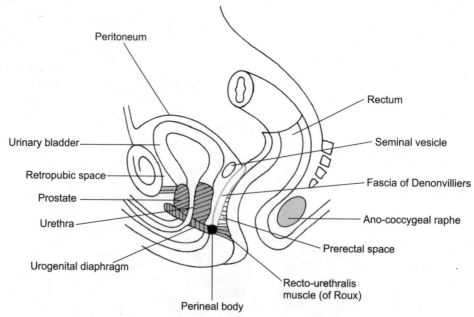

Fig. 9.16: Posterior relations of the urinary bladder in the male

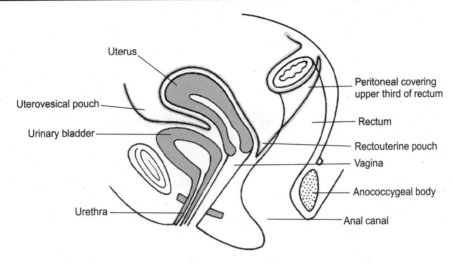

Fig. 9.17: Posterior relations of the urinary bladder in the female

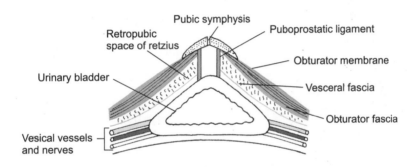

Fig. 9.18: Inferolateral surface of urinary bladder as related to retropubic space of Retzius

It lies below and is the lowest part of the bladder. When the bladder is distended, it is fixed at the neck because of ligamentous attachment and as it distends further it loses its surface contour and is more or less ovoid. As it rises up, it strips off the peritoneum from the anterior abdominal wall.

In the female the neck and the urethra are connected to the pubis by the **pubovesical ligaments**. In the male the neck is related to the prostate and the puboprostatic ligaments.

Ligaments of Bladder

The ligaments of the bladder help to support it and are classified as true and false.
- **True ligaments** are condensations of pelvic fascia (Fig. 9.11):
- **Pubovesical ligaments** are situated anteriorly between the pubis and bladder in the female. They correspond to **puboprostatic ligaments** of the male.
- **Lateral true ligaments** are attached laterally to the middle of the tendinous arch and medially to the inferolateral surface of the bladder.

- **Posterior true ligaments** stretch from the lateral borders of the base of the bladder to the internal iliac veins. They form a neurovascular pedicle for the bladder since they contain the vessels, nerve plexus and the ureter. In addition in the male they include the vas deferens also.

Posteriorly the bladder is reinforced by the rectovesical fascia (of Denonvilliers).
- **False ligaments** are formed by the peritoneal reflections:
- **Median umbilical ligament** is a peritoneal fold raised by the underlying urachus. It stretches from the apex of the bladder to the umbilicus.
- **Lateral umbilical ligaments** are formed by the reflection of peritoneum from the bladder to the side walls of pelvis.

The umbilical ligaments are bladder supports only in the sense that they act as guides in maintaining the bladder against the anterior abdominal wall when the bladder fills and rises out of the pelvis.

- **Posterior false ligaments** are formed by the peritoneum passing backwards to the sacrum. They are also known as **sacrogenital folds**.

Interior of Urinary Bladder (Fig. 9.19)

The mucous membrane of the bladder is loosely connected to the muscular coat and when the bladder is contracted it is thrown into a number of folds when the bladder is empty.

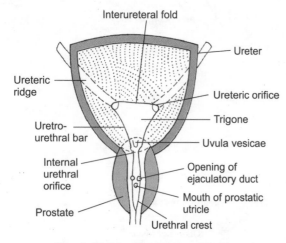

Fig. 9.19: Interior of urinary bladder

In a triangular area on the posterior surface outlined by the ureteric and urethral orifice the mucosa is firmly attached to the submucosa. This is the **trigone** of the bladder. The apex of the triangle is the **internal urethral orifice** while the base is the line joining the urethral orifices. Between the orifices of the ureter, there is a ridge called the **interureteric bar (of Mercier)** due to the presence of transverse bundle of fibres. It is curved so that it appears convex downwards and forwards. Lateral to the ureteric opening there is a ridge called **ureteric ridge (Bell's muscle)** produced by terminal intravesical parts of the ureter which pierces the muscle and mucosal walls very obliquely. The valve-like flap of mucosa, thus, produced prevents reflux of urine when intravesical pressure rises.

In the male immediately above and behind the internal uretheral orifice is a bulge known as **uvula vesicae**. It is produced by the median lobe of the prostate.

Structure of Urinary Bladder

The urinary bladder wall has the following linings:
- Mucous membrane is thick and folded and is lined by transitional epithelium at the trigone it is smooth and adherent to the muscle and not thrown into folds even in the empty slate.
- Lamina propria and submucosa are blended together. Muscularis mucosa is absent.
- **Muscle:** The bladder muscle is known as **detrusor**. It is made up of three layers of smooth muscle fibres:
- Outer longitudinal layer:
- Middle circular layer which is most prominent around the internal urethral orifice in the male to provide an internal urethral sphincter. It prevents seminal regurgitation into the bladder and has nothing to do with urinary incontinence and therefore, belongs functionally to the genital tract. In the female, the muscle in this region is arranged longitudinally so there is no internal sphincter.
- In both sexes the levator ani passes close to the urethra, it exerts a pincer action which can be used at will to interrupt the urinary stream.
- Inner layer consisting of separate longitudinal or oblique strands.

In the trigone in addition to the detrusor muscle there is a superficial triangular layer of muscle, **superficial trigonal muscle (of Bell),** which extends into the proximal urethra in both sexes. Its function is not clear but may be it helps to close the ureteral orifices.
- Serosa is a relatively thick connective tissue layer.

Blood Supply

- *Arteries* supplying the bladder are:
  - **Superior vesical artery** supplies the upper part of the bladder.
  - **Inferior vesical artery** supplies the base of the bladder and also neighbouring structures such as prostate and seminal vesicles.
  - **Obturator, inferior gluteal, uterine and vaginal arteries** give a small contribution to the lower part of the bladder.
  - *Veins:* The veins do not follow the arteries but form a plexus on the inferolateral surfaces of the bladder which drains backward across the pelvic floor to the internal iliac veins.

Lymphatic Drainage

Lymph vessels of the bladder drain into:
- **Internal iliac nodes** chiefly and;
- **External iliac nodes.**

Nerve Supply

The bladder is supplied by both sympathetic and parasympathetic components of the autonomic nervous system. Each of which contains motor (efferent) and sensory (afferent) fibres. The afferent fibres from the bladder are controversial.

Parasympathetic Supply

- The **efferent fibres** from S_2 to S_4 (pelvis splanchnic or nervi erigentes) convey motor fibres to the detrusor muscle and possibly inhibitory fibres to the trigone and the sphincter urethrae. They are concerned with emptying of the bladder since they contract the detrusor and relax the sphincter.
- The **afferent fibres** convey sensation of pain and bladder distension.

Sympathetic Supply

- The **efferent fibres** from $T_{11} - L_2$ segments pass by way of the hypogastric plexuses (presacral nerve) into the vesical plexus situated at the base of the bladder and are said to supply inhibitory fibres to the detrusor muscle and motor fibres to the trigone and sphincter urethrae. They are concerned with filling of the bladder since they relax the detrusor and close the sphincter.
- The **afferent fibres** carrying pain and perception of bladder fullness are conducted in sympathetic fibres located in the hypogastric nerves and reach $T_{12} - L_2$ segments.

The sympathetic contribution to bladder function is relatively unimportant because the bladder is not significantly affected by resection of the hypogastric nerves. Some authorities maintain that the sympathetic fibres are mainly vasomotor.

The **striated external sphincter urethrae** (circularly) arranged fibres of the deep transversus perenie muscle) and paraurethral striated muscles are supplied by the pudendal nerves (S_2 to S_4).

Development (Figs. 9.20 a, b, c and d)

The post-allantoic part of the hindgut dilates to form the **cloaca**. Caudally it ends blindly on the cloacal membrane, ventrally the allantois opens into it. The paired mesonephric ducts open into it at the sides. Further changes are as follows:

- **Urorectal septum,** a coronal mesodermal septum, extends caudally towards the angle between the allantois and the hindgut and fuses with the cloacal membrane.
- The cloaca is thus divided into a ventral part, the **primitive urogenital sinus** and a dorsal part, the **primitive rectum**.
- The cloacal membrane is also divided into a ventral part the **urogenital membrane** and a dorsal part, the **anal membrane**. The meeting point of the urorectal septum and the cloacal membrane is the **primitive perineal body**.
- The **mesonephric ducts (Wolffian)** open into the primitive urogenital sinus. The part of the sinus cranial to the opening of the ducts is called the **vesicourethral canal** and that caudal to it is known as the **definitive urogenital sinus**.
- The part of the mesonephric duct caudal to the origin of the ureteric bud, called the common excretory duct is gradually absorbed into the dorsal wall of the vesicourethral canal so that the ureters and the mesonephric ducts come to open independently.
- At first, the openings of the mesonephric ducts are cranial to those of the ureters, but with differential growth and absorption the ureteric openings shift laterally and cranially, while the mesonephric openings migrate distally to their adult levels (prostatic urethra) in the male. In the female the mesonephric ducts atrophy and vanish.
- The ureteric openings form the lateral angles, and the near midline mesonephric openings the caudal angle of the future trigone which receives epithelium of the common excretory ducts of mesodermal origin. The definitive bladder lining is wholly endodermal in origin.
- The **vesicourethral canal** is subdivided into a larger part, the **bladder** and a minor part, the **primitive urethra**.
- The vesicourethral canal originally opens to the exterior through the allantois which later is obliterated and becomes urachus.
- The bladder and urachus elongate proportionately as the infraumbilical abdominal wall forms.
- After birth the urachus forms a fibrous cord, the median umbilical ligament.

Micturition

The micturition is initiated by voluntary inhibition of the levator ani. This allows the bladder to descend and its outlet becomes funnel-shaped. Urine escapes into the urethra and

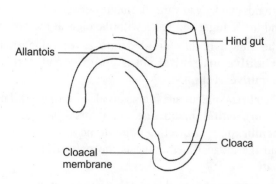

(a) Postallantoic part of the hindgut gets dilated to form cloaca.

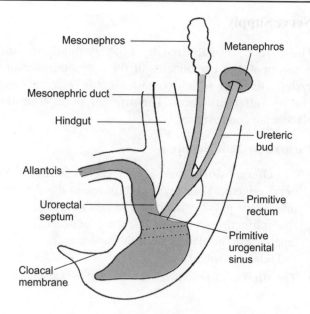

(b) A coronal urorectal septum extends caudally dividing cloaca into a ventral primitive urogenital sinus and a dorsal primitive rectum.

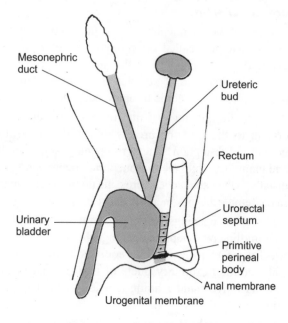

(c) The urorectal septum grows caudally to meet the cloacal membrane dividing it into a urogenital and anal membrane. The meeting point of urorectal septum and cloacal membrane is the primitive perineal body.

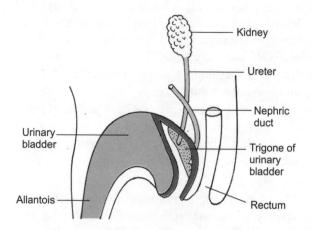

(d) The part of the mesonephric duct caudal to the origin of ureteric bud is gradually absorbed to form the trigone.

Fig. 9.20: Development of urinary bladder and rectum

mucosal afferents in the urethra relay to the detrusor centre in the pontine reticular formation, which responds by stimulating the sacral parasympathetic nucleus. Bladder emptying may be assisted by contraction of the abdominal wall, and the urethra is cleared by the bulbospongiosus muscles.

CLINICAL APPLICATION

- The interior of the bladder can be examined by passing an illuminated instrument (cystoscope) via the urethra. The process is known as **cystoscopy**. The trigone is seen as a smooth, pink triangular

- area; the ureteric orifices and interureteric bar are also clearly visible. The ureteric openings are seen ejecting drops of urine.
- The trigone has a large number of nerve endings carrying pain sensation. The pain is referred to the perineum via the pudendal nerves (S_2 to S_4) cancer involving this area and bladder stone eroding this area causes severe pain.
- Normally the bladder accommodates 250 to 300 mL urine. Distension becomes uncomfortable in the male at a volume 350 to 400 mL beyond which painful sensations are experienced.
- The urinary bladder is very prone to rupture in pelvic fracture, particularly when distended, with resulting intrapelvic and subperitoneal extravasation of urine.
- When the bladder distends, it rises up between the anterior abdominal wall and the peritoneum with its anterior aspect lifting quite above the pubic symphysis. This is taken advantage of in puncturing the bladder to relieve retention of urine without opening the peritoneum. The operation is known as **suprapubic cystostomy**.
- After difficult deliveries the bladder may be loosened from its attachment to the pelvic floor and may prolapse into the perineum, appearing at the vulva as a **cystocele**.
- In women urinary continence depends on the tone of the levator ani. Weakness of the levator ani is a common cause of incontinence. In men incontinence is caused only by the diseases involving the neck of the bladder or prostate.
- In women with multiple childbirths, repeated stretching of the pubococcygeus muscle causes the muscle to sag allowing the bladder and the uterus to descend (to prolapse). Descent of the bladder causes obliteration of the urethrovesical angle and the outlet becomes funnel-shapped at rest. In this condition a momentary increase in pressure (caused by sneezing or coughing, for example) may cause a jet of urine to be expelled (stress incontinence).
- Cortical control of the detrusor centre is not established until early in the second postnatal year. Until then, the detrusor centre empties the bladder every two to four hours, as the bladder fills.
- **Nocturnal enuresis** (bed-wetting) may occur in older children from loss of cortical control of the detrusor centre during sleep.

- The autonomic pathways to the sacral cord is interrupted by a lesion at any segmental level. During the stage of spinal shock, the bladder and rectum are atonic. Urine dribbles away from a distended bladder **(overflow incontinence)**. After four to eight weeks the bladder empties reflexly every four to six hours **(automatic bladder)**. However, automatic emptying does not develop if the conus is directly injured destroying many or all of the sacral segment neurons.
- Upper part of the bladder except the base are formed by the upper end of anterior division of cloaca while the base and the prostatic urethra are formed by the lower end of the Wolffian duct. These two portions fuse at the interureteric bar and so **congenital diverticula** and anomalies occur at the site of fusion.
- Defective development of the urachus may be responsible for (Fig. 9.21):
- **Patent urachus:** When it remains open in its whole length resulting in the discharge of urine at the umbilicus.
- **Lacunae of Luschka:** Small cavities remain in the urachus.
- **Cysts of urachus:** One of the lacunae enlarges to form a cyst which may be very large. It is below the umbilicus and central in position.

PELVIC PART OF URETERS

The abdominal and pelvic parts of the ureter are almost equal in length and so each is about 12.5 cm long. At the pelvic brim, it crosses just in front of the origin of the internal iliac artery. On the left at this point it underlies the **fossa intersigmoidea** of sigmoid mesocolon and is easily identifiable (Fig. 6.36). Each ureter descends retroperitoneally within the endopelvic fascia and passes backward and slightly downward on the side wall of pelvis following the anterior margin of the greater sciatic notch to reach the ischial spine. In this part of its course it is in front of the internal iliac artery (and behind the ovary in the female Fig. 9.24) and crosses in order from above downwards the following structures:
- Obturator nerve.
- Umbilical artery.
- Obturator vessels.
- Middle rectal.
- Inferior vesical (in the male) or uterine artery (in the female).

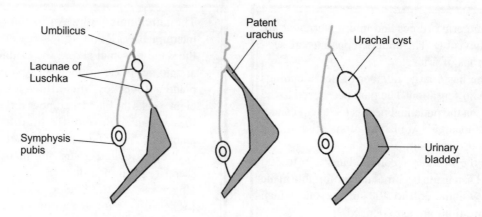

Fig. 9.21: Malformations of urachus

Reaching the ischial spine, it turns forward and medially to run just above the pelvic diaphragm to reach the base of the bladder where it enters its lateral angle. In this part of its course the relations are different in the two sexes.

In the Male (Figs. 9.15 and 9.22)

- The ductus deferens crosses the ureter superficially and then runs down medial to the bladder.
- The upper end of seminal vesicle lies just below the point where the ureter enters the bladder wall.

In the Female (Figs. 9.23 and 9.24)

- It lies in the base of the broad ligament.

- The uterine artery lies above and in front and then crosses the ureter to gain its medial side.
- Lower down under the broad ligament the ureter lies above the lateral vaginal fornix which separates it from the supravaginal portion of cervix before it enters the bladder (Fig. 9.24).
- Under the broad ligament it is at first on the surface of and then penetrates the **Mackenrodt's** ligament which is condensed tissue forming one of the supports of uterus.

Blood Supply

It is from all available arteries along its course. Abdominal part is supplied by:

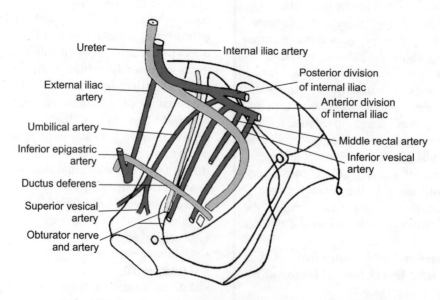

Fig. 9.22: Relations of ureter and ductus deferens in the male

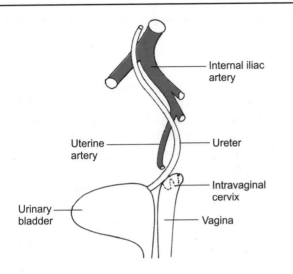

Fig. 9.23: The double relation of ureter to the uterine artery

- Renal and gonadal arteries.

  Pelvic part:
- Inferior vesical artery.

These vessels form a longitudinal anastomosis along the length of the ureter. Veins follow the corresponding arteries and terminate in corresponding veins.

Lymphatic Drainage

Abdominal part:
- Aortic and common iliac nodes.

  Pelvic part:
- External and internal iliac nodes.

Nerve Supply

Sympathetic supply is from T_{11} to L_2 spinal segments via coeliac and hypogastric plexuses. Pain fibres accompany sympathetic nerves.

  Parasympathetic fibres from S_2 to S_4 spinal segments come via pelvic splanchnic nerves.

  The functional significance of this innervation is not clear as urinary transport function is not dependent on this.

Development

Ureters are derived by a process of budding from the lower end of mesonephric duct **(Wolffian)** where it opens in the cloaca (Fig. 9.20 b).

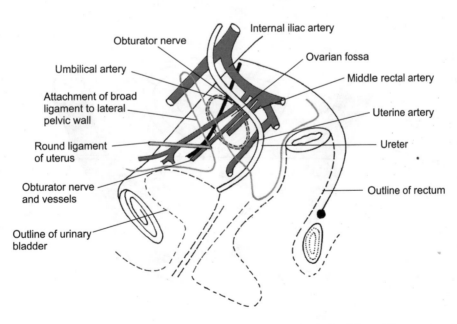

Fig. 9.24: Relations of ureter and round ligament of uterus and of attached margin of broad ligament and the fossa ovarica to the structures of the lateral pelvic wall

CLINICAL APPLICATION

- The ureters are very liable to injury during removal of uterus **(hysterectomy),** when the uterine arteries are ligated lateral to cervix and the ligaments are sectioned. The ureter are 2.5 cm lateral to cervix and are crossed by the uterine artery.

- The ureter is closely adherent to peritoneum. Stripping the parietal peritoneum from the ureter may cause avascular necrosis of the ureter by tearing off the vessel entering the ureter from the overlying peritoneum.

- The common sites of constructions of the ureter are:

- Pelviureteric junction.

- At the pelvic brim.

- Point of entry into the bladder. Ureteric orifice is narrowest of all. Renal stones get impacted at these sites causing intermittent contraction of smooth muscle to overcome obstruction. Sympathetic fibres carrying pain come from $T_{11} - L_2$ spinal segments and so the pain is referred to corresponding dermatome. Pain starts in the loin (T_{11} and T_{12}) passes around the flank and radiates downward towards the groin (iliohypogastric nerve, L_1) and testis (genitofemoral nerve, L_1 and L_2). This typical loin to groin radiation of intermittent pain is diagnostic of impacted ureteric stone and is called **'renal or ureteric colic'** which is purported to be among the most intense pains experienced by humans. The course of ureter in relation to the bony skeleton has to be taken into account when searching for a ureteric stone on a plain X-ray. It lies along the tips of the lumbar transverse processes, crosses in front of the sacro-iliac joint, lies against the ischial spine before passing medially to the bladder.

- The mesonephric duct may give off a double metanephric bud so that two ureters may develop on, one or both sides.

THE MALE PELVIC GENITAL ORGANS

THE PROSTATE

The prostate is a fibromuscular and glandular organ present only in the male. Its secretions add one-third to the volume of the semen. Paraurethral glands **(of Skene)** in the female are its **homologue.**

Situation

It is situated below the neck of the urinary bladder in the anterior and inferior part of the pelvic cavity (Fig. 9.25).

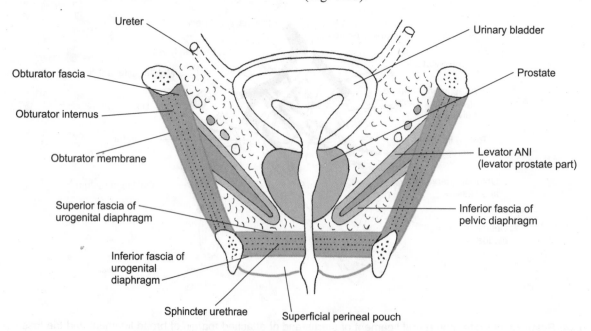

Fig. 9.25: Position and relations of prostate in the pelvic cavity

Shape and Size

It is cone-shaped resembling a chestnut. Its dimensions are 4 cm × 3 cm × 2 cm and weight about 8 g.

Capsules (Fig. 9.26)

The gland has two capsules:
- **True capsule** formed by the condensation of fibrous connective tissue on the periphery of the organ.
- **False capsule** formed by the condensation of visceral layer of pelvic fascia which splits to enclose both the prostate and the bladder in one sheath. Between the two capsules is the prostatic plexus of veins (Fig. 9.27).

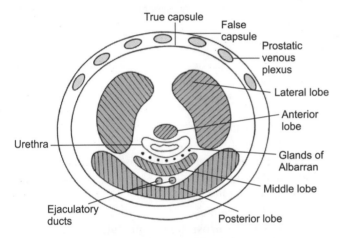

Fig. 9.26: Capsules and lobes of prostate

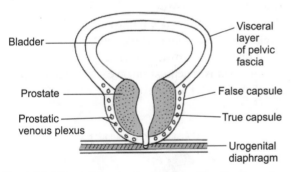

Fig. 9.27: Visceral layer of pelvic fascia splits to enclose both the prostate and the bladder and forms the false capsule of the prostate

Lobes (Fig. 9.26)

There are five lobes in the prostate:
- **Anterior lobe** is very small situated immediately in front of the urethra. It has little glandular tissue and is chiefly made of fibrous tissue.

- **Two lateral lobes** which lie on the sides of the prostatic urethra.
- **Posterior lobe** lies behind the prostatic urethra and below the ejaculatory ducts.
- **Middle (median) lobe** is wedge-shaped and lies between the prostatic urethra in front and the ejaculatory ducts behind (Fig. 9.28). It contains more glandular tissue than the other lobes. It produces two elevations (Fig. 9.30):
  - **The uvula vesicae** in the lower part of the trigone of urinary bladder.
  - The **urethral crest (verumontanum)** in the posterior wall of prostatic urethra.

Its posterior surface is marked by a vertical, midline shallow furrow which is palpable in rectal examination.

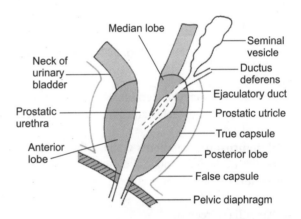

Fig. 9.28: Sagittal section of prostate to show the median lobe and the opening of ejaculatory ducts by the side of the utricle which occupies the median position

Surfaces and Relations

The prostate has a base, an apex and anterior, posterior and inferolateral surfaces. The relations are:
- **Base** or **the upper surface** is directed upwards and is related to the neck of bladder. The urethra passes from the bladder and perforates this surface and passes through the prostate, downwards and slightly near its anterior surface (Fig. 9.25).
- **Apex** lies inferiorly between the anterior edges of the levator ani and is related to (Fig. 9.25):
  - Superior fascia of urogenital diaphragm which separates it from sphincter urethrae.
  - Sphincter urethrae.

Sphincter urethrae

- **Anterior surface** is convex and rounded and is related to (Fig. 9.29):

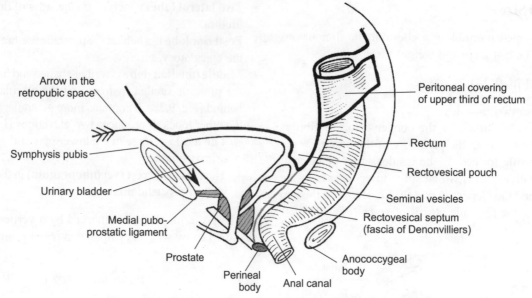

Fig. 9.29: Anterior, posterior and superior relations of prostate

- **Retropubic space of Retzius** which separates it from the lower part of pubis and is filled with retropubic pad of fat.
- **Puboprostatic ligaments** connect the surface to the bodies of the pubic bones below the cave of Retzius.
• **Posterior surface** is pierced by ejaculatory ducts and is related to (Fig. 9.29):
  - Ampulla of rectum.
  - **Rectovesical fascia (of Denonvilliers).** This fascia is formed due to the fusion of the anterior and posterior walls of a cul-de-sac of peritoneum which during intrauterine life extends to the pelvic floor and lies between the rectum behind and the urinary bladder and prostate in front. In the adult these two layers are attached to the floor of rectovesical pouch above and to the urogenital diaphragm and perineal body below. The anterior layer is firmly attached to the prostate but the posterior layer is not quite firmly blended with the fascial sheath of rectum. The potential space between the two layers is the **space of Denonvilliers**.
• **Inferolateral surface:**
  - Levator prostate part of levator ani clasps this surface (Fig. 9.25).

Prostatic Urethra

The prostatic urethra traverses the prostate from the base to the apex. It is about 3 cm long and is the most dilatable part of the urethra. It is narrow above and below but wider in the middle. Its posterior wall presents the following features (Fig. 9.30):
• **Urethral crest** or **verumontanum,** which is a vertical ridge in the midline.
• **Seminal colliculus,** which is a spherical swelling at the upper half of the crest.
• **Opening of the prostatic utricle,** (uterus masculinus) on the middle of the crest. The utricle is an embryological remnant resulting from union of the caudal ends of the paramesonephric (Mullerian) ducts. It is, thus, the homologue of the female uterus.
• **Openings of two ejaculatory ducts,** one on each side of the opening of prostatic utricle.
• **Prostatic sinus,** a depression on each side of the urethral crest, into which the ducts of the prostatic glands open.

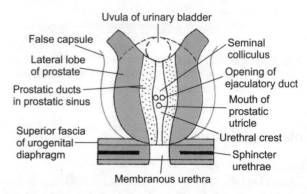

Fig. 9.30: The features on the posterior wall of the prostatic part of urethra

Blood Supply

The arteries supplying the prostate are:
- **Inferior vesical** mainly.
- **Middle rectal.**
- **Internal pudendal.**

The veins draining the prostate join the plexus lying between the true and false capsules (Fig. 9.27). This in turn joins the vesicoprostatic plexus situated in the groove between the prostate and the urinary bladder. This plexus drains into the internal iliac veins. The deep dorsal vein of penis drains into the prostatic venous plexus.

Nerve supply

- Sympathetic supply is from the inferior hypogastric plexus which contracts the muscle fibres in the prostate during ejaculation.
- Parasympthetic supply from the pelvic splanchnic nerves is not of much importance.

Lymphatic Drainage

It is into the:
- Internal iliac nodes.
- Sacral nodes.

Development

During intrauterine life 14 to 20 outgrowths mainly from the lateral aspect appear on the walls of the urethra just inferior to the bladder mostly caudal to mesonephric duct, about one-third cephalic to it. By process of budding these depressions are elaborated into a number of glandular masses or lobes which penetrate the surrounding mesoderm and connective tissue to form prostate (Fig. 9.31).

Structure

The prostate consists of (Fig. 9.32):
- Fibrous tissue stroma.
- Smooth muscle.
- **Glandular tissue:** The glands are of the tubulo-alveolar type and are distributed in two zones:
  - **Outer zone** contains the main glands which form the bulk of prostate. Their curving ducts open into the prostatic sinus.
  - **Inner zone** is periurethral. These are submucosal or mucosal. The submucosal like the glands of outer

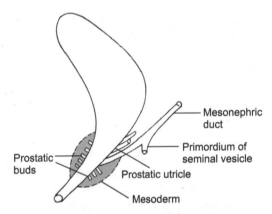

Fig. 9.31: Development of prostate

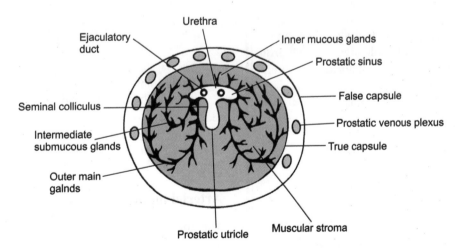

Fig. 9.32: T.S. of prostate showing the course of the prostatic ducts in the three concentric zones which are absent in the anterior part

zone, open into the prostatic sinus. The mucosal glands open on various points of the urethra.

Mucous glands, separate and distinct from the prostate, subtrigonal and subcervical in position lie in the middle lobe. These are known as **glands of Albarran.**

CLINICAL APPLICATION

- Surgical removal of an enlarged prostate does not attempt to enucleate the gland from its false capsule, with the attendant risk of bleeding from the prostatic plexus, but aims to shell it out from its true capsule.
- The middle lobe is clinically important since when affected by enlargement in old age, it elongates and obstructs the urethra causing retention of urine. It is the periurethral glands of inner zone which are involved in benign hypertrophy of prostate.
- The posterior and lateral lobes are commonest sites for cancer and the outer zone glands are involved and the retention of urine is not a feature.
- Enlargement of lateral lobes can be detected on rectal examination but middle lobe which is placed forward is not palpable.
- Very slight degree of enlargement of the glands of **Albarran** may lead to obstruction to the outflow of urine because of their intimate relation to the bladder neck.
- The prostatic venous plexus communicates with the lateral sacral veins which are connected with the vertebral venous plexus. This is the cause for the spread of cancer of prostate to vertebral column.
- Uvula vesicae, produced by the enlargement of the middle lobe, acts as a valve at the internal urethral orifice and also may produce, behind the orifice, a pocketing of the bladder in which urine collects and remains after micturition (residual urine).
- Palpable through digital examination per anus in the male are (Fig. 9.12):
- Membranous part of urethra.
- Posterior and lateral lobes of prostate.
- Rectovesical fosssa.
- Seminal vesicles if enlarged.
- Bladder base when distended.
- Ductus deferens when enlarged or displaced.

DUCTUS DEFERENS (VAS DEFERENS)

The ductus deferens conveys the sperms from the testis to the prostatic urethra. It begins from the tail of the epididymis and ends by joining with the duct of the seminal vesicle to form the ejaculatory duct which opens in the prostatic urethra. In its course it lies in the scrotum, the inguinal canal and the pelvis.

It enters the abdomen at the deep inguinal ring, hooks around the lateral side of the inferior epigastric artery and enters the pelvis by crossing the external iliac vessels. Its relations in the pelvis are:

- In the side wall of the pelvis it lies on the obturator fascia and is always covered by peritoneum. It crosses successively four parallel structures viz., (Fig. 9.22):
  - Umbilical artery.
  - Obturator nerve.
  - Obturator artery.
  - Obturator vein.
- The ductus reaches the posterior surface (base) of the bladder by curving medially and forwards (Fig. 9.33). It crosses in front of the lower end of the corresponding ureter and turns downward to lie by the side of its fellow near the midline medial to the seminal vesicle. It presents a dilatation known as **ampulla** before it joins the duct of the seminal vesicle to form the **ejaculatory duct**.

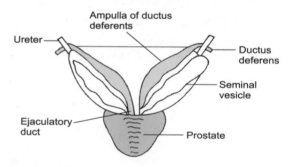

Fig. 9.33: Ampulla of ductus deferens and seminal vesicles lie on the posterior surface of urinary bladder

These structures are related to the rectum behind, but are separated from it by the **fascia of Denonvilliers** (Fig. 9.29).

Arterial supply

The artery to the vas is mainly from the inferior vesical artery.

Development

It develops from the mesonephric duct (Wolffian).

SEMINAL VESICLES

Each vesicle is a piriform, sacculated organ about 5 cm long, obliquely placed above the prostate (Fig. 9.33), in contact with the base of the bladder. It is a blind coiled duct about 15 cm long (Fig. 9.34). It is capped by the peritoneum of the rectovesical pouch. The upper end is near the entrance of the ureter into the bladder wall and the lower end is tapered and separated from its fellow by the two ductus deferens. From its lower end its excretory duct emerges to join ductus deferens to form the ejaculatory duct.

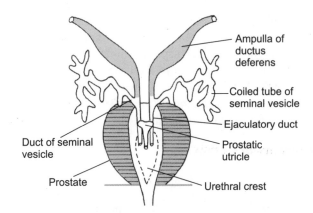

Fig. 9.34: The dissected seminal vesicle is a single convoluted blind tube with multiple diverticula

The ejaculatory duct is 2.5 cm long and runs through the substance of the prostate gland to open into the prostatic urethra lateral to the opening of the prostatic utricle.

The seminal vesicles produce about four-fifths of the seminal fluid which imparts motility to the sperms. They do not function for sperm storage.

Arterial Supply

By the branches of **inferior vesical** and **middle rectal arteries**.

Nerve Supply

Sympathetic fibres, coming from L_1 ganglion through the pelvic plexuses, are motor to the muscle wall.

Ejaculation is under the control of sympathetic system while the erection is controlled by parasympathetic system via the pelvic splanchnic nervi erigentes.

Development

Each develops as an outgrowth of the mesonephric duct (Fig. 9.31).

CLINICAL APPLICATION

- The ductus deferens may be double on occasion, an important factor if vasectomy for family planning is to be successful.
- The seminal fluid contains fructose and choline. Fructose is not produced anywhere else in the body and so it provides basis for the forensic determination of the presence of semen in cases of rape.
- A bilateral high lumbar sympathectomy results in sterility as ejaculation, which is controlled by L_1 sympathetic ganglion, is prevented.

FEMALE INTERNAL GENITAL ORGANS

THE UTERUS

Situation

The uterus is a hollow muscular organ situated in the pelvis between the rectum behind and the urinary bladder in front. The embryo and fetus normally develop and grow in it.

Shape and Size

The uterus is pear-shaped and is flattened anteroposteriorly. In adult nullipara, it is 7.5 cm long, 5 cm broad and 2.5 cm thick. Its average weight is 40 g. During pregnancy, it enlarges nearly ten times.

Axis and Angulation (Fig. 9.35)

- The long axis of the uterus is parallel to that of the pubic symphysis.
- The vagina passes upward and backward at an angle of 60° to the horizontal.
- The long axis of vagina is perpendicular to that of the uterus so that the whole uterus is bent forward at right angle to the vagina. This is called **angle of anteversion**.
- Just below the middle of the uterus is a constriction known as the **isthmus** which divides the uterus into a larger rounded upper part called the body and a smaller lower cylindrical part called cervix. The body is slightly bent forward on the cervix and this angle is known as **angle of anteflexion**.

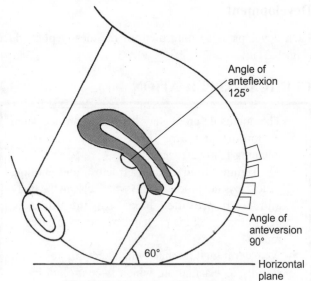

Fig. 9.35: Normal position of uterus

Parts and Surfaces

Uterus consists of the following parts (Fig. 9.36):

- **Fundus:** It is the convex upper portion above the openings of the fallopian tubes.
- **Body:** It is the upper two-thirds of the part of the organ below the fundus.
- **Cervix:** It is the lower one-third part below the body separated from it by a broad groove known as the **isthmus**. Cervix is inserted into the lumen of the vagina through the upper part of its anterior wall dividing the cervix into two halves:
  - **Supravaginal cervix** is the upper half.
  - **Vaginal cervix** is the lower half.

The uterus due to its flattening has following surfaces and borders:

- **Antero-inferior (vesical) surface.**
- **Posterosuperior (intestinal) surface.**
- **Right and left borders.**

Relations of the Body (Fig. 9.37)

- Antero-inferior surface is related to:
  - Uterovesical pouch of peritoneum.
  - Anterior two-thirds of the superior surface of the urinary bladder.
- Posterosuperior surface is related to:
  - Rectouterine pouch of peritoneum containing coils of small intestine and sigmoid colon.
  - Rectum separated by the pouch.
- Lateral borders give attachment to:
  - Fallopian tube.
  - **Broad ligament:** The uterus appears to have invaginated the pelvic peritoneum from below, so that a transverse fold is raised on each side, between the lateral borders and the side wall of the pelvis known as the **broad ligament** (Fig. 9.38).
  - Ovarian and round ligaments.

Relations of Cervix

Supravaginal Part (Fig. 9.38)

- To parametrium which is the connective tissue inferior to the broad ligament and around the cervix. Its anterior surface is related to the posterior one-third of the superior surface of the bladder and is not covered by peritoneum. The posterior surface is fully covered by peritoneum.

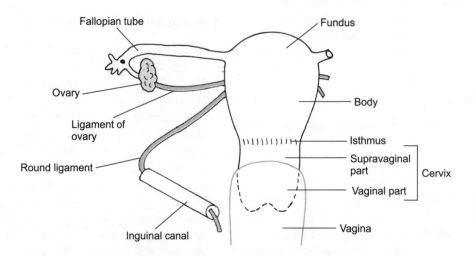

Fig. 9.36: The parts of uterus (seen from front)

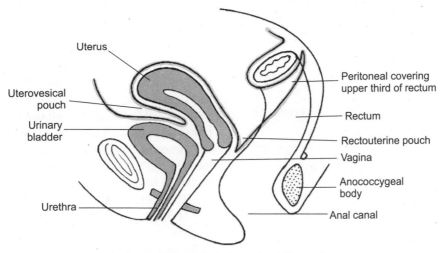

Fig. 9.37: Peritoneal and visceral relations of uterus

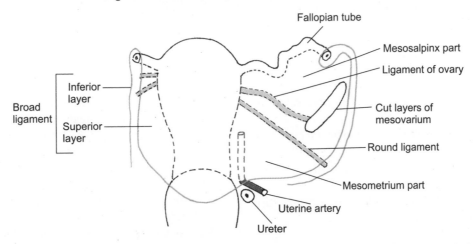

Fig. 9.38: A transverse fold of peritoneum, known as broad ligament, is attached to the lateral border of uterus its two parts are indicted (seen from behind)

- Ureter which passes forward in the parametrium to the bladder about 1.5 cm lateral to the supravaginal part of cervix.
  Uterine artery which runs medially to the side of supravaginal cervix and in front of the ureter.
- Lateral cervical ligament **(of Mackenrodt)** which passes from the lower part of the cervix and upper part of vagina to the side wall of pelvis (Fig. 9.42).

Vaginal Part

- This protrudes through the upper part of the anterior wall of vagina and is the lower half of the cervix. The parts of vagina clasping the cervix are called **fornices**. There are four fornices, one anterior, one posterior and two lateral. Their relations are described with the vagina (Page 156).

The Uterine Cavity (Fig. 9.39)

- Anteroposteriorly it is merely a slit because of the thickness of uterine walls.
- Transversely it is triangular in shape with base superiorly placed. It narrows below and becomes continuous with the canal of the cervix.
- The lumen of the cervix is spindle-shaped. The upper end is narrow and opens into the cavity of the body of uterus at the **internal os**. Its lower end opens into the lumen of the vagina at the **external os** which is a small transverse slit with smooth rounded lips before child bearing. The cervical canal has oblique ridges radiating from the midline on its anterior and posterior walls often referred to as **arbor vitae uteri**.

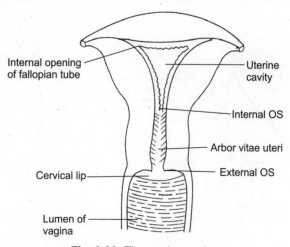

Fig. 9.39: The uterine cavity

Uterine Ligaments

Broad Ligament (Fig. 9.38)

It is the double fold of peritoneum with superior and inferior layers and like the body of the uterus has posterosuperior and antero-inferior surfaces.

- Medially the two layers are attached to lateral border of uterus and then separate to enclose it (Fig. 9.40 a).
- Laterally it is attached to the side wall of pelvis (Fig. 9.40 b).
- Inferiorly it is attached to the floor by a broad base hence the name.

- Superiorly the two layers are continuous around the uterine tube.

The ovary is suspended from the lateral part of the postero-superior surface by **mesovarium** (Fig. 9.38). The part of the broad ligament between the uterine tube and the mesovarium is called the **mesosalpinx**. The rest of the broad ligament is known as **mesometrium**. The part of the **mesometrium** between the lateral end of the uterine tube and the lateral pelvic wall is known as the **suspensory ligament of the ovary** (Fig. 9.41).

The contents of the broad ligament are (Fig. 9.41):

- **Uterine tubes** in the medial three quarters of its upper edge.
- **Round ligament** of the uterus.
- **Ligament of the ovary.**
- **Uterine artery** runs upward between the layers of the broad ligament adjacent to the uterus, then turns laterally below the uterine tube and anastomoses with the ovarian artery.
- **Ovarian vessels** after crossing the brim of the pelvis run medially in the suspensory ligament of the ovary. The part of the broad ligament between the lateral end of the uterine tube and the lateral pelvic wall is known as the suspensory ligament of ovary.

- **Vestigeal remains of the mesonephric duct** viz., epo-ophoron laterally, paro-ophoron medially and the duct of **Gartner** (Fig. 9.45 d).
- **Parametrium** which is the connective tissue.

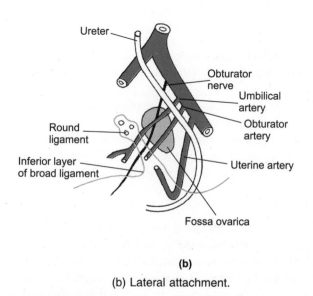

(a)

(a) Medial attachment.

(b)

(b) Lateral attachment.

Fig. 9.40: Attachments of broad ligament

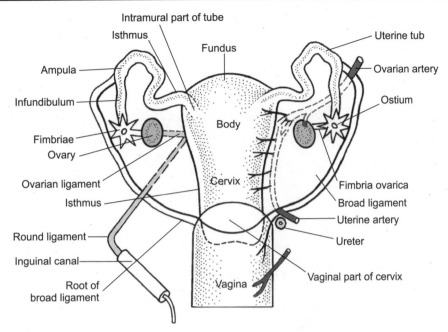

Ampula
Isthmus
Intramural part of tube
Fundus
Infundibulum
Uterine tub
Ovarian artery
Ostium
Body
Fimbriae
Ovary
Ovarian ligament
Cervix
Isthmus
Fimbria ovarica
Broad ligament
Uterine artery
Round ligament
Ureter
Inguinal canal
Root of
broad ligament
Vagina
Vaginal part of cervix

Fig. 9.41: Contents of the broad ligament

Round Ligament (Fig. 9.41)

Round ligament of the uterus is a fibromuscular band which commences from the upper part of the lateral border of the uterus, below and in front of the uterine tube, and passes through the inguinal canal to be attached to the labia majora. On its way to the deep inguinal ring, it crosses medial to the obturator vessels, the obturator nerve, the obliterated umbilical artery and the external iliac vessels (Fig. 9.23). At the deep ring it is lateral to the inferior epigastric artery. It is visible as a ridge on the inferior surface of the broad ligament (Fig. 9.40).

Ligament of the Ovary (Fig. 9.41)

Ligament of the ovary is attached below and behind the uterine tube. It is visible as a ridge on the superior surface of the broad ligament (Fig. 9.40).

Cardinal or Transverse Cervical Ligaments (of Mackenrodt) (Fig. 9.42)

These are thickenings of parametrium which pass laterally from the cervix and upper part of vagina to the lateral pelvic wall, where they have a wide attachment as they spread out towards it. They contain fibromuscular tissue. The ureter and the uterine vessels lie in the upper part of the ligament. They are one of the main structures maintaining the position of the uterus in the pelvis.

Uterosacral Ligaments (Fig. 9.42)

The uterosacral ligaments extend backwards from the posterior surface of the cervix, on either side of the rectum, to be attached to the sacrum.

Pubocervical Ligaments (Fig. 9.42)

They are bands extending from the side of the lower part of cervix towards the posterior surface of the body of pubis.

Supports of Uterus

It is not certain which of the supports and attachments of the uterus are functionally significant in maintaining the normal position of the uterus in the living person. Since, the cervix and vagina are connected, so the supports of both uterus and vagina are considered together. These are classified into upper and lower groups.

I. Upper Group

(a) Ligaments:

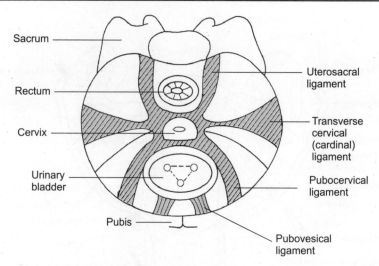

Fig. 9.42: The ligaments of uterus: The pubocervical, transverse cervical and uterosacral ligaments

- Cardinal or transverse cervical ligaments (of Mackenrodt).
- Uterosacral ligaments.
- Pubocervical ligaments.

(b) Pubovaginalis part of levator ani, some of whose fibres blend with the walls of vagina, support it and so assist in holding the cervix up.

(c) Broad ligament strictly speaking is not a ligament, but a mesentery for the uterus and the uterine tubes. It plays a little part in uterine support.

(d) Round ligament holds the uterus forward in anteflexion and anteversion especially when a distended bladder or any other force tends to push the uterus posteriorly.

(e) Fascial sheaths of uterine of vaginal arteries are continuous on each side with the transverse cervical ligament and act indirectly in the process of support.

II. Lower Group

(a) Urogenital diaphragm with its superior and inferior fascia.

(b) Perineal body which serves as a prop for the posterior vaginal wall.

(c) Intra-abdominal pressure.

(d) Weight of uterus and its direct attachment to vagina keep it in anteversion and anteflexion.

Blood Supply (Fig. 9.43)

Uterine Artery

The uterus is supplied mainly by the uterine arteries, which arise from the corresponding anterior division of the internal iliac. Each artery on its way to the supravaginal part of the cervix runs downward and forward to the base of the broad ligament, where it crosses the ureter about 2 cm away from the cervix. It then ascends up along the lateral border of the uterus and the fallopian tube between the layers of the broad ligament sending branches to the uterus and the tube. The artery takes a tortuous course within the broad ligament. The branches of the uterine artery include:

- The ascending branch, which gives off the tubal branch and anastomoses with the ovarian artery.
- The descending (vaginal) branch which anastomoses with other vaginal branches.

During pregnancy, the uterine artery becomes hypertrophic, with an enormous volume of blood flowing to the uterus and placenta. The tortuosity of the artery allows enlargement of the uterus during pregnancy.

Venous Drainage

The veins of the uterus, which correspond to the arteries, drain into the internal iliac vein.

Lymphatic Drainage (Fig. 9.44)

The lymphatic drainage of the uterus parallels the blood supply.

- Fundus and upper part of body drains into aortic nodes following the ovarian vessels.
- Lower part of body drains into:

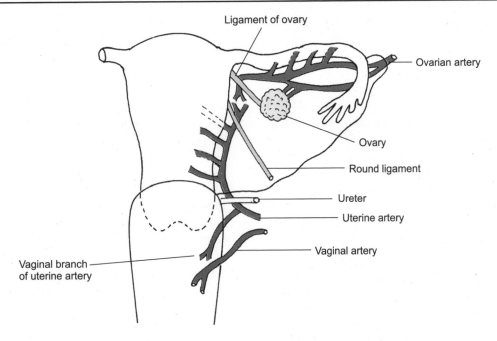

Fig. 9.43: Arterial supply of uterus and vagina as seen from behind

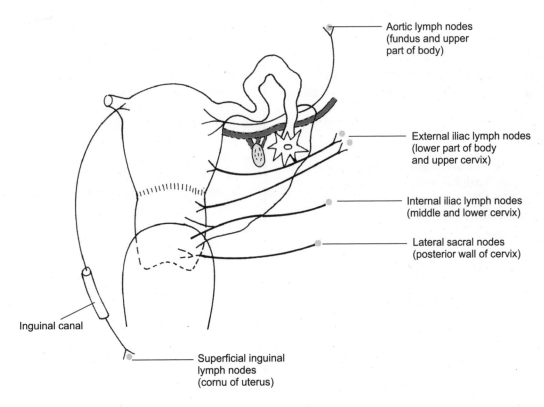

Fig. 9.44: Lymphatic drainage of uterus

– Internal iliac nodes by lymphatics accompanying the uterine vessels.
– Cornu of body into inguinal nodes by lymphatics following the round ligament.
• Cervix drains in three directions:
– Upper part into external iliac nodes, middle and lower part into internal iliac nodes by pathways through the parametrium.
– Posterior wall of cervix into sacral nodes by pathways through the sacrogenital folds.

Nerve Supply

The autonomic innervation to the uterus is derived as the uterovaginal plexus from the pelvic plexuses. The fibres accompany the uterine and vaginal arteries to supply this organ are both sympathetic and parasympathetic.

Sympathetic supply is from T_5 to T_{10} ganglia via the hypogastric and pelvic plexuses. The sympathetic nerves cause vasoconstriction and uterine contraction. Pain from the body of the uterus (labour pains), travels with the sympathetic fibres to the lowest thoracic segments of the cord and may be referred to T_{11} and T_{12} dermatomes.

Parasympathetic innervation is derived by the pelvic splanchnic nerves (S_2 to S_4 segments). They produce vasodilatation and an inhibition of muscular contraction. Pain from the cervix is carried by the parasympathetic nerves. Pain from the uterus arise as a result of ischaemia due to stretch.

The uterine muscle is very sensitive to hormonal influences and, so it is difficult to know about its motor pathways.

Development (Fig. 9.45)

The paramesonephric (Mullerian) ducts form most of the female genital tract. Each has three parts:
• Cranial vertical part.
• Intermediate horizontal part.
• Caudal vertical part.

The cranial part forms the uterine tube and its coelomic opening develops fimbriae. The intermediate parts of the two ducts expand and fuse to form the fundus and the body of the uterus. The caudal vertical parts fuse and form the cervix uteri.

As the paramesonephric ducts approach each other, the caudal part of the genital mesenteries are brought together which subsequently fuse with each other. The transverse peritoneal fold thus formed becomes the **broad ligament**.

In the female the mesonephric **(Wolffian)** duct, largely disappears, except for vestigeal tubular remnants lying in the mesosalpinx between the uterine tube and the ovary. These are as follows (Fig. 9.45 c):
• **Appendix vesiculosa** which is the persistent small cranial portion of the duct.
• **The duct and tubules of epoophoron** are formed by the persistent intermediate part of the duct along with those mesonephric tubules which are connected with the rete ovary. It lies above the ovary.
• **The paroophoron** are formed by more caudal tubules which end blindly. They lie medial to the ovary between the epoophoron and the uterus.
• **Gartner's duct** is formed by the caudal part of the Wolffian duct. It may be traced alongside the wall of the uterus and the vagina. It corresponds to the ductus deferens and ejaculatory ducts in the male.

The contribution of mesonephric ducts to the trigone of the urinary bladder and primitive urethra in the female is the same as in the male.

CLINICAL APPLICATION

• In 20% women the uterus is bent backwards on the cervix **(retroflexion)** and is itself bent backwards relative the vagina **(retroversion)**. Dysmenorrhoea (pain during menstruation), dyspareunia (pain on intercourse), sterility, abortion and backache may be due to this condition. The condition may exist without any sign or symptom.
• During pregnancy the isthmus is included in the body, **'taken up'** is the term used and constitutes the **lower uterine segment of obstetrics**.
• The relationship of the uterine artery to the ureter is kept in mind during hystectomy, as it is essential to avoid ureter while ligating the uterine artery.
• The strength of the pelvic floor depends on the integrity of the centrally situated perineal body, laceration of which during childbirth may lead to a descent of the upper part of vagina and then the uterus causing a **uterovaginal prolapse**. Ligaments of the uterus by themselves are unable to support the uterus.
• Any of the vestiges of the mesonephric **(Wolffian)** duct may form cyst in the broad ligament in adult life.
• Cancer of the cervix of the uterus is the commonest type of cancer in women. It spreads widely due to

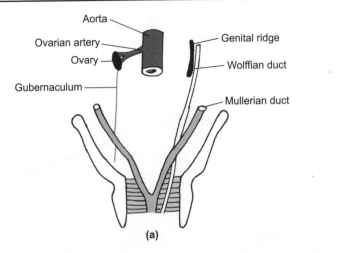

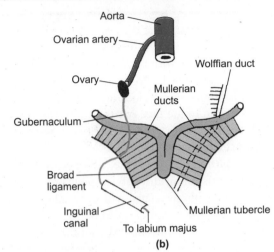

(a) The Mullerian duct at first courses lateral to the Wolffian duct, but more caudally crosses its ventral aspect to meet the Mullerian duct of the opposite side

(b) The two Mullerian ducts run longitudinally to end blindly on the dorsal wall of the urogenital sinus, between the Wolffian ducts, to produce an elevation termed the Mullerian tubercle.

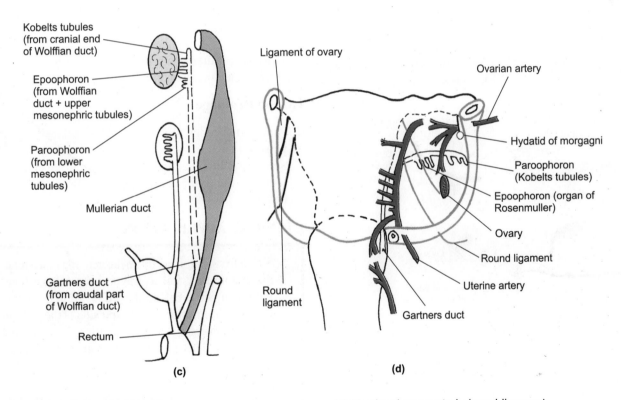

(c) Vestigeal remnants of Wolffian duct in the female.

(d) Vestigeal remnants in broad ligament

Fig. 9.45: Schematic development of female genitalia

widespread lymphatic drainage and so extensive lymphatic dissection is required.
- Pain associated with uterine spasm is referred to the dermatomes T_{12} to L_2 i.e., to midback, the inguinal and pubic regions and the anterior thigh. This is due to the fact that the course of visceral afferents from the body of uterus is parallel to sympathetic pathways.
- From the cervical region the course of the visceral afferents is along the pelvic splanchnic nerves. Thus, the pain associated with cervical dilation is referred to the sacral dermatomes S_2 to S_4 to the gluteal region, perineum, posterior thigh and leg.

THE UTERINE TUBES

Position

There is a uterine (fallopian) tube on each side of the uterus. It joins the uterus at its cornu and lies in the medial three quarters of the upper border of broad ligament (Fig. 9.46).

Extent

The uterine tube is 10 cm long. The medial end passes through the lateral wall of the uterus and opens into the

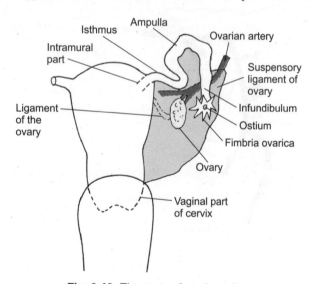

Fig. 9.46: The parts of uterine tube

upper lateral angle of the uterine cavity. At the lateral end it opens into the peritoneal cavity.

Parts

It is divided into four parts:

- Intramural part is narrow, 1-2 mm in diameter and is embedded in the lateral wall of the uterus.
- Isthmus is the narrow part following the intramural portion and next to it is.
- Ampulla the widest part, about 4 mm in diameter, is thin walled and tortuous.
- Infundibulum which is funnel-shaped and has finger-like processes called the fimbriae surrounding an opening known as ostium. The largest **fimbria ovarica,** is attached to the ovary. This fimbria is said to be concerned in transferring the ovum from the ovary after the rupture of the mature ovarian follicle. The ovum is usually fertilised at the lateral end of the tube. The lining of the tube is continuous with the lining of the peritoneal cavity, so that the female peritoneal cavity is in communication with the exterior via the tubes, uterus and vagina.

Blood Supply

The arterial supply comes from:
- Ovarian artery.
- Uterine artery.

The venous drainage is divided into:
- Ovarian and uterine veins.

Lymph Drainage

- Para-aortic nodes along with the ovarian lymphatic vessels.
- Superficial inguinal nodes drain the uterine end of the tube by the lymphatics which follow the round ligament.

CLINICAL APPLICATION

Since, fertilisation occurs in the ampulla of the tube, the zygote may fail to traverse the uterine tube, with resultant tubal implantation. Rupture of the tube with haemorrhage and expulsion of the embryo into the peritoneal cavity usually occurs in tubal pregnancy. This is a gynaecological emergency because the patient may die of internal haemorrhage.
- The exterior of genital tract in the female is in direct communication with the peritoneal cavity through the ostium of the uterine tube. This is a potential pathway for infection of the tube (salpingitis) and pelvic cavity (pelvic inflammatory disease).

OVARY

The ovary is a pair of organs producing the oocytes and important hormones act on the uterus.

Position (Fig. 9.47)

Ovary lies in the ovarian fossa on the side wall of the pelvis, between the ureter behind and the broad ligament in front.

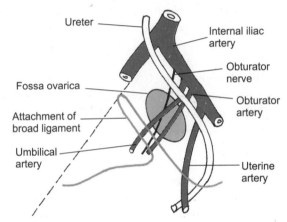

Fig. 9.47: Position of fossa ovarica and relations of the lateral surface of the ovary

Shape and Size

In nullipara, each ovary is a whitish gland shaped like an almond. It is 3 cm long, 2 cm wide and 1 cm thick. It has two ends (tubal and uterine), two surfaces (medial and lateral) and two borders (anterior and posterior). Its long axis is vertical.

Relations

- Tubal or superior end is closely related to the lateral end of the uterine tube, one of whose fimbria is attached to the ovary. This end is connected with the side wall of the pelvis by the suspensory ligament of the ovary which conducts the ovarian vessels and lymphatics (Fig. 9.46).
- Uterine or inferior end is connected with the lateral margin of the uterus near the fundus by the ligament of the ovary (Fig. 9.46).
- Medial surface is free and related to intestine and overlapped by the uterine tube.
- Lateral surface is in contact with the ovarian fossa and is separated by the pelvic peritoneum from the umbilical artery, obturator nerve and vessels and the obturator internus muscle (Fig. 9.47).
- Anterior (mesovarian) border is attached to the posterior layer of broad ligament by a fold of that layer, the mesovarium, containing the vessels and nerves of the ovary (Fig. 9.48).
- Posterior border is free and is related to the uterine tube.

Blood Supply

The ovarian artery is a direct branch of the aorta. After lying anterior to most of the structures on the posterior abdominal wall, it enters the suspensory (infundibulopelvic) ligament of ovary, then lies inferior to the uterine tube from where it gives off branches which go in the mesovarium to the ovary. It anastomoses with branches of the uterine artery.

- There is a plexus of veins around the ovary from which one vein is formed. The right ovarian vein joins the inferior vena cava while the left vein ends in the left renal vein.

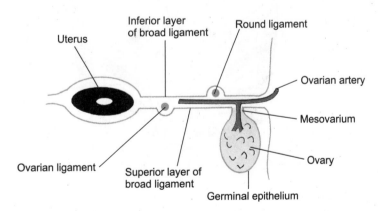

Fig. 9.48: Schematic diagram to show the entry of the ovarian artery and the relations of folds of ligament

Nerve Supply

The ovarian plexus is formed from the aortic and renal plexuses and from the inferior hypogastric plexus. The fibres are postganglionic sympathetic from T_{10} to T_{11} spinal segments and usually end in the walls of the blood vessels.

Lymphatic Drainage

Drainage is along the ovarian artery to the lumbar nodes.

Development (Fig. 9.45 a and b)

Medial to the mesonephros, in the intermediate mesoderm, a thickening known as **genital ridge** appears. This becomes larger, bulges into the coelomic cavity as a sessile body to ultimately form the ovary which lies in abdomen. As in male, a gubernaculum is present which connects it with the labium majus and pulls the ovary from the lumbar region to pelvic cavity. The gubernaculum gets attached to the paramesonephric ducts, from which the uterus develops and gets divided into the round ligament in front and the ligament of the ovary behind.

CLINICAL APPLICATION

- Visceral afferent fibres from the ovary run along the sympathetic pathways to T_{12} to L_2 spinal segments. Intractable ovarian pain may be alleviated by cutting the suspensory ligaments which contain these general visceral afferent fibres.
- An abnormally long mesovarium and suspensory ligament may cause ovarian torsion resulting in compression of blood supply. The resultant ischaemia causes pain referred to T_{12} to L_2 lumbar dermatomes.
- The normal caudal migration of the ovaries may continue so that the ovaries may descend to the deep inguinal ring or very rarely the labia majora.
- The ovaries which fail to descend are termed retroperitoneal. They are located on the posterior abdominal wall superior to the kidneys.
- Accessory ovarian tissue or ovaries may be seen in the broad ligament or mesovarium.
- One or both ovaries may be congenitally absent due to the defect of genital ridge.
- The ovary is extremely variable in its position and is frequently found prolapsed into the pouch of **Douglas** in perfectly normal women.

THE VAGINA

The vagina is the lower part of the female genital tract. It surrounds the cervix of the uterus from where it extends to open at the vestibule of the vulva (Fig. 9.49).

Shape

It is a tubular canal which is directed upwards and backwards. Its long axis makes an angle of about 90° with the long axis of the uterus (Fig. 9.35). The angle increases as the bladder distends. In its long axis it presents a slight forward concavity. Normally, the vaginal lumen is H-shaped as the walls of the canal are collapsed.

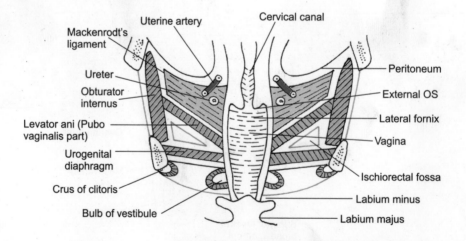

Fig. 9.49: Coronal section through vagina showing its relations

Length

The length of vagina is somewhat variable. Its anterior wall is about 7.5 cm while the posterior wall is longer and is 10.5 cm long. The upper vagina surrounds the lower cervix for a short distance above the external os. The four recesses around the cervix are known as anterior, posterior and lateral fornices related respectively to anterior, posterior and lateral walls of vagina.

Relations

The upper two-thirds of vagina is within the pelvic cavity and lower third is within the perineum (i.e., inferior to the pelvic floor).

- Anterior wall is related from above downward to (Fig. 9.37):
  - Cervix of uterus to upper part.
  - Base of urinary bladder to middle part.
  - Urethra to the lower part.
- Posterior wall from above downward to (Fig. 9.37):
  - Rectouterine pouch of **Douglas** to the posterior fornix of vagina. Strictly speaking the pouch is rectovaginal.
  - Rectum separated by the uterorectal septum.
  - Perineal body which separates the lower vagina from the anal canal.
- Lateral walls (Fig. 9.49):
  - Pubovaginalis part of levator ani.
  - Cardinal ligaments of uterus **(Mackenrodt's)** attached to the sides of vagina and cervix.
  - Ureters and uterine arteries lie close to the lateral fornices.
  - Urogenital diaphragm below the levator ani.
  - Greater vestibular glands.
  - Bulb of the vestibule covered with bulbospongiosus muscle.

Blood Supply

The arterial supply is from (Fig. 9.43):
- Vaginal artery.
- Vaginal branches of the uterine artery.
- Vaginal branches from the internal pudendal which reach vagina below the level of levator ani.

  The venous drainage is by:
- Vaginal venous plexus which drains into the internal iliac veins.

Lymphatic Drainage

- Upper third of vagina drains into external and internal iliac nodes.
- Middle third drains into the internal iliac nodes.
- Lower third drains into internal iliac nodes as well as into the superficial inguinal nodes.

Nerve Supply

- Upper two-thirds of vagina is supplied by sympathetic fibres from the uterovaginal plexus and parasympathetic fibres from the S_2 to S_4 nerves. The visceral afferent from this part travels along the nervi erigentes.
- The lower-third of vagina is supplied by pudendal nerve which mediates all cutaneous sensations.

Development

The vagina has a double origin:
- The upper three-quarter of vagina is developed from the fusion of the paramesonephric (Mullerian) ducts.
- The lower one-fourth is developed by the canalisation of the sinovaginal bulbs which form by the proliferation of the urogenital sinus.

Development Abnormalities (Fig. 9.50)

All stages of the original double mesonephric tubes may persist from a bicornuate uterus to a complete reduplication

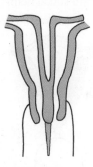

(a) Uterus didelphys (duplication of uterus, cervix and vagina) is due to failure of fusion of the Mullerian ducts which induce bilateral vaginal plates

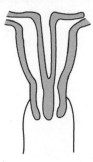

(b) Uterus bicornis bicollis. Failure of fusion of Mullerian ducts causing the body of the uterus to split into two equal parts with a single or double cervix and single vagina

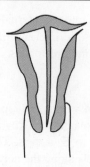

(c) Septate uterus due to non-disappearance of the septum between the fused Mullerian ducts. The uterus is normal outwardly.

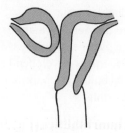

(d) Uterus unicornis caused by non-canalisation of one of the Mullerian ducts and consequent atrophy so that there is one horn.

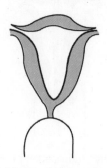

(e) Atresia of cervix

Fig. 9.50: Schematic representation of the main developmental abnormalities of the uterus and vagina

of the uterus and vagina. Alternatively, there may be absence, hypoplasia or atresia of the duct system on one or both sides.

CLINICAL APPLICATION

- Per vaginum (PV) digital examination is done by a finger introduced into the vagina. The following structures can be palpated:
- Through the anterior fornix the urethra, bladder and symphysis pubis are palpable.
- Through the posterior fornix the rectum and coccyx are palpable across the pouch of **Douglas**.
- Through the lateral fornices, the ovaries uterine tubes, side wall of the pelvis and occasionally the ureters are palpable.
- At the apex of the vagina the anterior and posterior cervical lips are palpable.
- Weakening of the pelvic support structures due to childbirth results in herniation of:
- Urinary bladder through the anterior vaginal wall into the vaginal lumen (**cystocele**).
- Rectum through the posterior vaginal wall into the vaginal lumen (**rectocele**).
- Vaginal duplication to variable extents and different types of fistulae occur as development anomalies.
- A ureteric stone lying in the part of ureter which is close to the lateral fornix can be palpated on vaginal examination.

  Pus or fluid accumulating in the pouch of **Douglas** can be drained surgically through the vagina, as there is peritoneal covering over the posterior fornix of vagina. The operation is known as **posterior colpotomy**.
- The pain from the upper two-thirds of vagina travels along the nervi erigentes and may be referred to the dermatomal distribution of S_2 to S_4 spinal segments.

10

The Perineum and the Joints of Pelvis

INTRODUCTION

The perineum is the region of the lesser pelvis below the pelvic diaphragm. On the surface, it presents as the inferior aspect of the trunk between the thighs.

SKELETAL FRAMEWORK (FIG. 10.1)

The skeletal and ligamentous boundaries of the perineum correspond to those of the pelvic outlet.

Anteriorly: Lower border of pubic symphysis.
Antero laterally: Ischiopubic rami.
Laterally: Ischial tuberosities.
Postero laterally: Sacrotuberous ligaments.
Posteriorly: Tip of the coccyx.

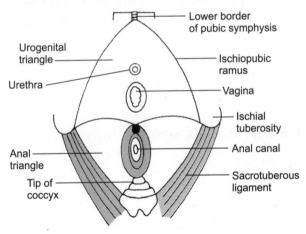

Fig. 10.1: Boundaries of perineum

Divisions

The perineum is divisible by an imaginary transverse line joining the anterior ends of the ischial tuberosities into two triangles (Fig. 10.1):
- Anal triangle posteriorly.
- Urogenital triangle anteriorly.

Contents

- The principal structures of the anal triangle are the anal canal and the ischiorectal fossa.
- The principal structures of the urogenital triangles are the external genitalia and urethra—superficial and deep perineal spaces (pouches) and their contents.

THE ANAL TRIANGLE

The contents of the anal triangle are:
- Anal canal in the centre.
- Ischiorectal fossae on either side.

ANAL CANAL

The part of the alimentary canal inferior to the pelvic diaphragm and contained in the anal triangle of perineum is called the **anal canal**. It is directed posteriorly and inferiorly from the rectum to the anal verge and is 3 to 4 cm long. Anus is its external opening.

Relations

Anteriorly (Figs. 10.2 and 10.3)

- Perineal body which separates it from bulb of penis.

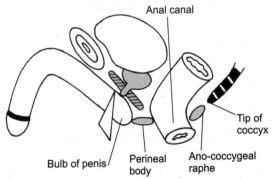

Fig. 10.2: Anterior and posterior relations of the anal canal in the male

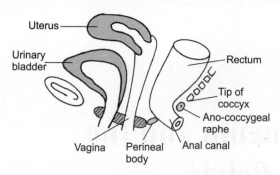

Fig. 10.3: Anterior and posterior relations of the anal canal in the female

- Bulb of penis in the male and lower one-third of vagina in the female.

Posterior (Figs. 10.2 and 10.3)

- Anococcygeal raphe which separates it from.
- The tip of coccyx.

Lateral (Fig. 10.4)

- Puborectalis part of levator ani.
- Sphincter ani externus.
- Ischiorectal fossa.

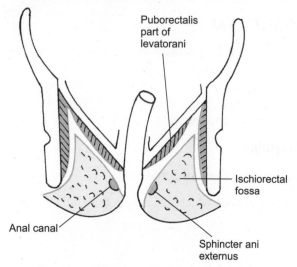

Fig. 10.4: Lateral relations of the anal canal

Interior of Anal Canal

It presents four landmarks (Fig. 10.5) :
- **The anocutaneous line** or the anal verge or rim. It is the external margin of the walls of the anus in its normal state of apposition. The epithelium superior to this line usually is thrown into folds by the action of an involuntary muscle known as **corrugator cutis ani**.

- **The intersphincteric groove** is palpable rather than visible. It marks the linear interval between the internal and external sphincters. This interval lies half way between the anal verge and the pectinate line. It does not represent other site of the embryonic cloacal membrane. Below the groove is a truly cutaneous area, continuous at the anal verge with the skin of the buttocks. The lining is stratified squamous keratinizing epithelium. It corresponds to **Hilton's white line** so described by Hilton on account of its relative avascularity. The line has never been clearly defined and the term has nearly been abandoned. It does not appear white in either the living or the dead.
- **The pectinate or the dentate line** is at the level of the anal valves. The band of tissue between the intersphincteric groove and the pectinate line has a smooth surface and a glossy shining appearance. It may be likened to a circular sawblade whose teeth point upward. These dentations interdigitate with the **columns of Morgagni** which are connected at their distal ends by valve-like folds **(the anal valves of Ball)** above which are **anal sinuses** into which 5-10 anal glands open. The appearance of this area with its dentations has resemblance to a comb and that is why it is known as **pecten** (comb). The lining of the pecten is stratified squamous epithelium, but is nonkeratinizing and there are no hair follicles, sebaceous glands or sweat glands.
- **The anorectal line** lies about 1.5 cm proximal to the pectinate line. The mucous membrane between the two shows upto a dozen longitudinal ridges, the anal columns.

Above the pectinate line the zone is lined with mixed columnar and stratified squamous epithelium, so there is no abrupt line of change to columnar intestinal cells of the rectum.

Sphincters of Anal Canal (Fig. 10.5)

There are two sphincters:
- Internal sphincter.
- External sphincter.

Internal sphincter is the distal continuation of the circular smooth muscle fibres of the rectum. It surrounds upper three-quarters of the anal canal and reaches the level of the pectinate line. It is surrounded by the deep and superficial parts of the external sphincter. It is innervated by the sympathetic and parasympathetic fibres. Sympathetic stimulation contracts the muscle, parasympathetic relaxes it. It is under a voluntary control similar to that of the smooth muscle of the urinary bladder. The sphincter is not

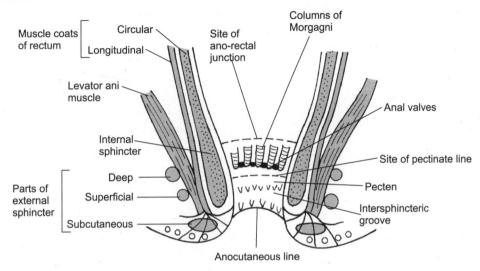

Fig. 10.5: Interior of anal canal and anal sphincters

competent alone, at least some of the deepest part of the external sphincter is necessary for complete continence of faeces and flatus.

The longitudinal muscle coat as it reaches the anorectal junction fuses with the fibrous part of the puborectalis to form a conjoint longitudinal sheet separating the internal sphincter from the external sphincter. Septa from this sheet penetrate the internal sphincter and the lower part of the external sphincter; some reach the fat of the **'ischiorectal fossa'** the perianal skin and the mucous membrane of the intersphincteric groove.

The septa which pass through the subcutaneous part of the external sphincter gain attachment to the skin around the anal orifice and form the **corrugator cutis ani muscle** which is considered part of the panniculus carnoses.

External sphincter is composed of striated muscle and has three parts:

- **Deep part** forms a complete sphincter to the upper end of the anal canal including the internal sphincter. It blends with the puborectalis part of the levator ani behind the anorectal junction. Thus, the anorectal junction is bounded by internal sphincter, deep part of external sphincter and puborectalis which collectively form the **anorectal ring** which is palpable on rectal examination. Rectal continence depends on this ring.

- **Superficial part** encircles the middle of the anal canal and is the only part of the sphincter with a bony attachment. It extends from the tip of the coccyx and the anococcygeal raphe to the perineal body in front. It overlaps the lower part of the internal sphincter.

- **Subcutaneous part** is a flattened circular band whose lower end curves inwards to lie below the lower end of the internal sphincter. This submucosal apposition of the two sphincters in the lower part of the canal gives rise to the palpable intersphincteric groove. The septa formed by the longitudinal muscle layer pass through the subcutaneous part to be attached to the skin around the anal orifice to form the **corrugator cutis ani**.

Arterial Supply

- **Superior rectal artery,** the continuation of the inferior mesenteric artery, travels in the medial limb of the pelvic mesocolon and supplies the upper end of the canal and terminates within the anal columns.

- **Middle rectal artery,** branch of anterior divisions of internal iliac artery, supplies a small part of the muscular wall.

- **Inferior rectal artery,** branch of the internal pudendal, crosses the ischiorectal fossa to supply the anal canal below the mucocutaneous junction.

- **Median sacral artery,** supplies a small part of the muscular wall of anal canal and the ampulla of rectum.

Venous Drainage

- At the level of the **(Hilton's line)** there is **portosystemic anastomosis**. Above the line, the anal canal is drained by the **superior rectal vein** which passes upward an inferior mesenteric vein to drain into splenic vein which is portal.

- **Middle and inferior rectal veins** drain the anal canal below the Hilton's line and go to the internal iliac vein which is systemic.

Lymphatic Drainage

The lymph drainage corresponds to the vascular pattern:
- The lymphatics above the pectinate line drain upwards to the internal iliac nodes.
- The lymphatics below the pectinate line pass to the superficial inguinal nodes.

Nerve Supply

The nerve supply to the upper part of anal canal is by the autonomic plexuses. The lower part is supplied by the somatic inferior rectal nerve a terminal branch of the pudendal nerve.

Development

The anal canal has a double origin:
- From an ectodermal invagination called the **proctodeum**.
- **The endodermal cloaca,** separated from the bladder by urorectal septum.

The cloacal or anal membrane separates these two parts initially, but breaks down subsequently to form a continuity between the two parts. The mucocutaneous junction of development is the pectinate line and not the **Hilton's line.**

CLINICAL APPLICATION

- The anal glands, 5-10 in number, either branch in the submucosal plane or more frequently penetrate the internal sphincter to end by branching in the intersphincteric plane between internal and external sphincter muscles. They are of considerable surgical importance in the development of anal abscesses and fistulae.
- The mucosa above the pectinate line has an autonomic nerve supply and is insensitive, whereas the skin below the line has somatic innervations and is acutely sensitive. A crack or fissure below the pectinate line causes severe pain on defecation, whereas an injection of an internal pile by a needle passing through the mucosa of the upper part of the canal is painless.
- The lymphatic drainage above the pectinate line is upwards to the lumbar nudes. Whereas, below this line the drainage is to the inguinal nodes. The

lymphatic spread of a carcinoma and of an infection in the two areas will differ.
- The lower rectum and upper anal canal are sites of portal systemic anastomosis. Varicosity of veins in this region is called **haemorrhoids**. The sites of varicose veins correspond to the three venous columns accompanying the three main branches of the superior rectal artery and are indicated by the 3, 7 and 11 O' clock positions in an imaginary clock face at the anal verge, when the patient is examined in the lithotomy position.
- Continence depends on the integrity of the sphincter mechanism and its nerve supply and on the maintenance of the anorectal angle. Incontinence may result from injury to pudendal nerve or damage to the sphincter. The external anal sphincter (striated) exerts temporary control of flatus and fluid faeces. The internal sphincter ani (smooth) has no supportive action: it responds to rectal filling by relaxation.

THE ISCHIORECTAL FOSSA

The ischiorectal fossa is a pyramidal shaped fat-filled space lateral to the anal canal shut off from the pelvic cavity by the pelvic diaphragm. The two fossae communicate with each other behind the anal canal.

Boundaries (Figs. 10.6 and 10.7)

- **Medial wall:**
  - External anal sphincter.

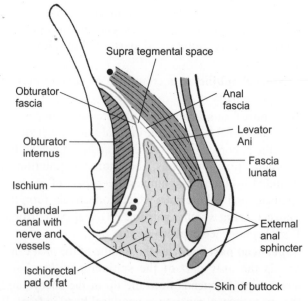

Fig. 10.6: Coronal section through the ischiorectal fossa showing its medial and lateral walls, roof and floor

– Levator ani (puborectalis) with its covering anal fascia which is continuous above with the inferior fascia of pelvic diaphragm.
- **Lateral wall:**
  – Ischium covered with obturator internus and lined with obturator fascia.
- **Anterior boundary:**
  – Posterior edge of the urogenital diaphragm.
- **Posterior boundary:**
  – Sacrotuberous ligament covered with the lower edge of gluteus maximus.
- **Roof:**
  – Meeting place of the levator ani and obturator internus muscles.
- **Floor:**
  – Skin of the buttocks.

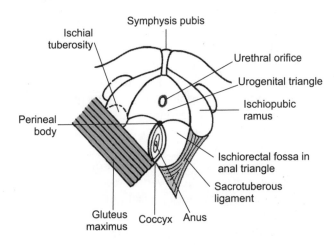

Fig. 10.7: Ischiorectal fossa from the perineal aspect showing its anterior and posterior boundaries

Contents (Figs. 10.6 and 10.8)

- **Ischiorectal pad of fat:** The deep fascia is separated from the skin by the whole thickness of this pad of fat which invaginates the fascia deeply. This fascia is named the **fascial lunata**.
- **Inferior rectal nerves and vessels** cross the middle of the fossa from lateral to medial side. They end in the sphincter ani externus and the perineal skin.
- **Perineal branch of** S_4 crosses the posterior corner of the fossa to supply the superficial part of the sphincter ani externus.
- Branches of posterior cutaneous nerves (S_2 and S_3) of thigh wind around the lower edge of gluteus maximus.

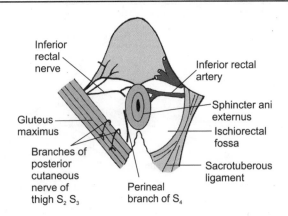

Fig. 10.8: Nerves and vessels of ischiorectal fossa

FASCIA LUNATA (FIG. 10.6)

Relations

- *Medial:* It covers the fascia on the levator ani (anal fascia) and ends at the lower end of levator ani.
- *Lateral:* It covers the obturator fascia on the obturator internus. The internal pudendal vessels and pudendal nerve are between these two layers which form the **pudendal canal**.
- *Anterior:* The fascia fuses with the urogenital diaphragm.
- *Superior:* The top of the fascial dome is referred to as **tegmentum** and space above as **suprategmental space** which contains fat.

PUDENDAL CANAL (ALCOCK'S) (FIG. 10.9)

The pudendal canal is an elongated cleft between the obturator fascia and fascia lunata. It runs forward on the lateral wall of the ischiorectal fossa. It starts at the lesser sciatic foramen, above the urogenital diaphragm, 3-4 cm above the lower margin of the ischial tuberosity and ends near the anterior end of the lateral edge of the urogenital diaphragm. In parts of its extent, its floor is formed by the falciform process of the sacrotuberous ligament, above the lower end of the ischial tuberosity.

The canal contains the pudendal nerve and internal pudendal vessels. The inferior rectal nerve and vessels pierce the fascia lunata to reach the anal canal and perineal nerve and vessels pierce it a little more anteriorly to reach the superficial perineal fascia close to the posterior edge of the urogenital diaphragm.

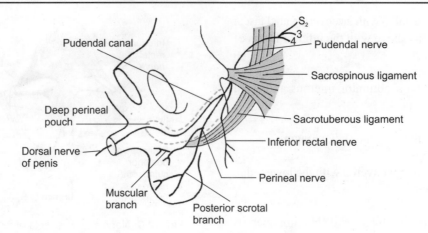

Fig. 10.9: The pudendal canal and deep perineal pouch with the course and branches of pudendal nerve

CLINICAL APPLICATION

- The ischiorectal pads of fat support the lower end of the rectum and anal canal. Loss of fat due to wasting diseases may lead to **prolapse of rectum**.
- There is great tendency of the ischiorectal fat to get infected due to poor blood supply thereby forming an **ischiorectal abscess**. The infection from one fossa spreads to the opposite side behind the anal canal above the sphincter ani externus (**"horseshoe" abscess**).
- The pudendal nerve may be injected with local anaesthetic solution through a needle passed up just medial to the ischial tuberosity where it crosses the ischial spine **(pudendal block)** to anaesthetize the perineum e.g., during the second stage of labour.
- Infection from the lining of anal canal may track through its wall into the ischiorectal fossa and may open through the skin on the surface at the side of the anus. This results in a condition known as **fistula-in-ano**.

UROGENITAL TRIANGLE

Skeletal Framework

The muscular and fascial attachments of the ischiopubic ramus is the key for the study of the urogenital triangle of the perineum (Fig. 10.10).

The ischiopubic ramus has external and internal surface and lateral and medial borders. The medial border along with the corresponding part of the other hip bone, forms the lateral boundaries of the urogenital triangle (Fig. 10.1). The lateral border forms the obturator foramen.

- Medial border gives attachment to:
  - Fascia lata (deep fascia) of the thigh.
  - Superficial fascia of the perineum.
- Internal surface is divisible into three areas by faint lines which are not easily discernible in every bone:
  - **Obturator internus** arises from the area adjoining the lateral border.
  - The faint ridge at the medial limit of the origin of obturator internus gives attachment to **obturator fascia and the superior fascia of the urogenital diaphragm.**
  - A second ridge extending from the medial margin of the ischial tuberosity to the lower limit of the symphyseal surface of the body of pubis gives attachment to the **falciform process of the sacrotuberous ligament posteriorly** and the **inferior fascia of the urogenital diaphragm** (perineal membrane) anteriorly.
- The medial border of the ischiopubic ramus as it is traced backwards, encroaches on the internal surface and meets the faint ridge giving attachment to the **perineal membrane**. Thus, the superficial fascia of the perineum fuses posteriorly with the perineal membrane. The area encloses between the two is the region of the **superficial perineal pouch**. It gives origin to the **ischiocavernosus** and **superficial transversus perenie** muscles posteriorly and is related to the **crus of penis** or **clitoris anteriorly**.
- The attachments of the superior and inferior layers of the urogenital diaphragm also fuse but more in front of

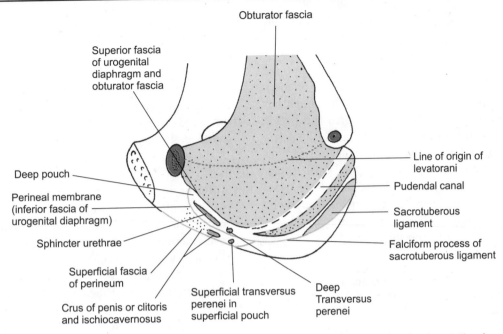

Fig. 10.10: Facial and muscular attachments of ischiopubic ramus which is the key for the study of perineum

the fusion for the superficial pouch. The area enclosed is the region of the **deep perineal pouch**. It gives origin to the sphincter urethrae and **deep transversus perenei muscles**.

Pouches of Urogenital Triangle

In the urogenital region, a muscular shelf stretches between the conjoint ischiopubic rami of the two sides; this is the urogenital diaphragm which serves as a foundation for the attachment of external genitalia. Three fascial layers attached to the conjoint ischiopubic ramus define two spaces (pouches) of considerable anatomic and clinical importance (Fig. 10.11).

- Superior fascia of urogenital diaphragm.
- Inferior fascia of urogenital diaphragm (perineal membrane).
- Superficial perineal fascial (of **Colle's**) which is the continuation of superficial fascia of the anterior abdominal wall (**Scarpa's fascia**). The space between the superior and inferior fascia of urogenital diaphragm is the **deep perineal pouch**. Both fascial layers of the

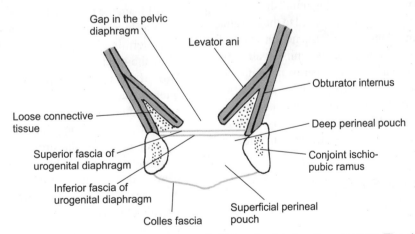

Fig. 10.11: Schematic transverse section through the urogenital triangle showing the pouches. The deficiency in the levator ani is compensated by the urogenital diaphragm

deep pouch are attached on either side to the ischiopubic rami. Anteriorly they are fused a short distance behind the pubic symphysis (Fig. 10.12).

Posteriorly also they fuse and are incorporated centrally in the perineal body. This pouch is a closed space. The central part of the roof of the pouch lies immediately below the anterior gap in the pelvic diaphragm and therefore immediately below the pelvic cavity. Lateral to this it is related to the anterior margins of the levator ani muscles (Fig. 10.12). Still further laterally, it forms the floor of a loose connective tissue space bordered medially by levator ani and laterally by the obturator internus. These spaces are continuous posteriorly with the ischiorectal fossae.

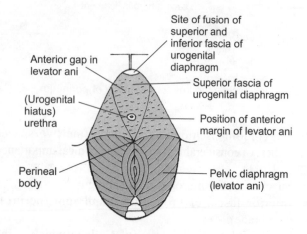

Fig. 10.12: The gap is the pelvic diaphragm as seen from the perineal aspect

The superficial perineal fascia (Colle's) is attached to the back of the inferior fascia of urogenital diaphragm (perineal membrane). Laterally, it is attached to the margins of the ischiopubic rami. Anteriorly it ascends in front of the pubic symphysis onto the anterior abdominal wall. This space between the Colle's fascia and the perineal membrane is the superficial perineal pouch. This pouch has no anterior wall and its anterior part is continuous through the interval between the deep pouch and the pubic symphysis and then through the anterior gap in the pelvic diaphragm with the pelvic cavity.

Pudendal Nerves (S$_2$ to S$_4$)

Course (Fig. 10.9)

Pudendal nerve, a branch of sacral plexus leaves the pelvis between piriformis and coccygeus muscles through the

lower part of the greater sciatic foramen and enters the gluteal region, crossing the sacropinous ligament close to its attachment to the ischial spine, being situated on the medial side of the internal pudendal vessels which lie on the ischial spine itself. It accompanies the internal pudendal artery through the lesser sciatic formamen into the pudendal canal on the lateral wall of the ischiorectal fossa (Fig. 10.9).

Branches (Figs. 10.9 and 10.13)

- **Inferior rectal nerve** is given off in the posterior part of the pudendal canal by piercing its medial wall. It crosses the ischiorectal fossa and supplies the sphincter and externus and the skin around the anus (Fig. 10.8).
- **Perineal nerve** is the inferior and larger terminal branch. It runs forward below the internal pudendal artery and accompanies the perineal artery. It divides into the following branches:
  - **Posterior scrotal (or labial) branches:** They are two, medial and lateral, which pierce or pass superficial to the inferior fascia of the urogenital diaphragm (perineal membrane) and run forward along the lateral part of the urogenital triangle in company with the scrotal branches of the perineal artery. They supply the skin of the posterior part of the scrotum or labium majus and communicate with the perineal branch of the posterior cutaneous nerve of the thigh and with the inferior rectal nerve. In the female they are known as posterior labial branches and supply the labium majus.
  - **Muscular branches** are distributed to the muscles in the superficial and deep perineal pouches and the anterior part of external sphincter and levator ani. A branch termed the nerve to the urethral bulb, is given off from the nerve to bulbospongiosus; it pierces this muscle and supplies the corpus spongiosum penis, its terminal fibres ending in the mucous membrane of the urethra.
- **Dorsal nerve of the penis** runs forward above the internal pudendal artery along the ramus of the ischium and accompanies the artery along the margin of the inferior ramus of the pubis on the deep surface of the inferior fascia of the urogenital diaphragm (perineal membrane). It gives a branch to the corpus cavernosum penis and at the apex of the membrane, passes through the lateral part of the gap between the structure and the lateral pubic ligament. It then runs forward, in company with the dorsal artery of the penis, between the layers of the suspensory ligament, to the dorsum of the penis and ends in the glans penis.

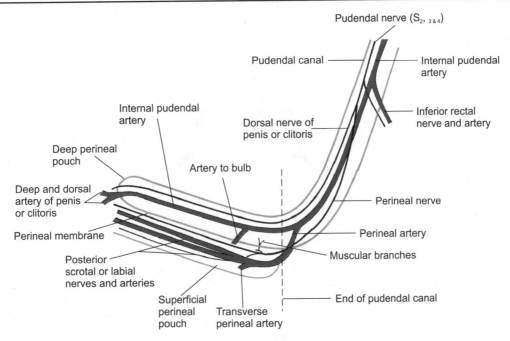

Fig. 10.13: Pudendal nerve and internal pudendal artery : Course and branches

In the female the corresponding nerve is very small, and supplies the clitoris.

The Internal Pudendal Artery (Fig. 10.13)

The internal pudendal artery is the smaller of the two terminal branches of the anterior division of the internal iliac artery. It leaves the pelvis between the ventral rami of S_3 and S_4 nerves. It exits through the greater sciatic foramen below the piriformis in company with the pudendal nerve. It follows a similar course to the nerve and gives off the following branches:

- **Inferior rectal artery** which accompanies the corresponding nerve to supply the lower part of the rectum and anal canal.
- **Perineal artery** is given off the internal pudendal artery near the anterior end of the pudendal canal. After giving off the **transverse perineal branch** which courses medially along the superficial transversus perenei muscle, divides into **medial** and **lateral scrotal** or **labial branches**.
- **Artery to the bulb** is given off in the deep perineal pouch. It pierces the perineal membrane to enter the bulb.
- **Deep artery of the penis or clitoris,** after piercing the perineal membrane, pierces the medial side of the crus and runs in the centre of the substance of the corpus spongiosum to supply it.

- **Dorsal artery of penis or clitoris** which after piecing the anterior part of the perineal membrane runs onto the dorsum of the penis or clitoris lying medial to the nerve.

MALE UROGENITAL TRIANGLE

Contents of Deep Pouch (Figs.10.14 and 10.15)

The contents of the deep pouch in the male are:
- Membranous part of urethra.
- Sphincter urethrae and deep transversus perenei.
- Two bulbourethral glands.
- Dorsal nerve of penis.
- Internal pudendal artery.
  - **Membranous part** of the urethra is continuous with the prostatic urethra through the superior fascia of urogenital diaphragm and with the penile urethra through the inferior fascia of the urogenital diaphragm (perineal membrane). It is a short segment and is the least distensible and narrowest part of the urethra.
  - **Sphincter urethrae** muscle surrounds the membranous urethra. It is attached laterally to the ischiopubic rami and passes medially to surround the membranous urethra. It is a voluntary muscle supplied by a muscular branch of the perineal nerve. It can be contracted voluntarily to interrupt micturition and is involved in expelling the last drops

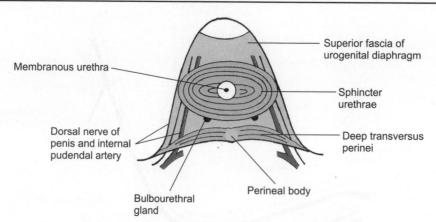

Fig. 10.14: The muscle of the deep pouch in the male

of urine. Note that the sphincter mechanism at the internal urethral orifice is involuntary.

- **Deep transversus perinei** muscles posterior to the sphincter pass from the rami of the ischium to midline where they are attached to the perineal body.
- **Bulbourethral glands** are two round glands, about 1 cm in diameter, which are embedded in the sphincter urethrae on each side of the membranous urethra. The single ducts of the glands pierce the perineal membrane, enter the bulb of the penis and open into the floor of the penile urethra. They secrete a small part of the seminal fluid (Fig. 10.15).
- **Dorsal nerve of penis** enters the pouch from the pudendal canal and runs forward along its bony lateral wall. It gives a branch to the corpus cavernosum penis, and then passes through the lateral part of the gap between the apex of the perineal membrane and the inferior pubic ligament. It then passes between the layers of the suspensory ligament, to the dorsum of the penis and ends in the glans penis (Figs. 10.15 and 10.16).

- **The internal pudendal artery** follows the dorsal nerve of penis into the deep pouch. It ends as three penile branches viz., bulbar, deep and dorsal, all of which pierce the perineal membrane to reach the penis in the superficial pouch (Fig. 10.16).

Contents of Superficial Pouch

The contents of the superficial pouch in the male are:
- Crura of the penis.
- Ischiocavernosus muscle covering the crura medially.
- Bulb of the penis containing the proximal part of the penile urethra.
- Bulbospongiosus muscle covering the bulb of the penis.
- Superficial transversus perenei muscle.
- Posterial scrotal branches of the perineal nerve.

The superficial fascia of the urogenital triangle **(Colle's fascia)** envelops the penis and sacrotum anteriorly and ascends in front of the pubic symphysis onto the anterior abdominal wall to become continuous with the membranous layer **(Scarpa's fascia)**. The superficial pouch has no structural anterior wall. Its anterior limit is arbitrarily regarded as being situated below the

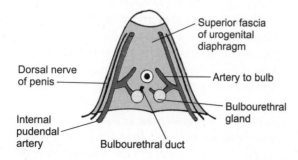

Fig. 10.15: The vessels and the nerves of the deep pouch in the male

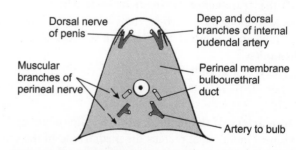

Fig. 10.16: The perineal membrane (inferior fascia of urogenital diaphragm) and the structures passing through

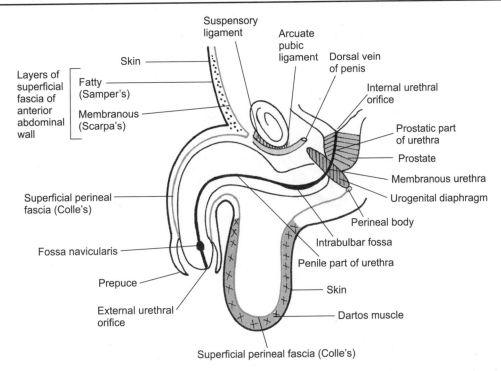

Fig. 10.17: The superficial fascia of the male urogenital diaphragm (Colle's fascia) and the parts of male urethra

pubic symphysis and beyond this it is directly continuous with the scrotum (Fig. 10.17).

- **Two corpora cavernosa** lie against the ischiopubic rami and gradually converge and come into contact below the pubic symphysis (Fig. 10.18).
- The single **corpus spongiosum** is situated in the midline, attached to the under surface of the perineal membrane. Posteriorly it ends in an expansion called the bulb of the penis, while anteriorly it comes to lie in the ventral groove between the corpora cavernosa. The ducts of the

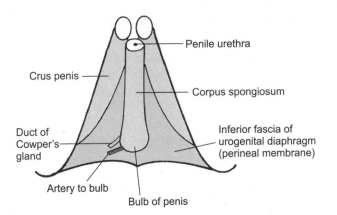

Fig. 10.18: Male organs of the superficial pouch after the reflection of the muscles

bulbourethral glands perforate the perineal membrane to enter the bulb of the penis. The bulbar arteries also enter the bulb after piercing the perineal membrane (Fig. 10.18).

- **The ischiocavernosus arises** from the corresponding ramus of the ischium to sweep over the crus of the penis and gain insertion into it. The two muscles help in the mechanism of erection of the penis by stopping the venous return (Fig. 10.19).
- **The bulbospongiosus** takes origin from median raphe on the inferior aspect of the corpus spongiosum. The fibres sweep dorsally to be inserted onto the corpus. These muscles help to empty the urethra of residual urine or semen. They also assist in the erection of penis (Fig. 10.19).
- **The superficial transversus perenei muscles** consist of two small slips arising from the ramus of the ischium on each side. They run transversely to be inserted into the perineal body which is a midline fibromuscular structure. They help to fix the perineal body and thus help to support the pelvic viscera (Fig. 10.19).
- **The perineal branch of the pudendal nerve** enters the superficial pouch by piercing the membranous layer of superficial perineal fascia close to its posterior

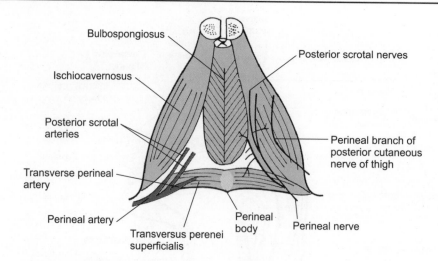

Fig. 10.19: Muscles, nerves and arteries of the superficial pouch in the male

attachment on each side. It divides into posterior scrotal nerves and muscular branches to all the muscles of the superficial and deep pouch. A branch, termed the **nerve to the urethral bulb** is given off from the nerve to the bulbospongiosus, it supplies the corpus spongiosum penis. The posterior cutaneous nerve of the thigh sends perineal branches to the skin of the perineum (Fig. 10.19).

- **The perineal branch of the internal pudendal artery** is given off in the vicinity of the posterior margin of the urogenital diaphragm and enters the superficial pouch. It almost immediately divides into transverse perineal and posterior scrotal branches which supply the subcutaneous tissue of the scrotum (Fig. 10.19).

THE MALE EXTERNAL GENITALIA

These include penis and scrotum. The scrotum contains the testes and the beginning of ductus deferens. The urethra runs longitudinally in the penis.

PENIS

The penis is the male copulatory organ. It is meant for the passage of both urine and the semen to the exterior.

Part (Fig. 10.20)

It has two parts:

- **Root of penis** is the fixed part and consists of two crurae one on each side and a bulb. They are made of erectile tissue and are attached to the inferior surface of the perineal membrane. They are situated in the superficial perineal pouch.

- **Body (shaft)** which is free cylindrical and pendulous measuring 7.5 cm to 10 cm in length. It consists of three parts, the two corpora cavernosa situated dorsally and corpus spongiosum lying ventrally and containing the penile urethra. The anterior end of corpus spongiosum is expanded dorsally and hollowed out of form the **glans,** a conical cop fitting over the blunt ends of corpora cavernosa.

Coverings (Fig. 10.21)

- **Skin:**
  - The skin is thin, delicate, dark and hairless. It is loosely connected to the underlying fascia, so as to allow free movement of the skin over the fascia. It is folded upon itself to form a hood over the glans called the **prepuce** (foreskin). The inner layer of the prepuce is continuous with the skin covering the glans at the neck of the penis. A triangular median sagittal septum called the **frenulum** stretches between the inner layer of the prepuce and the under surface of the glans. It contains small blood vessels which are apt to bleed when the prepuce is excised in the operation of circumcision.

The prepuce is a retractable fold of skin and the space between it and the glans is the **preputial sac.** There are preputial glands in the skin of the corona glandis, they secrete the smegma which collects in the preputial sac.

Beneath the skin in the midline is the superficial dorsal vein of the penis.

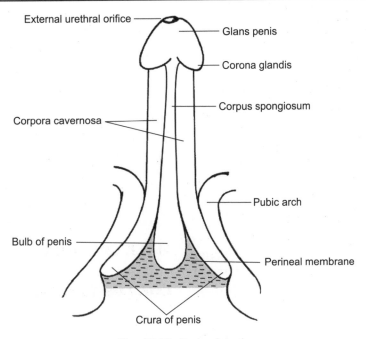

Fig. 10.20: Parts of penis

- **Fascia:**
  - The three corpora fused together are loosely surrounded by the **fascia of the penis (Buck's fascia),** a cylindrical prolongation of Colle's fascia beneath which lies the midline deep dorsal vein with a dorsal artery on each side and more laterally a dorsal nerve. Colle's fascia is the continuation into the perineum of the membranous layer of superficial fascia of the anterior abdominal wall **(Scarpa's fascia).**

Ligament of Penis

There are two ligaments:
- **Fundiform ligament:** It is sling of Scarpa's fascia which starts from the linea alba, splits to enclose the root of the penis and finally it is attached to the median raphe of the scrotum.
- **Suspensory ligament:** It is triangular in shape. Its base is attached to the front of the symphysis pubis while the apex is attached to the fascia of penis (Fig. 10.17).

Structures (Fig. 10.20)

- **Corpora cavernosa:** The anterior three-fourths of these two dorsal masses is composed of erectile tissue each contained in a strong fibrous capsule known as **tunica albuginea.** Proximally, the capsules of the adjacent sides of the corpora form a complete septum penis but distally the septum is incomplete. Posterior one-fourth of each corpus diverges as the **crus of the penis** which serves as attachment of the penis to the ischiopubic rami.
- **Corpus spongiosum:** This contains the urethra and has two expansions:

  Glans: It is a conical tip that forms the cap over corpora. The **corona glandis** is the widest, proximal portion.

  Bulb: It is the proximal enlargement entered by the urethra.

Arterial Supply (Fig. 10.21)

The arteries come from the internal pudendal artery.
- **Dorsal arteries** pierce the urogenital diaphragm, pass through the suspensory ligament to lie on either side of the deep dorsal vein beneath **Buck's fascia.**
- **Deep arteries** pierce urogenital diaphragm and enter the crura to run in the centre of corpora cavernosa.
- **Artery to bulb** pierces the urogenital diaphragm to enter the bulb of corpus spongiosum.

Venous Drainage (Fig. 10.21)

All the veins begin in the cavernous space of the erectile tissue.

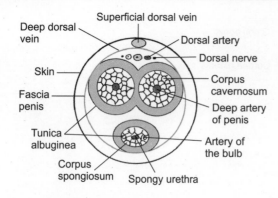

Fig. 10.21: The coverings of penis

- **Superficial dorsal vein** is a single vein which drains the prepuce and the skin, lies in the superficial fascia of the penis. It goes either to the right or the left to drain into the superficial external pudendal vein.
- **Deep dorsal vein** is also a single vein draining the erective tissue. It runs under the deep fascia **(Buck's),** between dorsal arteries, passes through the suspensory ligament enters the pelvis through the gap between the inferior pubic ligament and transverse perineal ligament. It drains into the prostatic venous plexus.

Lymphatic Drainage

- Excepting the glans the lymph vessels of penis drain into the medial group of **superficial inguinal nodes**.
- Glans drains into the **deep inguinal lymph nodes** (Cloquet's gland) and **external iliac nodes**.

Nerve Supply

Somatic

- **Dorsal nerve of penis,** a branch of the pudendal nerve, supplies the skin of the penis.
- **Perineal branch of pudenda nerve** supplies the ischiocavernosus and bulbospongiosus muscles.
- **Ilioinguinal nerve** (L_1) supplies the skin over the root of penis.

Autonomic

- **Parasympathetic:** Pelvic splanchnic (S_2 to S_4) are vasomotor and cause vasodilation of the arteries of the corpora producing engorgement of the cavernous spaces. This engorgement presses on the veins and prevents emptying of the spaces thereby causing erection of the penis.

- **Sympathetic:** From superior and inferior hypogastric plexuses (L_1) are vasoconstrictor. After ejaculation the parasympathetic stimulation ceases and with sympathetic stimulation producing vasoconstriction of the arteries the cavernous spaces empty and the erected penis returns to the flaccid state.

The sympathetic nerves are necessary for the initial stages of ejaculation. Ejaculation is also assisted by a rhythmic contraction of bulbospongiosum muscle which compresses the penile urethra and expels the semen. As bulbospongiosus has somatic nerve supply (pudendal nerve), so in ejaculation this nerve supply is also involved.

MALE URETHRA

Extent and Parts (Fig. 10.17)

The male urethra extends from the **internal urethral orifice** at the bladder neck to the **external urethral orifice** at the tip of the glans penis. It is about 20 cm in length. It is S-shaped, when the penis is hanging and has three parts which are:
- **Prostatic urethra** is the part lying within the prostate. It is about 3 cm in length and is the widest and most dilatable part of urethra. Its internal features have already been described with the prostate (Fig. 9.30).
- **Membranous urethra** is the shortest (1.25 cm), narrowest and least dilatable portion. It is so called because it lies between the two membranes i.e., superior and inferior fascia of the urogenital diaphragm. It pierces the inferior fascia (perineal membrane) 2.5 cm below and behind symphysis pubis and at once reaches the posterior part of superior surface of the bulb of corpus spongiosum which lies in contact with the membrane. It is surrounded by the sphincter urethrae muscle with a bulbourethral gland on either side of it.
- **Spongy** or **penile urethra** is the longest part measuring about 15 cm. It is so called as it lies in the corpus spongiosum penis and hence partly in the superficial pouch and partly in the body of the penis. It extends from the end of the membranous part to the external urethral orifice, which is the narrowest point in the urethral passage.

In its course it first ascends upwards and forwards in the superficial pouch upto the front of the lower part of the pubic symphysis and then descends down in the flaccid condition of the penis (Fig. 10.17). It shows two dilatations.

- **Intrabulbar fossa** lies in the bulb of the penis. Its floor is dilated but not the roof so that in cross-section it looks like a trapezium.
- **Fossa navicularis** lies within the glans.

In cross-section the lumen of the spongy urethra presents a transverse slit in the middle, but a vertical slit in the end.

Internal Features (Fig. 10.22)

- Internal features of the prostatic part have already been described.
- **Membranous part:** The interior presents no special features.
- Spongy or penile part presents the following features :
    - **Openings of small urethral glands (Littre's)** along its entire length.
    - **Openings of the ducts of bulbourethral glands** about 2.5 cm below the perineal membrane.
    - A number of pit-like depressions called **urethral lacunae** also open here.

Sphincter of Urethra

The urethra is surrounded by two sphincters:

- **Internal sphincter (sphincter vesicae),** which surrounds the bladder neck above the openings of the ejaculatory ducts. The muscle fibres are smooth, involuntary and innervated by the autonomic nerves from the vesical plexus.
- **External sphincter (sphincter urethrae),** which is situated in the deep perineal pouch, the muscle fibres are striated and innervated by the pudendal nerve (S_2 to S_4).

Arterial Supply

- Part above the opening of the ejaculatory ducts is supplied by inferior vesical, middle rectal and internal pudendal arteries.
- Rest of the part by the urethral branches of internal pudendal.

Venous Drainage

- Veins corresponding to arteries.

Lymphatic Drainage

- Prostatic and membranous part drain into internal and external iliac nodes.
- Spongy part into superficial and deep inguinal nodes.

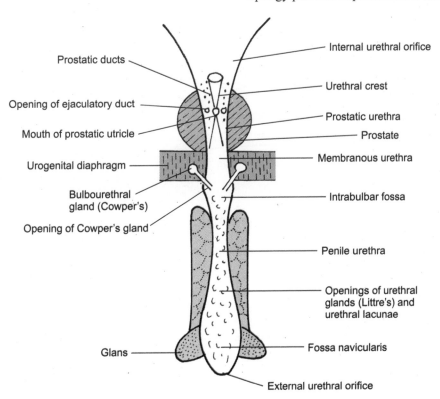

Fig. 10.22: Interior of male urethra seen straightened and laid open

CLINICAL APPLICATION

- The membranous part of urethra is short (1-2 cm long) and is relatively thin walled. Except for the external urethral meatus, this is also the narrowest and least distensible portion due to the tone of the surrounding sphincter urethrae muscle. Due to above factors and also due to the sharp angle between the penile and membranous portions, the membranous urethra is most likely to be ruptured by injury or passage of a catheter. The damage can occur above or below the urogenital diaphragm.
- If the damage is above the diaphragm, extravasation of urine is intrapelvic and extraperitoneal.
- If the damage is below the diaphragm, extravasations is within the superficial perineal pouch, with possible extension into the scrotum beneath the dartos muscle into the penis, superficial to Buck's fascia and up into the anterior abdominal wall beneath the Scarpa's fascia.
- Damage to penile urethra may result in extravasation of urine. The course taken by the urine will be as follows:
- If the Buck's fascia is not damaged, extravasation will be deep to this fascia.

- If the Buck's fascia is damaged, extravasation will be between the Buck's fascia and superficial penial fascia, with possible extension beneath the Colle's fascia into the superficial perineal pouch, beneath the dartos layer into the sacrotum and beneath the Scarpa's fascia up into the anterior abdominal wall.
- Introduction of instruments into the male urethra is done with care with the penis straightened into an approximately erect position, so that the angle between the membranous and penile part is made less acute.

SCROTUM

The scrotum is a bag of skin containing the testes and spermatic cords. It is usually divided into two halves by a spetum.

Layers

When the gubernaculum testis descends through the anterior abdominal wall to be attached to that part of skin which will form scrotum, it takes prolongation of each layer of the abdominal wall to form different layers of the scrotum. These layers are (Fig. 10.23):

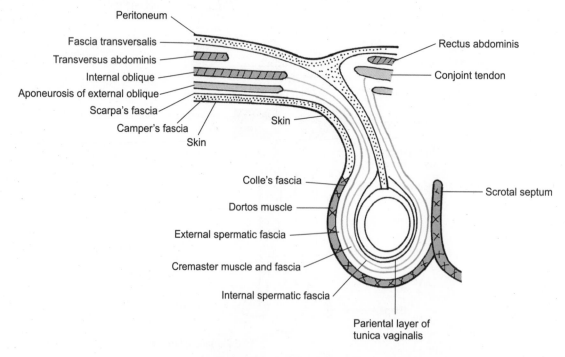

Fig. 10.23: Layers of scrotum

- **Skin** which is usually wrinkled and somewhat pigmented. It has hairs and sebaceous and sweat glands. Inferiorly there is a midline raphe continuous anteriorly with the raphe of the penis and posteriorly with that of the perineum.
- **Subcutaneous tissue containing the dartos muscle** but no fat. **Dartos muscle** is a part of panniculus cavernous and is nonstriped. It causes wrinkling of the scrotal skin. It is supplied by sympathetic fibres which reach by way of the genital branch of genitofemoral nerve. The muscle goes into contraction by cold or stroking.
- **Superficial fascia (Colle's fascia)** continuous with the superficial fascia of the penis and the perineum. In front it is continuous with Scarpa's fascia of the anterior abdominal wall.
- **The three fascial layers of the spermatic cord** spread out and line the scrotum (Fig. 10.24):
  - External spermatic fascia dragged down as part of the external oblique aponeurosis.
  - Cremaster muscle and fascia are prolongations of the internal oblique and transversus abdominis.
  - Internal spermatic fascia is the prolongation of the fascia transversalis beyond the deep ring.

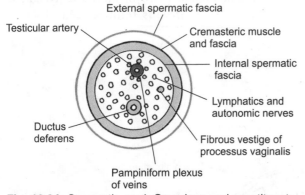

Fig. 10.24: Spermatic cord: Coverings and constituents

- **Parieteal layer of tunica vaginalis** dragged down by the gubernaculum.

The septum of the scrotum consists of all the layers except the skin.

Arterial Supply

- Superficial and deep external pudendal arteries from the femoral supply the anterior aspect.
- Scrotal branches from the internal pudendal and cremasteric branch of the inferior epigastric artery supply the posterior aspect.

Venous Drainage

- Veins correspond to the arteries and drain into the great saphenous vein.

Lymphatic Drainage

- Medial group of superficial inguinal nodes.

Nerve Supply (Fig. 10.25)

- Anterior one-third is supplied by the ilioinguinal nerve and the genital branch of the genitofemoral nerve (L_1 spinal segment).
- Posterior two-thirds is supplied by scrotal branches of perineal nerve (S_3 spinal segment) reinforced laterally by the perineal branch of the posterior cutaneous nerve of thigh (S_2 segment).

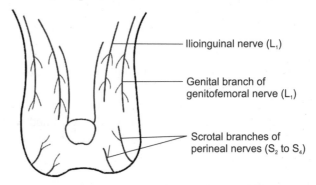

Fig. 10.25: Nerve supply of skin of scrotum

TESTIS

Testis is the male sex gland, one on each side. It is placed obliquely inside the scrotal sac, its upper extremity is tilted forward and laterally, possibly by the pull of the spermatic cord which suspends it from its posteromedial aspect.

Features (Fig. 10.26)

- It is ovoid in shape.
- It is about 4 cm long, 2.5 cm wide and 2 cm thick.
- Each gland has two poles—upper and lower, two borders–anterior and posterior and two surfaces—medial and lateral.

Relations (Fig. 10.26)

- Upper pole is related to the head of the epididymis, which is connected to it by the **efferent tubules of the testis**.
- Lower pole is related to the tail of the epididymis, which is connected to it by fibrous tissue.
- Anterior border is free.

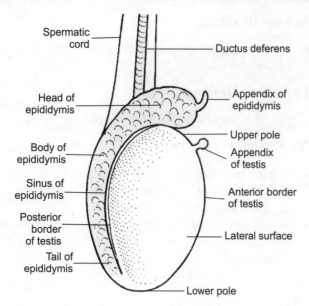

Fig. 10.26: Right testis and epididymis–lateral view

- Posterior border is related to the body of epididymis laterally and ductus deferens medially.
- Between the lateral surface of the testis and the body of the epididymis, there is an elongated cleft lined with visceral layer of tunica vaginalis known as **sinus of epididymis**.

Coverings (Fig. 10.23)

- All the layers of the scrotum.

- **Tunica vaginalis,** which is a serous membrane having a parietal and a visceral layer with a cavity in between (Fig. 10.27).
- Parietal layer lines the scrotum.
- Visceral layer clothes the testis except on the posterior border. It is reflected onto the parietal layer at the postero-medial aspect.
- **Tunica albuginea** a dense fibrous membrane immediately surrounding the testis and forming its coat.
- **Tunica vasculosa** is a vascular coat, consisting of plexus of blood vessels derived from branches of testicular artery, which lines the inner aspect of the tunica albuginea.

Structure (Fig. 10.27)

- At the posterior border of the testis the tunica albuginea projects into its substance forming an incomplete septum called **mediastinum testis**.
- The mediastinum testis contains a number of small channels called the **rete testis** and in addition, it is traversed by blood vessels and lymphatics.
- Numerous fine septa **(septula testis)** radiate from the mediastinum towards tunica albuginea dividing the testis into 2000 to 250 conical compartments **(lobules)**.
- Each lobule contains two or more highly coiled or **convoluted seminiferous tubules** each of which is over 60 cm long.

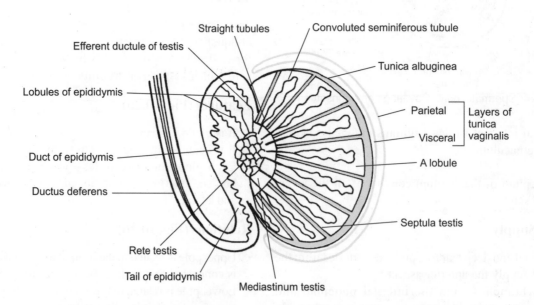

Fig. 10.27: Longitudinal section of testis and epididymis showing their structures

- As the seminiferous tubules approach the mediastinum, they join together to form a smaller number of tubes which finally become straighter to form the **straight seminiferous tubules**.
- The straight seminiferous tubules on entering the mediastinum anastomose to form a network known as **rete testis**.
- The rete testis communicate with the head of the epididymis by means of 15-20 **efferent ductules**.

Arterial Supply

- Testicular artery is a branch of abdominal aorta arising at the level of L_3 vertebra. It lies at the back of testis and from here the branches form the tunica vasculosa (Fig. 10.24).

Venous Drainage

Veins coming out of the testis form the **pampiniform plexus**. Testicular vein starts from the pampiniform plexus.
- Right testicular vein ends in the inferior vena cava.
- Left testicular vein ends in the left renal vein.

Lymphatic Drainage

- Aortic group of lymph nodes receive the lymphatics which run along the testicular artery.

Nerve Supply

The testis is supplied by sympathetic nerves and there is no parasympathetic supply. Sympathetic supply is both motor and sensory.

The preganglionic sympathetic fibres come from T_{10} segment of the spinal cord and travel in the lesser splanchnic nerve to the coeliac ganglion. Postganglionic fibres reach the testis via the testicular artery.

The motor fibres supply the blood vessels and smooth muscle found in the coverings of the testis. Painful sensations resulting from blows or squeezing of the testis run up through the coeliac plexus and lesser splanchnic nerve to cell bodies in posterior ganglion of T_{10} spinal nerve.

Development (Fig. 10.28)

The testis develops on the posterior abdominal wall from the genital ridge situated on the medial side of the mesonephros between the 10th and 12th dorsal segments of the embryo and then descends into the scrotum.

Descent of the Testis (Figs. 10.29 a and b)

The developing testis lies in front of the kidney in the lumbar

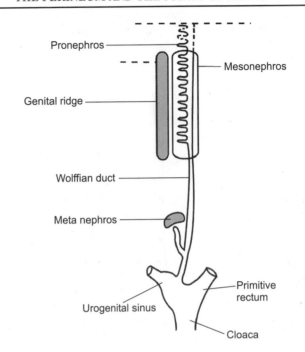

Fig. 10.28: Development of testis from genital ridge

region. It reaches the scrotum as a result of several factors which are:
- Increased intra-abdominal pressure which squeezes it through the inguinal canal.
- **Hormonal factors:** The gonadotrophic hormones of the anterior pituitary bring about the descent.
- Differential growth causing rapid elongation of the parietal peritoneum to which the developing testis is attached and failure of gubernaculum to elongate.
- **Gubernaculum testis:** It is a fibromuscular cord stretching from the lower end of the testis to the genital swelling where scrotum is developing. The testis is pulled down to the scrotum through the inguinal canal by the active contraction of the gubernaculum and is also controlled in its final stages by testosterone and maternal gonadotrophin.

The chronology of testicular descent is as follow:
- In third month, it descends from loin to iliac fossa.
- From the fourth to seventh month it rests at the deep inguinal ring.
- During the seventh month it travels through the inguinal canal.
- In the eighth month it lies at the superficial inguinal ring.
- In the ninth month or afterbirth it enters the scrotum to reach its base.

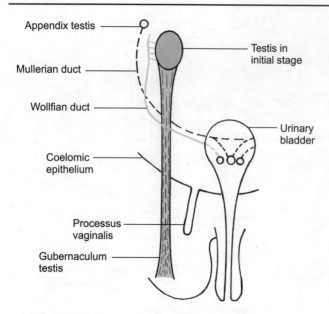

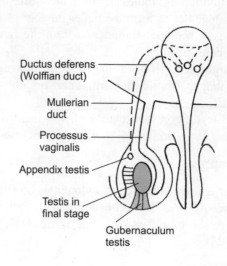

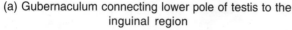

(a) Gubernaculum connecting lower pole of testis to the inguinal region

(b) Shift of the testis into the scrotum due to changes in the gubernaculum.

Fig. 10.29: The descend of testis

A diverticulum of the coelomic epithelium, called the **processus vaginalis** follows the path of the gubernaculum and invades the anterior abdominal wall forming the inguinal canal (Fig. 10.29).

Soon afterbirth, it becomes occluded at the deep inguinal ring and also just above the testis, cutting off the part of the sac in relation to the testis which forms the tunica vaginalis testis. The part of the sac between the two closures is the funicular process, which becomes obliterated, forming a fibrous cord, the rudiment of the processus vaginalis.

EPIDIDYMIS

The epididymis lies along the posterior margin of the testis with the ductus deferens to its medial side. It consists of (Fig. 10.26):
- **Head** which is attached to the upper pole of the testis.
- **Body** which lies along the posterior borders of the testis. The **sinus of epididymis,** a recesses of tunica vaginalis, lies between it and the lateral surface of the testis.
- **Tail,** which is attached to the lower pole of the testis and is continuous as the ductus deferens.

Structure (Fig. 10.27)

It consists of a single tube about six metres long, highly coiled and packed together by fibrous tissue.

The head receives 12-15 **efferent tubules** from the rete testes and is thus firmly attached to the testis. The body and the tail are firmly bound to the testis by fibrous tissue without any communication. In the tail the **duct** of the **epididymis** becomes thicker and straighter and emerges posteriorly at the **ductus deferens** which passes upward behind the epididymis through the scrotal sac to the superficial inguinal ring, where together with blood vessels and lymphatic vessels and nerves, it forms the spermatic cord.

Blood Supply

- A branch of the testicular artery which anastomoses with the artery to the ductus deferens.

Venous and Lymphatic Drainage

- As for the testis.

Nerve Supply

- Only sympathetic fibres from inferior hypogastric plexus supply it.

APPENDAGES OF TESTIS AND EPIDIDYMIS

There are vestigeal structures associated with the epididymis and the upper pole of the testis. They are remnants of mesonephros or the paramesonephric duct. The mesonephric (Wolffian) duct forms the single tube constituting the epididymis and the ductus deferens. It receives the efferent tubules of mesonephros. When mesonephros is replaced by the metanephros and disappears, some of its tubules remain attached to the testis and form the ductuli efferentes while some persist as paragenital tubules (Fig. 10.30 a).

Above and below the epididymis and blind at one or both ends (ductuli aberrantes superior and inferior), these vestiges are named as follows (Fig. 10.30 b):

- **Appendix of epididymis (Hydatid of Morgagni)** is formed by the most cranial ductuli aberrantes superior and sits on the head of the epididymis and is relatively constant.
- **Upper paradidymis (Organ of Giraldes),** formed by several caudal tiny tubules, lies at the lower end of the spermatic cord above the epididymis.
- **Lower paradidymis (Vas aberrans of Haller)** is a blind tube, which lies between the tail of the epididymis and commencement of the vas. Several of these tubules may exist. They are derived from inferior aberrant ductules.

The paramesonephric (Mullerian) duct disappears in the male except at its two ends which form:
- **Appendix testis** is formed by the upper end and sits on the upper pole of the testis (Fig. 10.30 a).
- **Prostatic utricle (uterus masculinus)** is formed by the conjoined lower ends of the two Mullerian ducts and opens in the prostatic part of urethra.

CLINICAL APPLICATION

- A patent processus vaginalis predisposes to **indirect (congenital) inguinal henia**.
- Partial occlusion of a processus vaginalis can result in fluid accumulation, **hydrocele,** which cannot be distinguished from a hernia or incompletely descended testis.
- Compression of the testicular vessels, as occurs in **torsion of testis,** leads to ischaemic necrosis of the testis within six hours leading to the loss of the testis.
- The pampiniform plexus is frequently affected by **varicocele** (dilation of veins) which are mostly on the left side. This is due to compression of the left testicular vein by the faeces loaded sigmoid colon.
- Pain originating in the testes is referred to the middle and lower abdominal wall as the afferent fibres travel to the spinal cord along the sympathetic pathways parallel to the testicular vessels. These then pass through the aorticorenal plexus, thence along the lesser and least splanchnic nerves to T_{10} to T_{12} spinal segments, as well as along the lumbar splanchnic nerves to L_1-L_2 spinal segments. The middle and lower abdominal wall has the same dermatomes.
- The testis may fail to descend **(cryptorchidism)** and may rest anywhere along its course in the abdomen, within the inguinal canal at the superficial ring or high in the scrotum (Fig. 10.31). Descend does not occur after the infant is one year old.

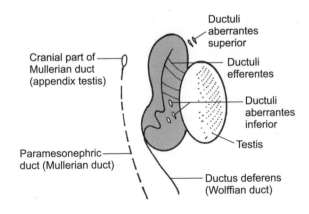

(a) The paragenital tubules.

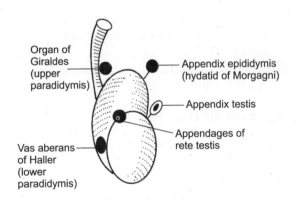

(b) Appendages of testis and epididymis.

Fig. 10.30: Vestigeal structure associated with testis and epididymis

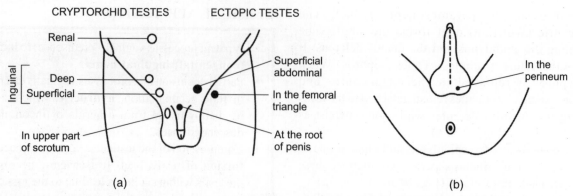

Fig. 10.31: (a) Common positions of cryptorchid testes (incomplete descent) and (b) of ectopic testes (maldescent) —in the perineum

- Occasionally the testis descends, but into an unusual **(ectopic)** position by deviation from the normal line of descend. An ectopic testis is always one which has successfully completed its intra-abdominal descent and has negotiated the inguinal canal and superficial ring. It is usually fully developed and may lie at the following sites (Fig. 10.31).
- Superficial abdominal after coming out of the superficial ring, it lies on the external oblique aponeurosis beneath the Scarpa's fascia.
- In front of the pubic at the root of penis.
- In the perineum.
- In the femoral triangle in the upper thigh.
- When the testis remains intra-abdominal spermatogenesis usually incomplete and the organ is more liable to malignant change.
- Pain originating in the epididymis, such as that accompanying epididymitis, is referred to the distribution of (S_2 to S_4) spinal segments, since the afferent nerves travel to these segment via nerve erigents.

FEMALE UROGENITAL TRIANGLE

Contents of the Deep Pouch

The contents of the deep perineal pouch are similar to those of the male except that the vagina traverses it in addition to the urethra.

- The deep muscles which are less well-defined than in the male (Fig. 10.32).
- Between the vagina and the anal canal is the perineal body which is much important in the female as the weight of the pelvic organs, especially the uterus is indirectly supported by it.

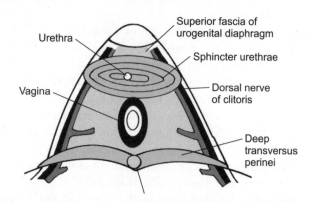

Fig. 10.32: Muscles and nerves of the deep perineal pouch in the female

- The inferior fascia of the urogenital diaphragm (perineal membrane) is wider than in the male, but weaker, since it is pierced in addition by the vagina, and gives no median support to the clitoris. It is pierced by (Fig. 10.33):
- Artery to the bulb of the vestibule on each side of the vagina.
- The internal pudendal artery and dorsal nerve of clitoris more anteriorly on each side.
- Small branches of the perineal nerves to the urogenital diaphragm.
- Duct of the greater vestibular gland behind the vagina, from below upwards.
- There is no structure corresponding to the bulbourethral gland of the male in the deep perineal pouch of the female.

Contents of the Superficial Pouch

The superficial perineal pouch is poorly demarcated due to the passage of vagina in the centre and urethra in front of it. Its contents are:

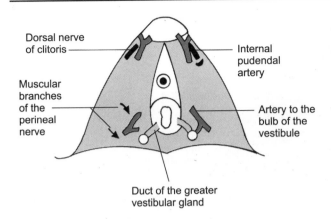

Fig. 10.33: Structures piercing the perineal membrane in the female

- Crura of clitoris.
- Vestibular bulbs.
- Greater vestibular glands (Bartholin's).
- Three pairs of muscles: Ischiocavernosus, bulbospongiosus and superficial transversus perenei.
- Labial vessels and nerve, dorsal and deep artery and dorsal nerve of clitoris.

Crura of Clitoris (Fig. 10.34)

The corpora cavernosa, paired bodies of vascular erectile tissue lie along the ischiopubic rami. They fuse to form the body of the clitoris and are homologous to the male corpora cavernosa.

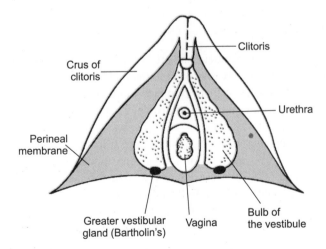

Fig. 10.34: Female superficial perineal pouch showing components of clitoris

Bulbs of the Vestibule (Fig. 10.34)

They are paired masses of vascular erectile tissue on the lateral sides of the vaginal wall under the labia minora, which they tend to spread and open the vaginal introitus. They are united in front of the urethral orifice to form the **commissure of the vestibule**. They are homologous to the fused halves of the bulb of the penis in the male.

- **Greater vestibular glands (Bartholin's):** These mucous glands are small rounded bodies lying beneath the posterior expanded ends of the bulbs of the vestibule. Their ducts open into the vestibule of the vagina. They are homologous to the bulbourethral glands in the male.
- The three paired muscles are similar to those seen in the male (Fig. 10.35):
- **Ischiocavernosus** lies over the clitoral crura. Each arises from the medial side of the ischial tuberosity and ischial ramus and is inserted into the margin of the pubic arch and into the crus of the clitoris.
- **Bulbospongiosus muscle** overlies the vestibular bulb. Each arises from the anterior portion of the perineal body. The medial fibres attach to the deep fascia of the dorsum of clitoris and the lateral one attach to the perineal membrane.
- **Superficial transversus perenei** arises from the anterior portion of the ischial tuberosity and is inserted into the perineal body which it stabilizes.
- The arteries of the superficial pouch come from the internal pudendal artery (Fig. 10.35).
- **Transverse perineal branch** runs parallel to the superficial transversus perineal muscle and gives off bulbar arteries, which supply the vestibule and erectile tissues of the bulb of the vestibule.
- **Posterial labial arteries** supply the posterior portion of the vulva.
- **Deep artery of the clitoris** is located within the corpora cavernosa and supplies its erectile tissue.
- **Dorsal artery of the clitoris** supplies its superficial aspect. It lies between the deep fascia of the clitoris and the tunica albuginea.
- The veins of the superficial pouch parallel the arteries with one exception which is:
- **Deep dorsal vein of the clitoris.** It passes between the arcuate and transverse ligaments of the urogenital diaphragm to drain into the vaginal venous plexus. The merging of the inferior and superior fascia of the urogenital diaphragm anteriorly forms the **transverse ligament**.

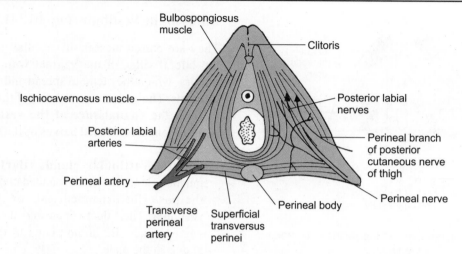

Fig. 10.35: Muscles, arteries and nerves of the superficial perineal pouch in the female

- The nerves of the superficial pouch come from the pudendal nerve and posterior cutaneous nerve of thigh (Fig. 10.35).
- **Posterior labial branches** supply the skin of the labia majora and minora.
- **Perineal branch** of the pudendal nerve supplies the muscles.
- **Perineal branches of the posterior cutaneous nerve of thigh** supply the posterolateral region.
- The lymphatics drain to the superficial inguinal nodes.

THE FEMALE EXTERNAL GENITALIA

The female external genitalia form the **vulva** or **female pudendum** and extend from the front of the **pubus** to the perineal body. The vagina opens externally in this region into the vestibule of the vagina. The vulva is the most obvious feature of the urogenital triangle.

- **The mons pubis** is the prominence in front of the symphysis pubis and is due to the underlying subcutaneous fat. At puberty the mons become covered with coarse hair which has a crescentic upper border just superior to symphysis.
- **The labia majora** are two folds of hairy skin, each supported by underlying fat pads. They define the boundaries of the pudendal cleft and over the symphysis pubis blend to form the **anterior commissure**. Across the midline anterior to the anus a fold connects the labia majora to form the **posterior commissure**.
- **The labia minora** are two small hairless folds located between the labia majora on either side of the space known as the **vestibule**.

Anteriorly each labium minora divides into a lateral and medial part. The lateral parts fuse superior to the clitoris to form the **prepuce of the clitoris,** while the medial parts fuse inferior to the clitoris to form the **frenulum of the clitoris**. A transverse fold, the **fourchette (frenulum labiorum)** connects the labia minora posterior to the vagina.

- **The vestibule** is the urogenital sinus bordered by the labia minora, frenulum of the clitoris and fourchette. The **introitus (vaginal opening)** is in the posterior region of the vestibule and is covered incompletely by the **hymen**. The external **urethral orifice** is located anterior to the vaginal opening about 2.5 cm below the glans clitoris.

The **fossa navicularis (vestibular fossa of the vagina)** is the region between the vaginal opening and the fourchette.

- The **greater vestibular glands (Bartholin's)** are a pair of glands in the superficial perineal pouch on either side of the vaginal opening.

They secrete mucus and are homologous to the **bulbo-urethral glands (Cowper's)** in the male.

The **para-urethral glands (Skene's)** open on either side of the external urethral orifice. They are homologous to prostate in the male.

- The **clitoris** is about 2.5 cm long. It has a body and a glans. The body is formed by three bodies of erectile tissue. The two corpora cavernosa fuse to form the body. The vestibular bulbs—two other bodies or erectile tissue unite to form the thread-like commissure of the clitoris, which terminates in an expansion, the glans clitoris. The clitoris is attached to the pubic symphysis by a suspensory ligament.

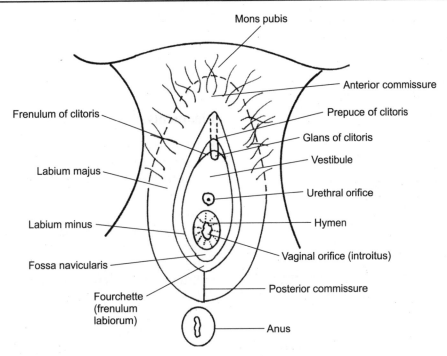

Fig. 10.36: Superficial features of female external genitalia (vulva)

CLINICAL APPLICATION

- The bulbovestibular glands are prone to infection (**Bartholin's cyst**).
- The perineum is sectioned prior to delivery to prevent uncontrolled tearing. The operation is known as **episiotomy**.

THE FEMALE URETHRA

Size of Extent

The female urethra is about 4 cm in length and passes downwards and forwards from the internal urethral orifice of the bladder to the external urethral orifice (meatus) which is in front of the vaginal opening and between the anterior ends of labia minora. Its diameter is about 5 mm but is dilatable to the extent of 1 cm.

Relations

It corresponds to the prostatic and membranous portions of the male urethra.
- Anteriorly the external orifice is 2.5 cm behind the glans clitoridis, while the internal orifice is about 3 cm behind the middle of the symphysis pubis (Fig. 10.3).
- Posteriorly it is fused to the adventitia of the anterior vaginal wall and is almost embedded in it.

- Fibres of the pubovaginalis part of levator ani lie adjacent to it and play some part in compressing it.

Interior

- The anterior and posterior walls are in apposition. The posterior wall has a prominent fold known as the **urethral crest**.
- Many small urethral glands open along its length and near the external orifice a group of these glands open by a common duct (the para-urethral duct) on either side of the orifice. These glands are known as **Skene's tubules** and are homologous with the prostate in the male.

Sphincters

- **Sphincter urethrae** muscle surrounds the urethra, where it passes through the urogenital diaphragm. It is a voluntary muscle supplied by the pudendal nerve.

The fibres of the deep transversus perinei muscle do not pass posterior to the urethra as it is embedded in the anterior wall of vagina; thus, the external sphincter is incomplete in the female. There is no internal sphincter of the female urethra. **Sphincter vesicae** surrounds the internal urethral orifice. It is an involuntary muscle supplied by sympathetic nerve fibres and vesical control appears to depend mainly on it.

- **Pubovesicalis** part of levator ani provides an important sphincter mechanism.

Blood Supply

- Vaginal arteries are the main source.
- Veins drain into the internal pudendal and internal iliac veins.

Nerve Supply

- The plexus around the vaginal arteries provides both sympathetic and parasympathetic fibres.
- Pudendal nerve innervates the distal part of the urethra.

CLINICAL APPLICATION

- There is much higher incidence of **stress incontinence** in the female as the external urethral sphincter is incomplete because the fibres of the deep transversus perinei do not pass posterior to urethra which is embedded in the anterior vaginal wall. Damage to the urogenital diaphragm during childbirth becomes the chief reason.
- Female urethra is very prone to injury during difficult childbirth due to its intimate relation to vagina. Injury results to **cystocele**.
- The mucosa of urethra herniates through the external meatus due to loss of tone in the sphincteric musculature permitting it to glide on the underlying tissue. This is known as **prolapsed of the female urethra**.

JOINTS OF THE PELVIS

SACROILIAC JOINT (FIG. 10.37)

Type

- Synovial joint of plane type.

Articular Surfaces

- Articular area on the lateral surface of the sacrum.
- Auricular area on the sacropelvis surface of the ilium.

There are irregular elevations and depressions in both surfaces which reciprocally fit with one another and provide a locking device which gives stability and strength to the joint. The joint has a synovial cavity and is reinforced by heavy ligaments.

Ligaments

- **Capsular ligament:** It is attached to the margins of the auricular surfaces.
- **Ventral sacro-iliac ligament** (Fig. 10.37): It is a thickening of the anterior and inferior parts of the capsular ligament. It is a strong ligament and more so in females. The preauricular sulcus which is sometime present in front and below the auricular surface of ilium is an indentation produced by this ligament.
- **Interosseous sacro-iliac ligament:** It is very strong and thick. It fills the large space immediately above and behind the joint cavity, between the iliac tuberosity laterally and sacrum medially (Fig. 10.38).

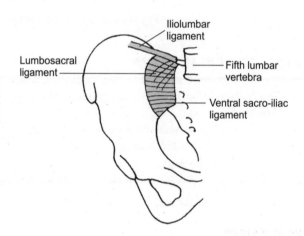

Fig. 10.37: Ligaments of sacro-iliac joint

- **Dorsal sacro-iliac ligaments:** It lies over the interosseous sacro-iliac ligament. Its fibres stretch obliquely from the intermediate and lateral crests of the sacrum to the posterior superior iliac spine. It is not separable from the interosseous ligaments (Fig. 10.39). The **sacrotuberous** and **sacrospinous ligaments** are also a source of strength and stability to the joint (Fig. 10.39).

Nerve Supply

Superior gluteal nerves and twigs from S_1 and S_2 supply it.

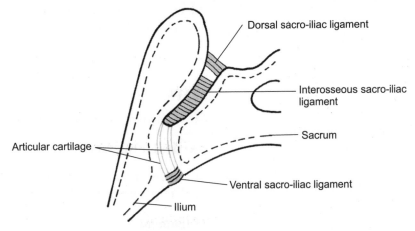

Fig. 10.38: Ligaments of sacro-iliac joint

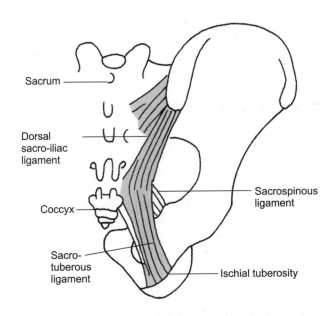

Fig. 10.39: Right sacro-iliac joint with posterior ligaments

Movements

Two types of movement occur at these joints.

- Tilting of the upper part downwards and forwards of about 5° when standing.
- Downward movements of the whole scrum about 2 mm when standing as compared with lying. The sacrotuberous and sacrospinous ligaments anchor the lower end of the scrum, thereby resist rotation of sacrum between the hip bones.

CLINICAL APPLICATION

- Sudden bending can result in tearing of the posterior ligaments or even minor dislocation of the adjacent joint surfaces. This results in extreme pain in flexion movements of the trunk.
- These joints lie in the line of weight transmission. The weight of the body tends to displace the sacrum downwards but this is prevented by the arrangement of the ligaments and the structure of the joint. The upper part of the sacrum also tends to tilt downward and forward but this is prevented by the sacrotuberous and sacrospinous ligaments.
- During pregnancy the ligament is made lax by the influence of **relaxin** hormone secreted by placenta and ovary, rendering the locking mechanism of the joint less efficient and permitting greater rotation of the hip bone. This facilitates delivery.

SACROCOCCYGEAL JOINT

Type

- Secondary cartilaginous joint:
  - Lower surfacing the body of last sacral vertebra.
  - Upper surface of first coccygeal vertebra.

Ligament

- Cornua of two bones are joined together by feeble ligaments.

Movement

- Considerable movement is possible.

PUBIC SYMPHYSIS

Type

- Secondary cartilaginous joint (symphyseal).

Articular Surfaces

- Medial surfaces of the bodies of the two pubic bones which are covered by hyaline cartilage.
- A fibrocartilaginous interpubic disc intervenes between the articulating surfaces.

Ligaments are present above, below and in front (Fig. 10.40).

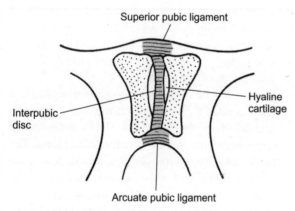

Fig. 10.40: Coronal section through pubic symphysis

- **Superior pubic ligament** extends between the pubic tubercles connecting the two pubic bones.
- **Inferior (arcuate) pubic ligament,** connects the lower borders of the symphyseal surfaces of the pubic bones.
- **Anterior pubic ligament** covers the joint anteriorly.

Movement

The ligaments, together with the structure of the joint, produce an immobile joint which resists separation of the hip bones.

LUMBOSACRAL JOINT

Type

- Secondary cartilaginous joint.

Articular Surfaces

- Lower surface of fifth lumbar vertebra.
- Upper surface of first piece of scrum.

Ligament

- Some as between two typical vertebrae viz. :
    - A fibrous intervertebral disc which is the largest.
    - Anterior and posterior longitudinal ligaments.
    - Ligaments flava.
    - Supraspinous and interspinous ligaments.
    - Synovial joints between the articular processes.

Accessory Ligaments (Fig. 10.37)

- **Iliolumbar ligament** connects the transverse process of L_5 vertebra with the inner lip of the iliac crest. It is a strong band and is directed upwards and laterally.
- **Lumbosacral ligament** formed by the lower fibres of iliolumbar ligament extends from the lower border of that ligament to the ala of sacrum. It merges with the ventral sacro-iliac ligament.

Nerves supply filaments from L_4 and L_5.

CLINICAL APPLICATION

- The fifth lumbar vertebra slips forwards on the first sacral vertebra causing pain and a feeling of weakness at the lumbosacral region. The condition is known as **spondylolisthesis**.

SECTION—II
LOWER LIMB

11 The Bones of the Lower Limbs

The bones of the lower limb consist of the *innominate* or *hip bone* which along with the sacrum forms the pelvis, the *femur* or the bone of the thigh, the *tibia* and the *fibula* which form the bones of the leg and the *tarsals, metatarsals* and the *phalanges* which form the bones of the foot.

THE HIP BONE

The hip bone is a large, flat bone of irregular shape which articulates with the sacrum and with its fellow of the opposite side to form the bony pelvis. It also articulates with the femur.

IDENTIFICATION OF SURFACES: Its *lateral surface* is identified by the presence of a large cup-shaped depression, the acetabulum, its *upper end* by a long and curved upper border, the iliac crest and the *posterior aspect* by the presence of an ear shaped articular surface, the auricular surface, on the posterior and upper part of the medial surface. *Below and in front* of the acetabulum is a wide gap which is the *obturator foramen.*

PARTS: It has *three parts* the ilium, pubis and ischium which meet at the acetabular cavity and are joined in a child by a Y-shaped cartilage. In the fully ossified bone, however, the three parts are united.

- The *illum* forms the upper part of the acetabulum and the fan-shaped bone above it.
- The *pubis* constitutes the anterior part of the acetabulum and the part of the bone associated with it.
- The *ischium* rest of the bone. The latter two parts are also united medially to the obturator foramen to form the ischiopubic ramus.

ANATOMICAL POSITION: In the normal anatomical position, the symphyseal surface of the pubis is in the sagittal plane and the anterior superior iliac spine and the pubic crest occupy a common vertical plane.

THE ILIUM

GENERAL FEATURES (FIGS. 11.1 & 11.2)

The ilium is that part of the hip bone which forms most of the skeletal framework of the gluteal region and of the false pelvis.

It possesses
- *two ends* which are upper and lower
- *three borders* which are anterior, posterior and medial and
- two surfaces named lateral or gluteal and medial. The latter is subdivided into the iliac fossa and sacropelvic surface by a medial border.

ENDS

UPPER END: It is the expanded end opposite the acetabulum. Viewed from the side it is convex in outline but seen from the top it is sinuously curved (S-shaped). It is limited anteriorly and posteriorly by projections termed the *anterior* and *posterior superior iliac spines* and is divisible into ventral and dorsal segments, the former constituting a little more than the anterior two-thirds of it. The ventral segment is bounded by *outer* and *inner lips* enclosing between them an *intermediate area.* The outer lip exhibits projection about 5 cm behind the anterior superior spine and is known as the *tubercle of the iliac crest.* The dorsal segment possesses lateral and medial sloping surfaces separated by a prominent ridge.

LOWER END: The lower end forms a part of the acetabulum.

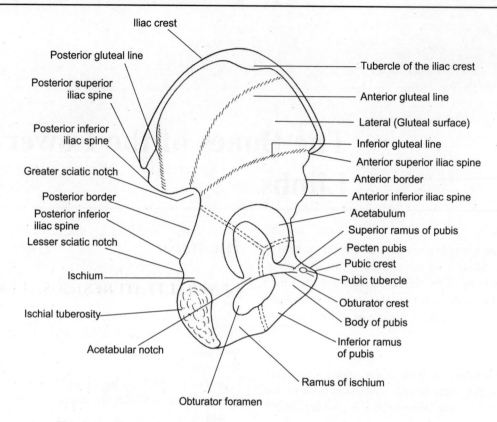

Fig. 11.1 : The dorsal aspect of the right hip bone showing general features.

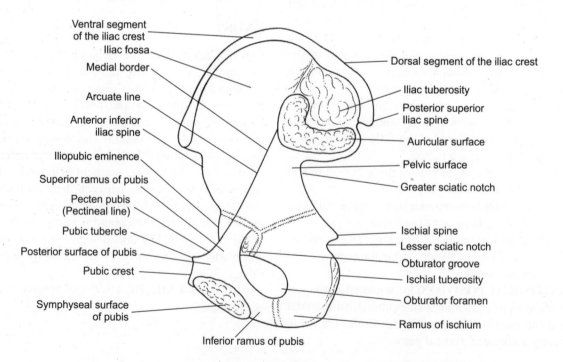

Fig. 11.2 : The ventral aspect of the right hip bone showing general features

BORDERS

ANTERIOR BORDER: It extends between the anterior superior iliac spine and the acetabulum. Just above the latter is marked by a rough projection, the *anterior inferior iliac spine.*

POSTERIOR BORDER: This is longer and irregularly curved. Commencing at the posterior superior iliac spine it first runs downwards and forwards terminating in a small projection which is the *posterior inferior iliac spine.* Thereafter it proceeds horizontally forwards and then turns abruptly downwards and backwards, thereby forming the *greater sciatic notch.* Finally, it becomes continuous with the posterior border of the ischium.

MEDIAL BORDER: It is present on the medial surface of the bone and separates the iliac fossa from the sacropelvic surface. Rough and indistinct in the upper part, it becomes sharp where it forms the anterior boundary of the sacral articular surface and finally smooth and rounded where it forms the iliac part of the *arcuate line* (boundary line between the false and the true pelvis). It ends at the *iliopubic (iliopectineal) eminence.*

SURFACES

GLUTEAL SURFACE : This is the lateral surface of the bone, provides attachments to the major muscles of the gluteal region and is bounded by the anterior and posterior borders, the iliac crest and the acetabulum. It is divided into *four areas* by *three ridges,* the posterior, middle and inferior gluteal lines.

The *posterior gluteal line* is the shortest of the three and extends from the outer lip of the iliac crest about 5 cm in front of the posterior superior spine to a little in front of the posterior inferior spine.

The *anterior gluteal line* is the longest and extends from the middle of the greater sciatic notch to a little in front of the tubercle of the iliac crest. It has a curved course.

The *inferior gluteal line* is the least conspicuous of the three and runs upwards and forwards from the apex of the greater sciatic notch to a point a little above and behind the anterior inferior iliac spine.

MEDIAL SURFACE

ILIAC FOSSA: It is the smooth hollowed out anterior and upper part of the medial surface of the bone limited by the anterior border in front, medial border behind and the ventral part of the iliac crest above. It forms the lateral wall of the false pelvis.

SACROPELVIC SURFACE

It forms the lower and posterior part of the medial surface and is bounded below and behind by the posterior border, above and in front by the medial border and above and behind by the dorsal segment of the iliac crest. It is distinguishable into *three areas* which are:
- **Iliac tuberosity:** It is the rough area just below the iliac crest.
- Auricular surface situated below and in front of the iliac tuberosity.
- Pelvic surface: It is the smooth area in front of and below the auricular surface. It forms the lateral wall of true pelvis. A sulcus known as preauricular sulcus is present between the inferior margin of the auricular surface and the greater sciatic notch.

ATTACHMENTS AND RELATION

UPPER END

Anterior Superior Iliac Spine (Fig. 11.3): It forms an important bony landmark and has the following attachments:
- Above: Lateral end of the *inguinal ligament.*
- Below this: Origin of *sartorius* muscle which extends to the anterior border.

Ventral segment of the iliac crest (Fig. 11.3): The attachments and relations are:
- **Outer lip** (from outwards within):
(a) Along whole length: *Fascia lata* (deep fascia) of the thigh.
(b) In front of the tubercle: Origin of *tensor fascia lata muscle.* (Fig. 11.4)
(c) Anterior two-thirds: Insertion of *external oblique muscle.*
(d) Posterior to (c) : Origin of *latissimus dorsi muscle.*
(e) A small interval exists between the last two attachments and the bone over this small segment forms the base of the *lumbar triangle.*
- **Intermediate area** (11.3) : Origin of *internal oblique* muscle over the whole extent.
- Inner lip (From within outwards)
(a) *Fascia transversalis* over the extent of the attachment of the transversus abdominis (see below) and *anterior lamella of thoracolumbar fascia* behind this.
(b) Origins of (i) *transversus abdominis* muscle from the anterior two-thirds, and (ii) *quadratus lumborum* muscle behind this.
(c) Quadratus lumborum is enclosed by the *anterior* and

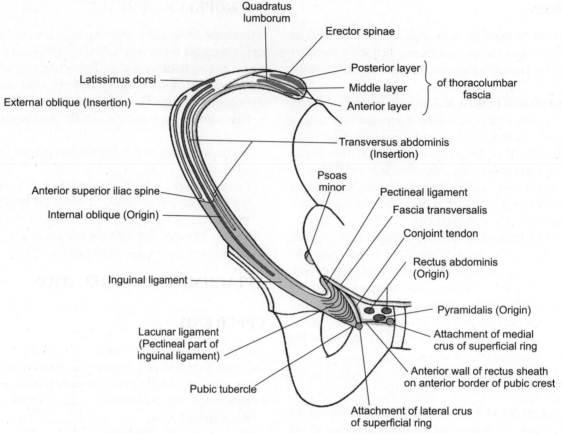

Fig. 11.3 : Attachments of iliac crest, pubic tubercle and pubic crest

middle lamellae of the thoracolumbar fascia which are attached to the bone over here. Traced posteriorly, the attachment of the middle lamella passes between those of the quadratus and the erector spinae.

Dorsal segment of iliac crest

- **Lateral slope:** Origin of *gluteus maximus* muscle. (Fig. 11.4)
- **Medial slope:** Origin of *erector spinae* muscle.
- **Intervening ridge:** Attachment of *posterior lamella of thoracolumbar fascia*. (Fig. 11.3)

ANTERIOR BORDER (FIG. 11.4)

Anterior *inferior iliac spine* gives origin to the *straight head of rectus femoris* muscle above and attachment to the *iliofemoral ligament* below.

POSTERIOR BORDER (FIG. 11.4)

- **Between the two spines:** Attachment of *sacrotuberous ligament*.

- **Upper border of greater sciatic notch:** (between the posterior inferior spine and the apex of the notch): Origin of *piriformis* muscle (encroaches on the gluteal surface).
- **Apex of greater sciatic notch:** *Related* to superior gluteal vessels and nerve. (Fig. 12.4).
- **Lowermost part** (between the apex and the ischium): Related to the piriformis muscle and the sciatic nerve at the lower border of the muscle. (Fig. 12.4).

GLUTEAL SURFACE (FIG. 11.4)

The attachments on this surface are as follows:
- **Areas behind posterior gluteal line:** (a) Origin of *gluteus maximus* muscle from the upper rough part and (b) attachment of *sacrotuberous ligament* below this.
- **Area between posterior and middle (anterior) gluteal lines:** Origin of *gluteus meatus* muscle.
- **Area between middle (anterior) and inferior gluteal lines:** Origin of *gluteus minimus* muscle.
- **Area below inferior gluteal line**
(a) Groove above acetabulum: Origin of *reflected head of rectus femoris* muscle.

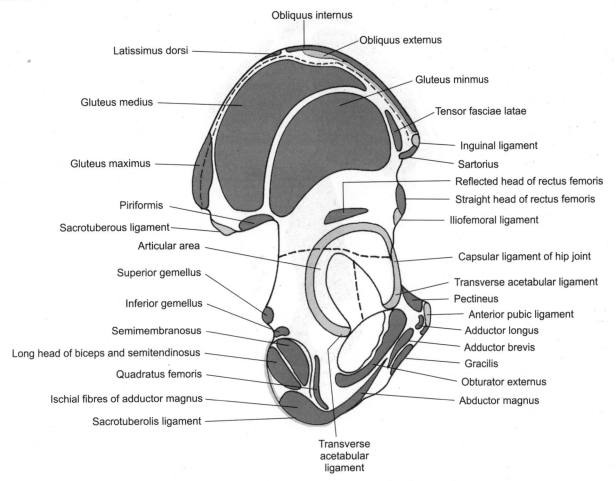

Obliquus internus
Latissimus dorsi
Obliquus externus
Gluteus minmus
Gluteus medius
Tensor fasciae latae
Inguinal ligament
Gluteus maximus
Sartorius
Reflected head of rectus femoris
Straight head of rectus femoris
Piriformis
Iliofemoral ligament
Sacrotuberous ligament
Articular area
Capsular ligament of hip joint
Superior gemellus
Transverse acetabular ligament
Inferior gemellus
Pectineus
Anterior pubic ligament
Semimembranosus
Adductor longus
Long head of biceps and semitendinosus
Adductor brevis
Quadratus femoris
Gracilis
Ischial fibres of adductor magnus
Obturator externus
Abductor magnus
Sacrotuberolis ligament
Transverse
acetabular
ligament

Fig. 11.4 : The dorsal aspect of the right hip bone showing attachments

(b) Margin of acetabulum: Attachment of *capsular ligament of hip joint.*

(c) Posterior part of the surface: *Related* to the piriformis muscle and some of the structures emerging from the greater sciatic foramen below this muscle. (Fig. 12.4).

• **Gluteal lines:** Attachment of fascia covering the different gluteal muscles.

MEDIAL SURFACE
ILIAC FOSSA (FIG. 11.5)

The attachment and relations of this surface are:

• **Margin adjoining the iliac crest:** Attachment of *fascia iliaca.*

• **Upper two-thirds of the surface:** Origin of *iliacus* muscle.

• **Lower one-third of the surface:** *Related* to iliacus muscle and iliolumbar artery.

Groove between the anterior inferior iliac spine and the iliopubic eminence: *Related* to iliacus muscle and the tendon of psoas major which are separated from the bone by a bursa.

• **On the musculofascial bed** of the iliac fossa are *related*—the ileocaecal region of the gastrointestinal tract on the right side and the descending colon on the left.

SACROPELVIC SURFACE (FIG. 11.5)

Iliac tuberosity provides attachments to the (a) *dorsal sacro-iliac ligament* below the attachment of the erector spinae, (b) *interosseous sacro-iliac ligament* behind the auricular surface and (c) *iliolumbar ligament* below the attachment of quadratus lumborum muscle.

Auricular surface *articulates with the sacrum.* Its anterior and inferior borders are sharp and provide attachment to the *anterior sacro-iliac ligament.* The articulation with the sacrum usually occupies the upper

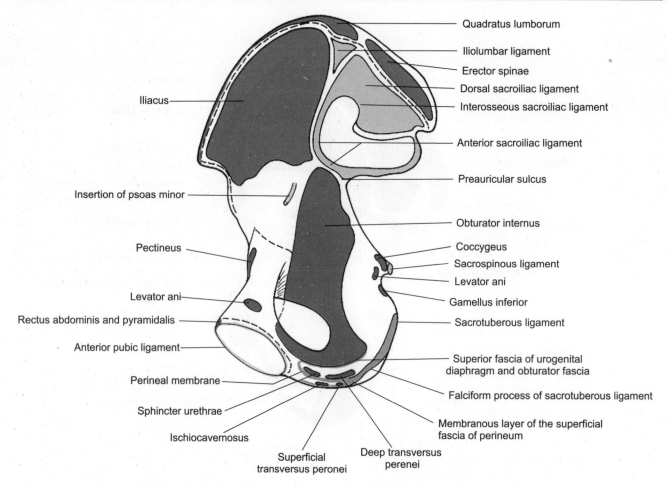

Quadratus lumborum

Iliolumbar ligament

Erector spinae

Dorsal sacroiliac ligament

Interosseous sacroiliac ligament

Anterior sacroiliac ligament

Preauricular sulcus

Obturator internus

Coccygeus

Sacrospinous ligament

Levator ani

Gamellus inferior

Sacrotuberous ligament

Superior fascia of urogenital diaphragm and obturator fascia

Falciform process of sacrotuberous ligament

Membranous layer of the superficial fascia of perineum

Deep transversus perenei

Superficial transversus peronei

Ischiocavernosus

Sphincter urethrae

Perineal membrane

Anterior pubic ligament

Rectus abdominis and pyramidalis

Levator ani

Pectineus

Insertion of psoas minor

Iliacus

Fig. 11.5 : The ventral aspect of the right hip bone showing attachments

two and part of the third piece of the latter although in females it is slightly extensive.

Pelvic surface

(a) It forms part of the *lateral wall of the true pelvis.*
(b) The *preauricular sulcus* gives attachment to the lower fibres of the ventral (anterior) sacro-iliac ligament.
(c) Lateral to the sulcus: Origin of a few fibres of *piriformis* muscle.
(d) Rest of the surface: Origin of *obturator internus* muscle.

THE PUBIS

GENERAL FEATURES (Figs. 11.1 & 11.2)

The pubis constitutes the anterior part of the hip bone. It possesses a *body,* which articulates with the pubis of the opposite side to form the pubic symphysis, a *superior ramus* which is directed upwards and backwards to meet the ilium at the acetabulum, and an *inferior ramus* which runs

backwards, downwards and laterally (forming the medial boundary of the obturator foramen) to meet the ramus of the ischium and constitute the ischiopubic ramus.

BODY

It is flattened anteroposteriorly, forms the anterior wall of the true pelvis and has *three surfaces* which are anterior, posterior and medial or symphyseal and an upper border termed the *pubic crest.*

Anterior surface : Directed downwards, forwards and laterally.

Posterior surface : It is smooth, faces upwards and backwards and forms the anterior boundary of the true pelvis and of the retropubic space.

Symphyseal surface : It is oval in shape, covered with cartilage in the recent state and forms the *symphysis pubis* with the opposite bone.

Pubic crest: It is the rounded upper border of the body which ends laterally in a blunt projection termed the *pubic tubercle.* The crest has anterior and posterior borders which enclose a surface and meet at the pubic tubercle.

SUPERIOR RAMUS

The superior ramus extends upwards, backwards and laterally from the upper lateral part of the body to the acetabulum. It has *three surfaces,* pectineal, pelvic and obuturator, enclosed between *three borders, viz.* the pecten pubis (pectineal line), obturator crest and inferior border.

Pecten pubis (pectineal line) : It is the easiest to find because it is the sharpest of the three borders and extends from the pubic tubercle to the arcuate line. Together with the pubic crest it forms the pubic part of the arcuate line.

Obturator crest : Most rounded and situated anterior to the pectineal line, it extends from the pubic tubercle to the acetabulum.

Inferior border : It forms the anterior margin of the obturator foramen.

Pectineal surface : Limited by the pecten pubis behind and the obturator crest in front.

Pelvic surface : It is bounded above by the pectineal line and below by the inferior border.

Obturator surface : Bounded by the obturator crest in front and the inferior border behind, it exhibits the *obturator groove* which runs from behind, downwards and forwards. The groove is converted into the *obturator canal* by the obturator externus in front, obturator internus behind and the obturator membrane in between and transmits the *obturator vessels nerve* from the pelvis to the thigh.

INFERIOR RAMUS

It arises from the lower and lateral part of the pubis and runs downwards, backwards and slightly laterally forming the inferior boundary of the obturator foramen. It joins the ramus of the ischium and they are known together as the *ischiopubic ramus.*

ATTACHMENTS AND RELATIONS

BODY

Anterior Surface (Fig. 11.4)

- Medial part of the surface: Attachment of *ventral (anterior) pubic ligament.*
- Angle between upper part of this attachment and the pubic tubercle: Origin of the tendon of *adductor longus.*
- Close to the lower part of the symphyseal surface and extending to the inferior ramus : Origin of *gracilis* muscle.

- Lateral to above :
  Origin of *adductor brevis.*
- Lateral to above : Origin of *obturator externus* muscle.

Posterior Surface (Fig. 11.5)

In the middle : Origin of *anterior fibres of levator ani* muscle.

Lateral to above : Origin of *obturator internus* muscle.
Medially : Attachment of *puboprostatic ligaments.*

Whole surface above the attachment of levator ani : *related* to urinary bladder but separated by the retropubic pad of fat.

Symphyseal Surface

Forms the symphysis pubis with the opposite bone.

Pubic Crest (Fig. 11.3)

Pubic tubercle: It is an important landmark.
- Attachments : (a) Medial end of the *inguinal ligament* and (b) ascending limb of the *loops of cremaster* muscle.
- Relations: (a) Lies in the floor of the superficial inguinal ring and (b) is crossed by the *spermatic cord* in males which can be roled on the tubercle.
- *Anterior border of pubic crest :* Attachment of (a) *anterior wall of rectus sheath* and the (b) *conjoint tendon* which becomes continuous with (a) and forms its major constituent.

Enclosed surface

Laterally : Origin of lateral head of *rectus abdominis* and *pyramidalis muscles*
Medially : Related to the medial head of rectus abdominis muscle.

ANTERIOR RAMUS

Pecten pubis (pectineal line) (Fig. 11.3)

- Medially : (a) *Pectineal part of the inguinal ligament* (lacunar ligament) anteriorly and (b) *conjoint tendon* behind this. The former becomes continuous with the inguinal ligament at the pubic tubercle and the latter with the attachment of the anterior wall of the rectus sheath at the pubic crest.
- Along its whole extent: *Pectineal ligament.*
- At its middle: Insertion of *psoas minor* when this muscle is present.

Obturator crest

Its lateral end gives attachment to some fibres of the pubofemoral ligament.

Pectineal Surface (Fig. 11.4)

It gives origin to the pectineus muscle from its medial part and along a linear area below the pectineal line. The rest of the surface is covered by the muscle.

Pelvic Surface (Figs. 9.22 & 9.24)

In general, this surface is *covered by peritoneum* with extraperitoneal tissue intervening. It is crossed by *lateral umbilical ligament* (obliterated umbilical artery) and the *vas deferens* in males and round ligament of uterus in females.

THE ISCHIUM

GENERAL FEATURES (FIG. 11.1 & 11.2)

The ischium constitutes the lower and posterior part of the hip bone and consists of a *body* and a *ramus*. The latter extends upwards, forwards and medially from the lower part of the body, forms the lower boundary of the obturator foramen and meets the inferior ramus of the pubis to form the ischiopubic ramus.

BODY

The body has *two ends,* upper and lower and *three borders, viz.,* dorsal of posterior, lateral and the margin of the obturator foramen. They enclose between them *three surfaces* which are, femoral, dorsal and pelvic.

    Upper end : It forms a part of the acetabulum.

    Lower end : It is free and forms the ischial tuberosity.

    Femoral surface : It is the lateral surface of the body and is limited anteriorly by the margin of the obturator foramen and posteriorly by the lateral border.

    Dorsal surface : It is a continuation downwards of the gluteal surface of the ilium. The upper part of the surface is convex and smooth. This is followed by a grooved area. The lower part is continued into the *ischial tuberosity.*

    Pelvic surface : This surface is bounded in front by the margin of the obturator foramen and behind by the posterior border.

    Posterior border : It is a continuation downwards of the posterior border of the ilium and separates the dorsal from the pelvic surface. It runs at first downwards and backwards to complete the lower margin of the greater sciatic notch. It then forms a projection termed the *ischial spine* below which it forms the *lesser sciatic notch.*

    Greater sciatic notch : This notch is converted into the greater sciatic foramen by the sacrotuberous and sacrospinous ligaments. Its upper, anterior and inferior margins are bony. The lower boundary is formed by the ischial spine anteriorly and the sacrospinous ligament posteriorly. The posterior boundary is formed by the sacrotuberous ligament.

    Lesser sciatic notch : It is situated below the greater sciatic notch and is converted into a foramen by the sacrospinous and sacrotuberous ligaments. It is bounded above by the ischial spine and the sacrotuberous ligament, in front by the body of the ischium and behind by the sacrotuberous ligament.

RAMUS

The ramus of the ischium arises from the lower part of the body and passes upwards, forwards and medially to meet the inferior ramus of the pubis to form the ischiopubic ramus.

ISCHIOPUBIC RAMUS

It has external and internal surfaces and lateral and medial borders. The medial border, along with the corresponding part of the other hip bone, forms the lateral boundaries of the urogenital triangle. The lateral border forms the margin of the obturator foramen.

ATTACHMENTS AND RELATIONS

BODY

Femoral Surface (Fig. 11.4)

- Close to the obturator foramen : Origin of a part of *obturator externus muscle.*
- On and close to the lateral border opposite the ischial tuberosity : Origin of *quadratus femoris* muscle.
- Rest of the surface : *Covered* by obturator externus muscle.

Dorsal surface (Fig. 11.4)

- *Convex part* : This part of the dorsal surface lies *in relation* with piriformis muscle but is partially separated from it by the sciatic nerve and the nerve to quadratus femoris (Fig. 12.4)
- *Grooved area :* It is related to the obturator internus and gemelli muscles (Fig. 12.4).

- *Ischial tuberosity* (Fig. 11.4) : It is divided by a near transverse ridge into an *upper quadrilateral* area and a *lower triangular* one. The former is further subdivided by a diagonal line into upper lateral and lower medial areas. The triangular part is also divisible into lateral and medial areas.

(a) Upper lateral area : Origin of *semi-membranous* muscle.

(b) Lower medial area : Origin of *long head of biceps* and *semitendinosus* muscle.

(c) Lateral area of triangular part : Origin of ischial fibres of *adductor magnus* muscle.

(d) Medial area of triangular part : *Related* to fibrofatty tissue and the ischial bursa of the glutenus miximus muscle. This part of gluteus miximus muscle. This part of the bone supports the body weight to the sitting posture and is palpable.

(e) Curved ridge on the medial margin of the tuberosity : Attachment of the *sacrotuberous ligament* and its falciform process (Fig. 11.5).

(f) Wide groove above and medial to tuberosity : Is *related* to the tendon of the obturator internus muscle. The bone is covered by a layer of cartilage and is further protected by a bursa.

(g) Lower margin of the groove near the tuberosity : Origin of *inferior gemellus* muscle.

(h) Upper margin of the groove close to the ischial spine : Origin of *superior gemellus* muscle. (Fig. 11.4)

Pelvic Surface (Fig. 11.5)

- *Its upper part:* Partly gives origin to a part of the *obturator internus* muscle and the rest of the area is covered by it.

- *Its lower part :* Forms the lateral wall of the ischiorectal fossa but is covered by the obturator internus muscle.

Ischial Spine

Ischial spine : It has the following attachments and relations :

- *Tip :* Attachment of the *sacrospinous ligament* (Fig. 11.5).

- *Dorsal surface :* (Fig. 11.5) : *Related* to (a) internal pudendal vessels medially and (b) nerve to the obturator internus laterally. (Fig. 11.5)

- *Pelvic surface :* Gives origin to the (a) most posterior fibres of *levator ani* and (b) *coccygeus* muscles. (Fig. 11.6).

Greater sciatic notch (Fig. 12.4)

Transmits a number of structures from the pelvis to the gluteal region. *The piriformis muscle, as it comes out through* the foramen, divides it into an upper and a lower compartment. Through the upper compartment (above the piriformis) come out the

- superior gluteal nerve and
- superior gluteal vessels.
- The structures coming out of the *lower compartment* (below the piriformis) are,
- sciatic nerve,
- inferior gluteal nerve,
- nerve to obturator internus,
- nerve to quadratus femoris,
- pudendal nerve,
- posterior femoral cutaneous nerve,
- internal pudendal and
- inferior gluteal vessels.

Lesser sciatic notch

Transmits the tendon of the obturator internus from the pelvis to the gluteal region and the nerve to the obturator internus, pudendal nerve and internal pudendal vessels from the pelvis to the perineum *via* the gluteal region. (Fig. 12.4).

Ischio-pubic ramus

External surface : It gives attachment to the muscles of the thigh. (Fig. 11.4)

- *Close to the medial border :* (Extending from the level of the middle of the symphyseal surface to a little in front of the ischial tuberosity) : Origin of *gracilis* muscle.
- *Lateral to above :* extending from the ischial tuberosity to a little above the lower limit of the symphyseal surface: Origin of *adductor magnus* muscle.
  - *Between the above two :* Origin of *adductor brevis* muscle, (inferiorly) extends only slightly into the ischial part of the joint ramus and in its upper part overlaps the lower half of the attachment of adductor longus).
  - *Lateral to adductor magnus :* Origin of *obturator externus* muscle.

Medial border : It gives attachment to the *fascia lata* (deep fascia) of the thigh and *membranous layer* of the superficial fascia of the superficial fascia of the perineum.

Internal Surface : This surface is divided into areas by faint lines which are *not easily discernible in every bone.*

- An area adjoining the lateral border : Gives origin to *obturator internus* muscle.
- The medial limit of this attachment shows a *faint ridge:* Gives attachment to the *obturator fascia* and *superior fascia of the urogenital diaphragm* (both are in continuity).

- *Another faint ridge* extending from the medial margin of the ischial tuberosity to the lower limit of the symphyseal surface of the body of the pubis : Gives attachment to *falciform process of the sacrotuberous ligament* posteriorly and *inferior fascia of the urogenital diaphragm* (perineal membrane) anteriorly.

The medial border of the ischiopubic ramus, as it is traced backwards, encroaches the internal surface and meets the faint ridge described above but somewhat in front of the ischial tuberosity. Thus, the membranous layer of the superficial fascia of the perineum fuses posteriorly with the perineal membrane.

The area of the internal surface enclosed by the attachments of the membranous layer and perineal membrane is the region of the *superficial perineal pouch.* It gives origin to the *ischiocavernosus* and *transversus perinei* muscles posteriorly and is related to the crus penis (or clitoris) anteriorly.

The attachments of the superior and inferior layers of the urogenital diaphragm also fuse but more in front of the fusion described above. The area enclosed is the *deep perineal pouch.* It gives origin to the *sphincter urethrae* muscle posteriorly and more anteriorly is related to the dorsal nerve of the penis and the internal pudendal vessels.

ACETABULUM

GENERAL FEATURES (FIG. 11.1)

The acetabulum is a cup-shaped cavity on the lateral aspect of the hip bone which has a contribution from all the three components of the bone. It is surrounded by a projecting margin, the *rim of the acetabulum,* except inferiorly where there is a deficiency termed the *acetabular notch.* The anterior, superior and posterior parts of the cavity are occupied by a horseshoe shaped articular surface for the head of the femur. The inferior aspect and the floor are rough and nonarticular and are termed the *acetabular fossa.* The pubis forms the anterior one-fifth of the articular surface; the ischium contributes to the acetabular fossa and a little more than the posterior two-fifths of the articular surface while the remainder is formed by the ilium.

ATTACHMENTS AND RELATIONS (FIG. 11.4)

- **Margins of acetabular notch :** Gives attachment to the *transverse ligament of the acetabulum* which deepens

the socket inferiorly for the head of the femur. The ligament converts the notch into *acetabular foramen* through which acetabular branches of the obturator and medial circumflex fermoral arteries enter the joint. The margins also provide attachment to the ligament of the head of the femur.
- **Acetabular rim :** Gives attachment to the cartilaginous *acetabular labrum.*
- **Attachment of the capsular ligament :** Above, it is attached to the margin of the acetabulum 5 or 6 mm away from the acetabular labrum; in front and behind, to the labrum and inferiorly to the transverse ligament.
- **Acetabular fossa :** It lodges a pad of fat which is covered by the synovial membrane of the hip joint.
- **Articular surface :** It is covered with articular cartilage.

OBTURATOR FORAMEN

It is a gap in the hip bone, below and in front of the acetabulum. It is bounded above and in front by the superior ramus and body of the pubis, medially and below by the ischiopubic ramus, behind by the body of ischium and above by the inferior margin of the acetabulum. It is large and oval in the male but smaller and triangular in the female in the recent sate it is occupied by the *obturator membrane* which is attached to the margins of the foramen except superiorly where there is a gap. The gap forms the *obturator canal* for the passage of the obturator nerve and vessels from the pelvis to the thigh. The outer and inner surfaces of the membrane provide origin for the obturator externus and internus muscles respectively.

OSSIFICATION

Primary Centres : There are three in number.
    For illum : Appears during 2nd month IUL.
    For ischium : Appears during 3rd month IUL.
    For pubis : Appears during 4th month IUL.
Secondary Centres

For iliac crest : 2 centres	Appears at puberty, fuse
For acetabulum : 2 centres	latest by 25th yr.
For ischial tuberosity : 1 centre.	
For anterior inferior iliac spine : 1 centre	*Occasional:* Appear at puberty, fuse latest by 25th yr.
For symphyseal surface including pubic crest and tubercle : 1 centre.	

SEX DIFFERENCES

	Female	Male
Greater sciatic notch	Nearly a right angle	Less
Ischial spine	Not inverted	Inverted
Ischiopubic ramus	Not everted	Everted
Obturator foramen	Triangular	Oval
Acetabular diameter	Usually less than 5 cm	Usually more
Distance between pubic tubercle and acetabular margin	Greater than the diameter of the acetabular cavity	Equal or less

N. B. The usual statement that the pre-auricular sulcus is absent in males in not always correct.

CLINICAL APPLICATION

> * The weakest part of the hip joint is its inferior aspect because of the absence of the acetabular rime at this site. Hence, in traumatic dislocation of the head of the femur the primary displacement is downwards and anteriorly.
> * The blood vessels to the upper part of the head of the femur reach it through the ligament of the head of the femur. Hence, a trauma involving this ligament may cause an avascular necrosis of the upper part of the head.

THE FEMUR

GENERAL FEATURES (FIGS. 11.6 & 11.7)

The femur is the skeleton of the thigh and is the longest and strongest bone of the body. It has *two ends,* upper and lower, joined by a *shaft.*
* The upper end consists of a *head* joined to the rest of the bone by a *neck.* At the junction of the neck with the shaft are two projections, the *greater* and *lesser trochanters.*
* The lower end of the bone is expanded and is partly separated to form the *lateral* and *medial condyles.*

ANATOMICAL POSITION : In the normal erect posture, the lower end of the two femora approximate each other at the mid-line. Hence, the bone occupies an oblique position so that the lower surfaces of the two condyles *lie in the same horizontal plane.* To demonstrate the anatomical position, either hold the bone upright on the surface of the table so that the lower surfaces of the two condyles touch the table surface or suspend the bone in air by placing the head of the bone on the extended index finger.

DETERMINATION OF SIDE : When the bone is held in a way that the lower end points downwards, the convexity of the shaft faces anteriorly and the head faces medially, the side to which it belongs is opposite the side to which the head points.

UPPER END

The upper end consists of a head, a neck, a greater and a lesser trochanter.
* **HEAD :** It is globular and directed upwards, medially and slightly forwards. Otherwise smooth, it presents a rough depression or *fovea* a little below and behind its centre.
* **NECK :** It connects the head with shaft with which it forms an angle (140° in child, 125° in adult male and less in females). It has anterior and posterior surfaces.

Anterior surface

* It is *intracapsular* and covered with the synovial membrane of hip.

Posterior surface

It is smooth and its junction with the shaft forms the *intertrochanteric crest.*

Intertrochanteric crest presents a *quadrate tubercle* below its middle.

GREATER TROCHANTER : It possesses anterior, lateral and medial surfaces and a free upper border.

LESSER TROCHANTER : Situated behind the lower end of the intertrochanteric line, it presents a summit, a slightly rough anterior surface and a smooth posterior surface.

SHAFT

The shaft is narrow in the middle but expanded at the *two ends.*
* *Three surfaces,* anterior, medial and lateral, are present in its middle third bounded by
  - *three borders,* lateral, medial and posterior.

BORDERS

The former two are indistinct but the posterior border is very prominent and is termed the *linea aspera* which consists of a central rough part limited on either side by medial and laterl lips.

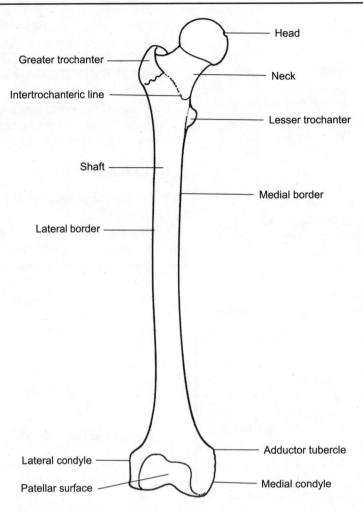

Fig. 11.6 : The general features of the right femur—anterior view

- The upper and the lower thirds possess a *fourth surface* each, bounded by the bifurcation of the lips of the linea aspera.
- The *fourth surface* of the upper part, known as the posterior surface, is triangular and limited by the *gluteal tuberosity* laterally and the *spiral line* medially.
- That in the lower part, termed the *popliteal surface,* is also triangular and is bounded by the *medial* and *lateral supracondylar lines* which are the continuation downwards of the medial and the lateral lips respectively of the linea aspera.

SURFACES

ANTERIOR SURFACE : Situated between the ill defined medial and lateral borders.

LATERAL SURFACE : It is situated between the lateral and posterior borders. The latter is replaced by the gluteal tuberosity above and by the lateral supracondylar line below.

MEDIAL SURFACE : It lies between the medial and the posterior borders. The spiral line in the upper third of the shaft and the medial supracondylar line in the lower third replace the posterior border.

GLUTEAL TUBEROSITY : It is the tipward continuation of the lateral lip of the linea aspera and has a central area flanked by medial and lateral lips.

SPIRAL LINE : It extends from the medial lip of the linea aspera to the lower end of the intertrochanteric line.

POSTERIOR SURFACE : It is a triangular surface limited between the spiral line and the gluteal tuberosity.

LINEA ASPERA : It is the posterior border of the shaft of the femur which forms a linear ridge having medial and lateral lips.

MEDIAL SUPRACONDYLAR LINE : It is the

condyles which are united anteriorly and are continuous with the shaft as one mass. Posteriorly, however, they are independently continuous with the shaft being separated from each other by the *intercondylar fossa (notch)*. The lower end articulates with the patella and the tibial condyles. The articular areas for the two are continuous and occupy anterior, inferior and posterior aspects of each condyle.

LATERAL CONDYLE : It presents lateral, medial, anterior, posterior and inferior surfaces.

MEDIAL CONDYLE : It possesses medial, lateral, anterior, posterior and inferior surfaces.

INTERCONDYLAR FOSSA (NOTCH) : It separates the posterior and inferior parts of the two condyles. It is limited anteriorly by the inferior margin of the patellar articular area and posteriorly from the popliteal surface of the shaft by the *intercondylar line.*

PATELLAR ARTICULAR SURFACE (FIG. 11.8): The articular surface for the patella occupies the anterior surfaces of both the condyles and forms a continuous area which is slightly grooved in the middle and is concave from side to side. It extends higher on the lateral condyle and is separated from the tibial articular surfaces by two grooves. Each groove is related to the repective meniscus

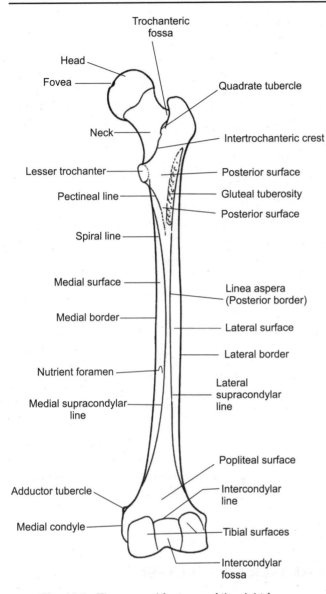

Fig. 11.7 : The general features of the right femur posterior view

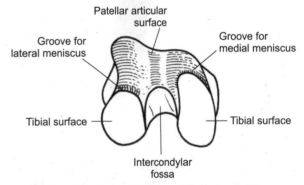

Fig. 11.8 : Articular surfaces of lower end of femur

during full extension of the knee. The groove on the medial condyle is deficient near the intercondylar fossa where a semilunar facet is present for articulation with the patella during full flexion of the knee joint.

TIBIAL ARTICULAR SURFACES (FIG. 11.11) : These are meant for articulation with the condyles of the tibia. They are limited anteriorly by the grooves for the menisci and are separated from each other by the intercondylar fossa. Each surface is convex from side to side as well as anteroposteriorly. The anteroposterior curve is more sharp posteriorly in both condyles, longer in the medial condyle and more gentle in the lateral condyle. These features have important bearings on the movement and stability of the knee joint.

downward continuation of the medial lip of the linea aspera. Inconspicuous in its upper two-thirds, it becomes better defined lower down and terminates in the *adductor tubercle.*

LATERAL SUPRACONDYLAR LINE : It is the downward and lateral continuation of the lateral lip of the linea aspera.

POPLITEAL SURFACE : It is bounded by the medial and lateral supracondylar lines.

LOWER END

The lower end is widely expanded, more in the transverse axis; further, it projects posteriorly. It consists of *two*

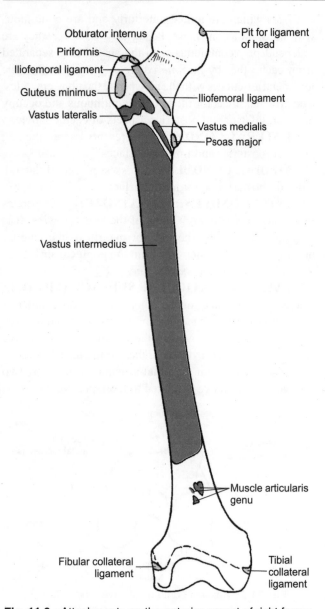

Fig. 11.9 : Attachments on the anterior aspect of right femur

ATTACHMENTS AND RELATIONS

- **HEAD (Fig. 11.9)**

  Fovea : Gives attachment to the *ligament of the head of the femur* which conveys the acetabular branches of the obturator and medial circumflex femoral arteries to supply the upper one-fourth of the head.

  Margin of fovea : Gives attachment to the *synovial membrane* covering the ligament.

  Rest of the surface : *Covered* with hyaline cartilage and articulates with the acetabulum.

- **NECK**

  Anterior Surface (Fig. 11.9)

- The *capsular ligament* is attached along the intertrochanteric line which marks the junction of the anterior surface with the shaft.
- Capsular fibres containing blood vessels run upwards and medially from the intertrochanteric line to form *retinaculae* which supply the neck and lower three-fourths of the head.
- A *tongue-shaped smooth area* close to the head to covered by cartilage.

  Posterior Surface (Fig. 11.9)

- The *capsular ligament* is attached along a line just beyond its medial half.
- *Area above capsular attachment :* Covered by synovial membrane.
- *Area below capsular attachment* : Related to the tendon of obturator internus.

  Intertrochanteric line (Fig. 11.9) : It gives attachment to the

- *Capsular ligament* along its whole length.
- Upper and lower strong bands of the *iliofemoral ligament* to the upper and lower parts of the line and to the weak central band in between.
- *Vastus lateralis* muscle (origin) from the upper part
- *Vastus medialis* muscle (origin) from the lower part.

  Intertrochanteric Crest (Fig. 11.10)

- On the tubercle : Insertion of quadratus femoris muscle.
- Part above tubercle : *Related* to gluteus maximum muscle.
- Part below Tubercle : *Related* to quadratus femoris and adductor magnus muscles.

GREATER TROCHANTER

Anterior surface (Fig. 11.11)

- A ridge on the lateral aspect : Provides insertion to *gluteus minimus* muscle.
- Area medial to ridge : *Related* to gluteus minimus muscle but separated by the trochanteric bursa of gluteus minimus.
- **Lateral surface :** It is divided into two areas by a ridge which runs downwards and forwards to meet the lower end of the ridge on the anterior surface.
- On the ridge : Insertion of *gluteus medius* muscle (Fig. 11.11).
- Area in front of it : *Related* to gluteus medius muscle but separated by the trochanteric bursa of gluteus medius.

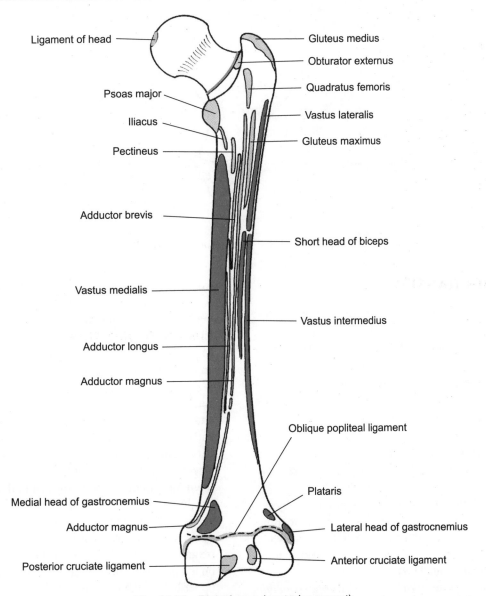

Fig. 11.10 : Right femur (posterior aspect)

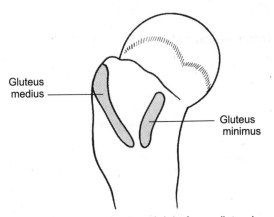

Fig. 11.11 : Greater trochanter of right femur (lateral aspect)

– Area behind it : *Related* to gluteus maximus muscle. Trochanteric bursa of the muscle sometimes intervenes.

Medial surface : It is conspicuous by the presence of the trochanteric fossa (Fig. 11.12).

– Trochanteric fossa : Insertion of *obturator externus* muscle.

– Oval impression above and in front of it : Insertions of *obturator internus, gemellus superior* and *gemellus inferior.*

– Upper border : It provides insertion to the *piriformis* muscle.

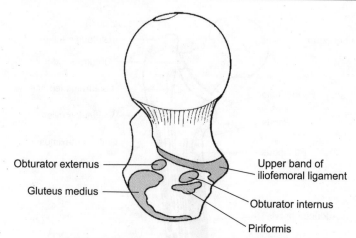

Fig. 11.12 : Right femur (superior aspect)

LESSER TROCHANTER

Summit and medial part of the anterior surface : Insertion of *psoas major* muscle (Fig. 11.10).

- **Rest of the anterior surface :** Insertion of *illiacus* muscle (inclines slightly backwards).
- **Posterior surface** : *Related* to adductor magnus muscle with an occasional bursa intervening.

SHAFT

Anterior surface (Fig. 11.9)
- **Upper three-fourths :** Origin of *vastus intermedius* muscle.
- **Below this :** Origin of *articularis genu* muscle by 5-6 small slips. It is a detached part of vastus intermedius.
- **Lowest 5 cm :** *Related* to the suprapatellar bursa which communicates with the synovial cavity of the knee joint.
Lateral surface (Fig. 11.9)
- **Upper three-fourths :** Origin of *vastus intermedius* muscle.
- **Below this :** *Covered* by vastus intermedius.
Medial surface (Fig. 11.10) : It is covered only by the vastus medialis muscle.
- **Gluteal tuberosity (Fig. 11.10)**
- **Central area :** Provides insertion to *gluteus maximus* muscle.
- **Lateral lip :** Gives origin to *vastus lateralis* muscle.
- **Medial lip :** Provides insertion to the pubic fibres of *adductor magnus* muscle.
- **Spiral line (Fig. 11.10) :** Gives origin to the vastus medialis muscle.
Posterior surface (Fig. 11.10) : Provides insertion to the pectineus muscle from the root of the lesser

trochanter to the linea aspera which it just encroaches. Adductor brevis is inserted laterally and extends upto the upper half of the linea aspera.
Linea aspera (Fig. 11.10)
Medial lip : Origin of *vastus medialis* muscle medially and attachment of *medial intermuscular septun* lateral to it.
Lateral lip : Origin of *vastus lateralis* muscle laterally, attachment of *lateral intermuscular septum* medial to it and origin of *biceps femoris* muscle still more medially.
Intervening area :
- The insertion of *adductor magnus* continues down from the medial lip of the gluteal tuberosity and gradually inclines medially to find the medial supracondylar line.
- *Adductor brevis* muscle is inserted medial to the adductor magnus. It extends half way up the insertion of pectineus on the posterior surface (lateral to it) and down upto the upper half of the linea aspera.
Adductor longus muscle is inserted medial on the same plane as the insertion of pectineus but below it. It thus occupies only the linea aspera.
Medial Supracondylar Line (Fig. 11.10)
- **Upper two-thirds :** Origin of *vastus medialis* muscle.
- **Lateral** to (1) : Attachment of *medial intermuscular septum.*
- **Whole line lateral** to (2) : Insertion of *adductor magnus* muscle which is aponeurotic except in the lowermost 4 cm of the line.
- **The upper part of the line** shows an ill-defined groove where popliteal artery lies in contact with the bone as it passes from the adductor canal to the popliteal fossa through the aponeurotic insertion of the adductor magnus.

Adductor tubercle : Insertion of ischial fibres of *adductor magnus* muscle.
Lateral supracondylar line (Fig. 11.10)
- **Whole line :** Attachment of the *lateral intermuscular septum.*
- **Upper two-thirds :** Origin of short of head of *biceps femoris.*
- **Lowermost part :** Origin of *plantaris* muscle (extends on popliteal surface).

Popliteal Surface (Fig. 12.18)

It is related to the *popliteal artery* with fat intervening. The *superior medial* and *superior lateral genicular arteries,* which are branches of the popliteal, run across this surface arching over the medial and lateral condyles of femur respectively and are separated from the bone by the origins of the *medial head of the gastrocnemius and plantaris* muscle in respective cases.

LATERAL CONDYLE

Lateral surface (Fig. 11.13) : It presents :
- An elevation termed the **lateral epicondyle :** Attachment of *fibular collateral ligament* of knee joint.
- **Smooth impression above and behind the above :** Origin of lateral head *of gastrocnemius* muscle.
- **Groove** between lateral epicondyle and postero-inferior part of articular margin : Origin of *popliteus* muscle from the anterior part; posterior part lodges the tendon of the muscle during full flex on of the knee joint. *The origin of the muscle is intracapsular.*
- **Along a line about 1 cm away from the articular margin :** Attachment of the *capsular ligament* of the knee joint. The intracapsular part of the bone is covered with synovial membrane.

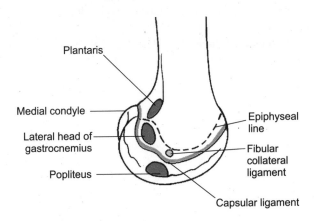

Fig. 11.13 : Latera surface of lateral condyle of right femur

Medial surface : It forms the lateral boundary of the intercondylar fossa (notch).
Anterior surface : It forms part of the patellar articular surface.
Posterior surface : It articulates with the lateral condyle of the tibia during full flexion of the knee joint.
Inferior surface : It articulates with the same part of the tibia during extension.

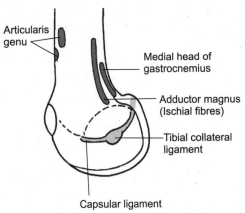

Fig. 11.14 : Medial surface of medial condyle of right femur

MEDIAL CONDYLE
Medial surface (Fig. 11.14) It presents :
- The **medial epicondyle** (most prominent part of the surface) : Attachment of the *tibial collateral ligament* of the knee joint.
- Above and behind medial epicondyle is the **adductor tubercle :** Receives insertion of the ischial fibres of the *adductor magnus* muscle.
- **Along a line about 1 cm away from the articular margin :** Attachment of the *capsular ligament.*
Lateral surface : It forms the medial boundary of the intercondylar fossa (notch).
Anterior surface : It forms part of the patellar articular surface (Fig. 11.8).
Posterior surface : It articulates with the tibia during full flexion of the knee joint (Fig. 11.8).
Inferior surface : It articulates with the medial condyle of the tibia during extension of the knee (Fig. 11.8).
- **Intercondylar fossa (Fig. 11.10)**
- It is intracapsular but mostly extrasynovial.
- **Impression at the upper and posterior part of the lateral wall :** Attachment of the upper end of the *anterior cruciate ligament* of the knee joint.

Impression on the anterior part of the medial wall: Attachment of the upper end of the *posterior cruciate* and *meniscofemoral ligaments* of the knee joint.

Intercondylar line : Attachments of (a) *capsular ligament* in its whole extent and (b) *oblique popliteal ligament* in the lateral part. (Fig. 12.17)

Anterior border : Attachment of the *infrapatellar fold of the synovial membrane* of the knee joint.

ATTACHMENT OF CAPSULAR LIGAMENT OF KNEE (FIG. 11.9, 11.10, 11.13, 11.14) : It is attached *posteriorly* to the intercondylar line and the margins of the condyles immediately beyond the articular areas, *laterally* and *medially* to the lateral and medial surfaces of the respective condyles 1 cm away from the articular margin, *anteromedially* and *anterolaterally,* the capsule blends with the medial and lateral patellar retinaculae (which are expansions of the vastus medialis and lateralis to which the deep fascia of the thigh also contributes) which are attached to the two margins of the patella, while *anteriorly* the capsule is entirely deficient as a result of which the synovial membrane projects above the joint as the suprapatellar bursa.

N.B. The intracapsular nonarticular parts of the condyles are covered by synovial membrane and the origin of the popliteus muscle is intracapsular.

OSSIFICATION

The femur is ossified from five centres, one primary for the shaft and the rest are secondary for the two ends.

Centre	Appearance	Fusion with shaft
Shaft	7th week IUL	–
Head	Within 6 months after birth	17th year
Greater trochanter	4th year	After puberty
Lesser trochanter	12th–14th year	After gr. troch.

Lower Shortly before birth About 20th year

EPIPHYSEAL LINE (Shown dotted): The epiphyseal line of the head runs along the articular margin and is thus wholly intracapsular. The epiphyseal lines of the trochanters run along their bases. That of the greater trochanter in its upper part includes a small part of the neck. This epiphysis is therefore mostly extracapsular but partly intracapsular. The epiphyseal line for the lesser trochanter is, however, wholly extracapsular.

The epiphyseal line of the lower end runs almost transversely through the adductor tubercle. It is extracapsular on all sides except anteriorly where the synovial covered surface (intracapsular) extends into the diaphysis.

NUTRIENT ARTERY : The nutrient artery to the femur is derived from one of the perforating arteries (branches of profunda femoris artery), usually the second. It enters the bone at the linea aspera. The nutrient foramen points to the upper end; hence the lower end of the bone is the growing end. (Fig. 11.7).

CLINICAL APPLICATION

The arterial supply to the upper one-fourth of the head is derived from the branches of the obturator and medial circumflex femoral arteries which are conveyed through the ligament of the head of the femur. Hence, an injury to this ligament as a result of dislocation of the head may interrupt the blood supply and cause subsequent necrosis of the area of supply.

The arterial supply to the rest of the head and the neck is derived from capsular blood vessels. These are conveyed through the retinaculae and pass upwards and medially. A fracture of the neck nearer the head is liable to tear the retinaculae and damage the finer blood vessels causing delayed union or nonunion of the fracture.

THE PATELLA

GENERAL FEATURES

The patella is a *sesamoid bone* (the largest in the body) which has developed in the tendon of the quadriceps femoris and lies in front of the knee joint. It is triangular in shape and flattened anteroposteriorly. It presents anterior and posterior surfaces, superior, lateral and medial borders and an apex which is directed inferiorly.

Anterior Surface (Fig. 11.15) : It is featureless except that numerous vascular foramina are present. It is

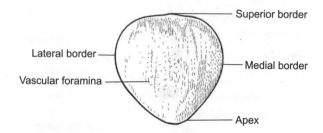

Fig. 11.15 : Anterior surface of right patella

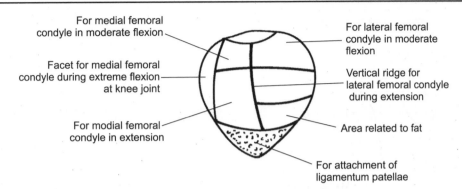

Fig. 11.16 : Posterior surface of right patella

subcutaneous but is separated from the skin by the *subcutaneous prepatellar bursa* and an expansion from the superficial fibres of the quadriceps tendon which becomes continuous with the ligamentum patellae.

Posterior Surface (Fig. 11.16) : It has an upper oval articular area and a lower rough area.

Oval articular area : It has the following features:

- A *vertical ridge* divides the area into two large facets of which the lateral is larger. The ridge fits into the groove on the patellar area of the femur.
- The *medial part of the medial facet* forms an elongated strip which comes in contact with the femur during extreme flexion.
- The *rest of the medial surface* is indistinctly divided into an upper and a lower area. The former remains in contact with the femur in *moderate flexion* and the latter in extension.
- The *lateral articular area* is larger and is indistinctly divisible into three areas from above downwards. The upper and middle areas are in contact with the femur, the former during moderate flexion and the latter during extension. The lowermost area is related to fat.

ATTACHMENTS

Rough area

- Its lower part gives attachment to the ligamentum patellae.
- Its upper part is related to the infrapatellar pad of fat.

SUPERIOR BORDER : It gives insertion to that part of the *quadriceps femoris* which is derived from the rectus femoris and vastus intermedius tendons.

LATERAL AND MEDIAL BORDERS : These provide insertion to the lateral and medial parts of the *quadriceps femoris* (derived from the vastus lateralis and medialis muscles respectively).

DETERMINATION OF SIDE: The surface, borders and the apex are easily distinguished. The medial side of the bone is recognised by the presence of the vertical strip on the posterior surface or by the smaller size of the medial articular area. When the patella is made to rest with its posterior surface on the table and the apex away from you it inclines to the side to which the bone belongs.

THE TIBIA

GENERAL FEATURES

The tibia is the medial and stronger bone of the leg. It transmits the weight of the body from the femur to the foot. The bone has a shaft connecting the upper and lower ends. The upper end is more massive and expanded to form the medial and lateral condyles, the upper surfaces of which are smooth and separated from each other by an *intercondylar area*. The lower end projects medially to form the *medial malleolus*. The most conspicuous feature of the shaft is its sharp anterior border.

Anatomical Position : The bone lies vertically and the upper surfaces of the two condyles lie in a horizontal plane.

DETERMINATION OF SIDE : A tibia is assigned to its proper side by holding the bone vertically so that condyles face upwards, the sharpest border of the shaft is anterior and the medial malleolus is medial.

UPPER END

The upper end of the bone is expanded transversely and more projecting posteriorly, specially in individual who are habitual squatters. It consists of a *medial* and a *lateral condyle* (which however are not separated as in the case of the lower end of the femur) and a small projection termed the *tuberosity of the tibia*. The medial condyle is characterised by a groove on its posterior and posterior

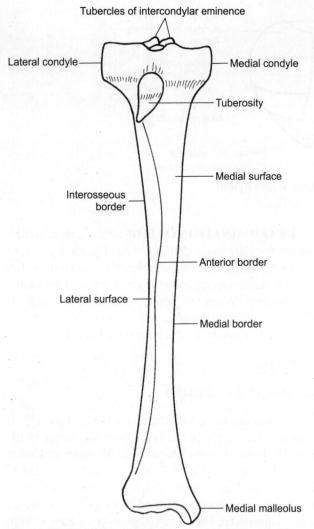

Fig. 11.17 : Right tibia: anterior aspect showing general feature

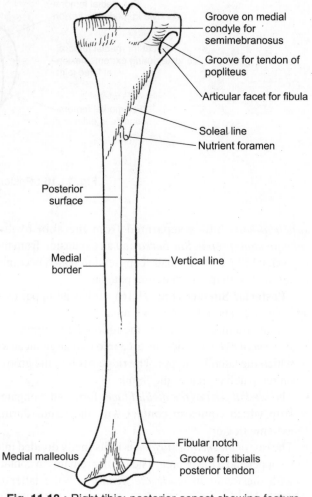

Fig. 11.18 : Right tibia: posterior aspect showing feature

part of the medial aspects while the lateral condyle possesses a circular articular facet for the head of the fibula on the posterolateral part of its inferior aspect. The upper surfaces of the two condyles are separated by an intercondylar area which has two eminences in its middle.

Medial Condyle : It has upper, posterior, medial and anterior surfaces.

Lateral Condyle : It has upper, posterior, lateral and anterior surfaces.

Intercondylar Area (Fig. 11.19) : It is the nonarticular area between the upper surfaces of the condyles and is marked by an intercondylar eminence in the middle formed by the medial and lateral intercondylar tubercles which divide the area into anterior and posterior parts.

TUBEROSITY OF THE TIBIA : It is situated at the

junction of the anterior surfaces of the shaft and upper end. It is divided into two parts by a faint transverse line into an upper and a lower part.

SHAFT

The shaft of the tibia is triangular on section and possesses three borders, viz., anterior, interosseous and medial, which enclose three surfaces, medial, lateral and posterior.

Borders

ANTERIOR BORDER : It extends from below the tuberosity to the anterior border of the medial malleolus and is sinuously curved.

INTEROSSEOUS BORDER : It extends from below and in front of the fibular facet (at the upper end) to the anterior border of the fibular notch at the lower end.

MEDIAL BORDER: It extends from the medial end of the groove for the semimem branosus to the posterior

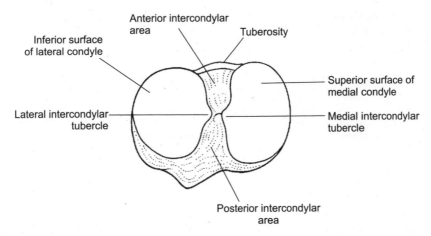

Fig. 11.19 : Articular surface of right tibia

border of the medial malleolus. The meeting of the soleal line divides it into two parts.

Surfaces

MEDIAL SURFACE : It is enclosed by the anterior and medial borders and is mostly subcutaneous.

LATERAL SURFACE : It is bounded by the anterior and interosseous borders. Above it faces laterally but curves forwards lower down.

POSTERIOR SURFACE : Bounded by the medial and interosseous borders, the posterior surface is divided into an upper (triangular) and a lower area by the soleal line which is a rough ridge running from above downwards and medially. The lower area is further subdivided by a vertical line in its upper three-fourths into a medial and a lateral area.

LOWER END

The lower end is expanded and is roughly quadrangular. Its medial aspect projects downwards as the *medial malleolus* which is continuous above with the medial surface of the shaft. The lower end possesses anterior, posterior medial, lateral and inferior surfaces.

ANTERIOR SURFACE

It is transversely grooved in the lower part.

POSTERIOR SURFACE : It is continuous above with the posterior surface of the shaft.

MEDIAL SURFACE : It is subcutaneous and is continuous above with the medial surface of the shaft and below with that of the madial malleolus.

LATERAL SURFACE : It presents a rough triangular area called the fibular notch which forms the inferior tibiofibular syndesmosis by articulating with the lower end of the fibula.

INFERIOR SURFACE : It is covered with hyaline cartilage and articulates with the superior surface of the body of the talus.

MEDIAL MALLEOLUS : It has four surfaces, anterior, posterior, medial and lateral and an inferior border.

ATTACHMENTS AND RELATIONS

UPPER END

MEDIAL CONDYLE

Upper surface (Fig. 11.20)

- Smooth and oval in shape, its long axis is directed anteroposteriorly and is concave in both diameters.
- The lateral border projects upwards to form the *medial intercondylar tubercle.*
- The anterior, medial and posterior margins are related to the *medial meniscus* for which there is a C-shaped impression.
- The posterior part of the impression is wider.
- The entire surface articulates with the medial condyle of femur.

Posterior surface (Fig. 11.21) : It is grooved.
Upper margin of the groove : Attachment of *capsular ligament* of knee joint and posterior fibres of the *tibial collateral ligament* of the knee joint.

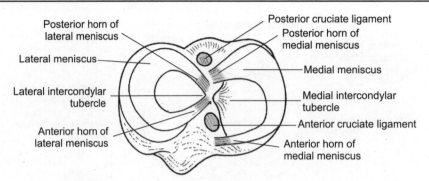

Fig. 11.20 : Attachments on upper surface of right tibia

Groove and its lower margin : Insertion of *semimembranosus* muscles.

Medial and anterior surfaces (Fig. 11.21) : These surfaces are rough. They give attachment to the *medial patellar retinaculum* which is an expansion of the aponeurosis of vastus medialis. The groove of the posterior surface extends to the posterior part of the medial surface and has the same attachments.

LATERAL CONDYLE

Upper surface (Fig. 11.20)

- Smooth and circular in shape, it is gently concave in all diameters.
- The medial border is raised to form the *lateral intercondylar tubercle.*
- The anterior, lateral and posterior borders are related to the *lateral meniscus.* The cartilage (unlike the medial) is of uniform width and forms almost a complete circle.
- Whole of the surface *articulates* with lateral condyle of the femur.

Posterior surface (Fig. 11.22) : It presents:
- **A groove :** Related to the *tendon of popliteus* but a *bursa* intervenes which communicates with the synovial cavity of the knee joint.
- **Below and lateral to groove :** A *circular articular facet* articulates with the head of the fibula.
- **Margins of facet :** Attachment of *capsular ligament* of the superior tibiofibular joint.

Lateral and anterior surfaces

They are not demarcated from each other, are rough and separated from the shaft by a sharp margin.

Sharp margin : Attachment of the *deep fascia of leg*.

- **Upper end of sharp margin terminates in an oval area :** Attachment of the *iliotibiat tract* (Fig. 11.21).
- Area above upper two : Attachment of the *lateral patellar retinaculum* which is an expansion of the aponeurosis of vastus lateralis.
- Area below and in front of the fibular facet : Origin of (a) *extensor digitorum longus* and (b) *peroneus longus* (occasional muscles. A part of the biceps *femoris* is inserted above and in front of the fibular face (11.21).

Intercondylar area (Fig. 11.20)

Anterior intercondylar area : It has the following attachments:
- Anteriormost part : *Transverse ligament* connecting the menisci.
- Anteromedial part : Anterior horn of *medial meniscus.*
- Behind the anterior horn of medial meniscus : Lower end of *anterior cruciate ligament.*
- **Lateral to above :** Anterior horn of *lateral meniscus.*

Posterior intercondylar area: The attachments here are:
- Behind the lateral intercondylar tubercle : Posterior horn of *lateral meniscus.*
- Behind the above and behind the medial intercondylar tubercle : Posterior horn of *medial meniscus.*
- Posteriormost sloping area : Lower end of *posterior cruciate ligament.*

TUBEROSITY OF THE TIBIA (FIG. 11.21)

Upper smooth part : Attachment of the *ligamentum patellae.*

Lower rough part : It is subcutaneous and forms an important bony landmark. It is separated from the skin by the *subcutaneous infrapatellar bursa.*

Area above the ligamentum patellae is related with the *deep infrapatellar bursa.*

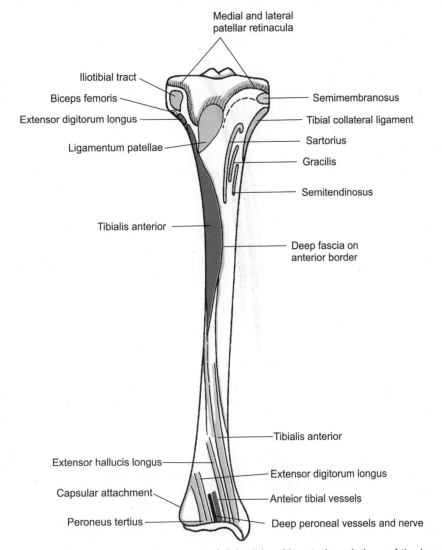

Fig. 11.21 : Attachments on anterior aspect of right tibia with anterior relations of the lower end

Labels in figure:
- Medial and lateral patellar retinacula
- Iliotibial tract
- Biceps femoris
- Extensor digitorum longus
- Ligamentum patellae
- Tibialis anterior
- Semimembranosus
- Tibial collateral ligament
- Sartorius
- Gracilis
- Semitendinosus
- Deep fascia on anterior border
- Tibialis anterior
- Extensor hallucis longus
- Capsular attachment
- Peroneus tertius
- Extensor digitorum longus
- Anteior tibial vessels
- Deep peroneal vessels and nerve

SHAFT

ATTACHMENTS (FIGS. 11.21 & 11.22)

Anterior Border

It is *subcutaneous* and gives attachments to the *superior extensor retinaculum* for about an inch above the medial malleous and deep fascia of the leg along the rest of its extent.

Interosseous Border

- **Along the whole length** (except the upper and lower ends) : *Interosseous membrane.*
- **At the lower end : Anterior tibiofibular ligament.**
  Above the free upper margin of the interosseous memberane the *anterior tibial vessels* pass forwards from the popliteal fossa to the anterior compartment of the leg.

Medial Border (Fig. 11.22)

- **Part above the soleal line :** Provides attachments to posterior fibres of the *tibial collateral ligament*, an expansion of the *semimembranosus muscle* (insertion) and fascia covering the *popliteus muscle*, in that order from before backwards.
- **Below the soleal line :** Provides origin of soleus muscle in its upper part, attachment to *fascia covering the deep muscles of the back of leg* in its whole extent.

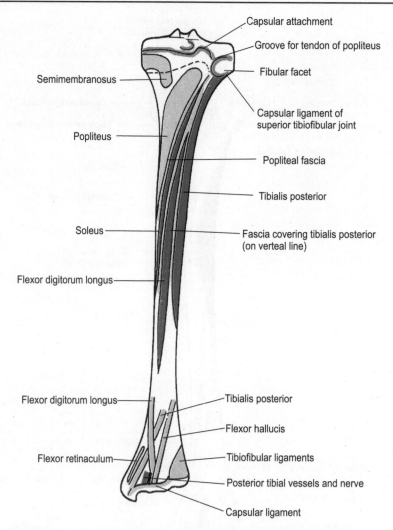

Capsular attachment

Groove for tendon of popliteus

Fibular facet

Capsular ligament of superior tibiofibular joint

Popliteal fascia

Tibialis posterior

Fascia covering tibialis posterior (on verteal line)

Semimembranosus

Popliteus

Soleus

Flexor digitorum longus

Flexor digitorum longus

Tibialis posterior

Flexor hallucis

Tibiofibular ligaments

Flexor retinaculum

Posterior tibial vessels and nerve

Capsular ligament

Fig. 11.22 : Attachments on posterior surface of right tibia with posterior relations of the lower end

MEDIAL SURFACE (FIG. 11.23)

Its upper part gives insertion anteriorly to *sartorius, gracilis* and *semitendinosus* muscles in that order from before backwards. The insertion of the sartorius is inverted. J-shaped and the hook, overlook the insertion of the other two muscles. Posteriorly, it provides attachment to anterior fibres of the tibial collateral ligament of the knee joint (for which there is an elongated impression) and an expansion of the semimembranosus muscle (insertion).

Its lower part is subcutaneous and is related with the *great saphenous vein*.

LATERAL SURFACE (FIG. 11.21)

- Its upper two-thirds is hollowed out for the origin of tibialis anterior muscle.

- Its lower one-third is related to tibialis anterior, extensor hallucis longus, anterior tibial vessels, deep peroneal nerve, extensor digitorum longus and peroneus tertius in that order mediolaterally.

Opposite the ankle joint they lie undercover of the superior extensor retinaculum.

POSTERIOR SURFACE (FIG. 11.22)

Triangular area : Provides insertion to *popliteus muscle.*

Soleal line : Gives attachments to the (a) *fascia covering popliteus muscle*, (b) *fascia covering soleus muscle*, (c) *soleus* muscle (origin), and (d) *fascia covering the deep muscles* of the back of the leg in that order from above downwards. The upper lateral end of the line gives

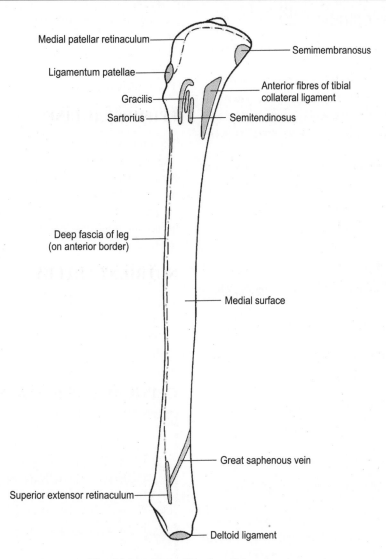

Fig. 11.23 : Right tibia (medial surface)

attachment to the medial end of the *tendinous arch* of origin of the soleus muscle. The fascia covering the deep muscles of the back of leg forms an intermuscular septum separating the soleus, gastrocnemius and plantaris from the flexors digitorum and hallucis longus.

Vertical line : Gives attachment to the *fascia covering the tibialis posterior* muscle. It forms an intermuscular septum between the flexors and the tibialis posterior.

Medial area : Provides origin to *flexor digitorum longus* muscle.

Lateral area : Provides origin to *tibialis posterior* muscle.

Lower one-fourth of posterior surface : It is *related*

to (a) tibialis posterior, (b) posterior tibial vessels (c) tibial nerve and (d) flexor hallucis longus.

The flexor digitorum longus muscle crosses the tibialis posterior from the medial to the lateral side and is therefore not related directly to the bone.

LOWER END

ANTERIOR SURFACE (FIG. 11.21)

- **Transversely grooved lower part :** Attachment of the *capsular ligament* of ankle joint.
- **Whole surface :** *Related* to tendons, nerve and vessels of the anterior (extensor) compartment of the leg already enumerated earlier.

POSTERIOR SURFACE (FIG. 11.22)

Vertical groove at the medial end : *Related* to the tendon of tibialis posterior.

    Area lateral to above : Related to the (a) tendon of flexor digitorum longus, (b) posterior tibial artery with its venae comitantes, (c) tibial nerve, and (d) tendon of flexor hallucis longus in that order from medial to lateral side and running from above downwards.

    Lower margin : Attachment of the *capsular ligament* of ankle joint.

MEDIAL SURFACE

It is subcutaneous.

LATERAL SURFACE

- **Anterior border of notch :** Attachment of the *anterior tibiofibular ligament.*
- **Posterior border of notch :** Attachment of the *posterior tibiofibular ligament.*
- **Upper part of the floor of notch :** Attachment of the *interosseous tibiofibular ligament.*

INFERIOR SURFACE

It is covered with hyaline cartilage to articulate with talum.

MEDIAL MALLEOLUS

Anterior surface : Attachment of the *capsular ligament* of the ankle joint.

    Posterior surface : It presents a groove which lodges the tendon of *tibialis posterior.* The medial margin of the groove gives attachment to the *flexor retinaculum* (Fig. 11.22).

    Medial surface : It is *subcutaneous.*

    Lateral surface : It has a *comma-shaped facet* for articulation with the malleolar facet on the medial surface of the talus.

    Inferior border : It is pointed anteriorly but depressed behind. It gives attachment to the *capsular ligament* and *deltoid ligament* of the ankle joint.

OSSIFICATION

The tibia ossifies from three centres, one primary for the shaft and two secondary centres, one for each end.

Centre	Appearance	Fusion with shaft
Primary	7th week IUL	–
Upper end	Shortly before birth	18th year
Lower end	1st year	17th year

The tuberosity of the tibia ossifies as a tongue-shaped projection of the upper epiphysis but the lower part of the tuberosity may ossify from a separate centre which appears at 10-12 years and soon joins the tongue-shaped projection. The medial malleolus may also have a separate centre.

EPIPHYSEAL LINE

The epiphyseal line of the upper end is represented by a line which runs parallel to but between the attachment of the capsule and the patoellar retinaculae. Anteriorly it cuts the tuberosity of the tibia.

    At the lower end, the epiphyseal line runs transversely across the bone above the capsular attachment of the ankle joint.

NUTRIENT ARTERY

The nutrient artery of the tibia is a branch of the posterior tibial and enters its posterior surface. The foramen is directed inferiorly, hence the upper end is the growing end of the bone.

CLINICAL APPLICATION

- The lower third of the tibia has a relatively poor blood supply because of the absence of periosteal blood vessels, there being no attachment of muscles in this part. Hence, this part of the bone is notorious for nonunion of fracture.
- An eversion injury causes an avulsion of the deltoid ligament with a fracture of the tip of the medial malleolus.
- An inversion injury causes a transverse fracture of the medial malleolus at its base.

THE FIBULA

GENERAL FEATURES (FIGS. 11.24, 11.25, 11.26 & 11.27)

The fibula is the lateral bone of the leg. It is slender and does not take any part in the transmission of body weight. It articulates with the tibia and the talus. It has two ends, the upper or the head and the lower or the lateral malleolus, connected by shaft. The upper end is identified by the presence of a circular articular facet and a projection termed the styloid process. The lower end presents, on one of its surfaces, a triangular articular facet and a depression called the malleolar fossa.

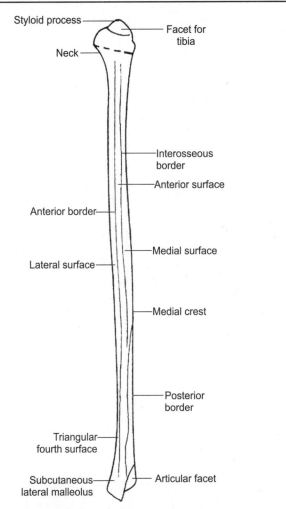

Fig. 11.24 : Right fibula: anterior aspect

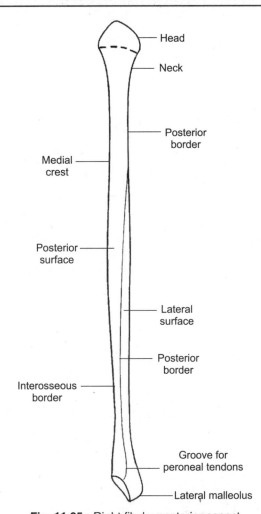

Fig. 11.25 : Right fibula: posterior aspect

ANATOMICAL POSITION : Vertical.

DETERMINATION OF SIDE : The upper and the lower ends are easily identified. When the lower end is kept downwards in such a way that the malleolar fossa lies behind the triangular facet, the bone will belong to the side opposite to which the facet points.

HEAD

The head of the fibula is expanded in all diameters and overlooks the shaft anteriorly, posteriorly and laterally. Its upper surface possesses a *roughly circular* facet which is sloping medially and downwards. The posterolateral part of the head forms a projection known as the *styloid process*. The remaining surfaces of the head are continuous with the shaft.

SHAFT

The shaft of the fibula has got three borders, viz., anterior,

interosseous and posterior which enclose three surfaces which are posterior and lateral. In its lower part, however, there is a triangular fourth surface enclosed by the bifurcation of the anterior border.

BORDERS

Anterior border (Fig. 11.24) : It extends from the anterior aspect of the head and traced downwards is seen to bifurcate to enclose the fourth surface which is continuous with the lateral surface of the malleolus.

INTEROSSEOUS BORDER (FIG. 11.24) : It lies closely medial to the anterior border and terminates below in a rough triangular area.

POSTERIOR BORDER (FIG. 11.25) : It extends from the posterior aspect of the head to the medial margin of the groove (for peronei) at the posterior surface of the lower end.

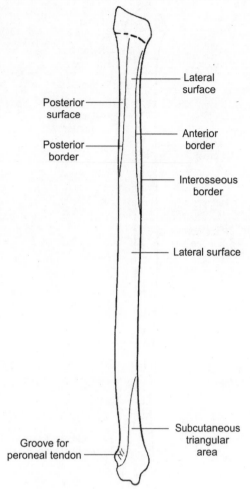

Fig. 11.26 : Right fibula: lateral aspect

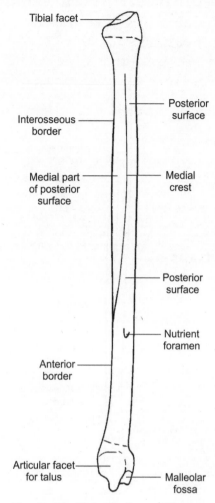

Fig. 11.27 : Right fibula: medial aspect

SURFACES

MEDIAL (EXTENSOR) SURFACE (FIG. 11.24) : It is placed between the anterior and interosseous borders and is very narrow.

POSTERIOR (FLEXOR) SURFACE (FIGS. 11.25 & 11.27) : It is the widest of the surfaces and is bounded by the interosseous and posterior borders. Its upper two-thirds is divided into two areas, lateral and medial, by a sharp crest, termed the medial crest, which runs at first downwards and then inclines forwards to meet the interosseous border (Fig. 11.24). The posterior surface itself presents a rough triangular area in its lower part. It has the following attachments:

LATERAL (PERONEAL) SURFACE (FIG. 11.24) : Enclosed between the anterior and posterior borders, its lower fourth part inclines posteriorly and its terminal part becomes continuous with the groove on the posterior surface of the lateral malleolus.

TRIANGULAR FOURTH SURFACE : It is subcutaneous (Fig. 11.24).

LOWER END

Also known as the lateral malleolus, it projects lower down than the medial malleolus of the tibia and articulates with the talus. It has medial, lateral, anterior and posterior surfaces.

ATTACHMENTS AND RELATIONS

HEAD

- In general, the head is subcutaneous and forms an important bony landmark.
- **Articular facet :** Articulates with the superior fibular articular facet of the tibia.
- **Margins of articular facet :** Give attachment to the

capsular ligament of the superior tibiofibular joint (Fig. 11.28).

- **Anterior sloping surface of styloid process:** Provides attachment to the *fibular collateral ligament* of the knee joint (Fig. 11.30).
- **Area surrounding the anterior sloping surface or styloid process anteriorly,** laterally and posteriorly; Insertion of the tendon of biceps femoris (Fig. 11.30).
- **Anterior surface :** Origin of the uppermost fibres of extensor digitorum longus muscle (Fig. 11.28).
- **Lateral surface :** Origin of peroneus longus muscle (Fig. 11.28).
- **Posterior surface :** Origin of *soleus muscle* (Fig. 11.30)
- The constriction below the head is known as the neck and it is related laterally to the common peroneal nerve which at this site divides into its terminal branches, the superficial and deep peroneal.

SHAFT

Anterior Border

- **Upper three-fourths :** Anterior intermuscular septum of the leg which separates the extensor from the peroneal compartment.
- **Anterior border of triangular surface :** Superior extensor retinaculum.
- **Posterior border of triangular surface :** Superior peroneal retinaculum.

Interosseous Border

- **From a little below its origin to the rough area :** Attachment of the *interosseous membrane.*
- **Upper part :** Related to the anterior tibial artery as it passes from the popliteal fossa to the anterior compartment of the leg.

Posterior border

It provides attachment to the posterior intermuscular septum of leg (except at the lower part) which separates the peroneal from the flexor compartment.

Medial (Extensor) Surface (Fig. 11.28)

- **Whole of upper fourth and anterior part of middle two-fourths :** Extensor digitorum longus muscle.
- Posterior part of **middle two-fourths :** Extensor hallucis longus muscle.
- **Whole of lower one-fourth :** Peroneus tertius muscle.

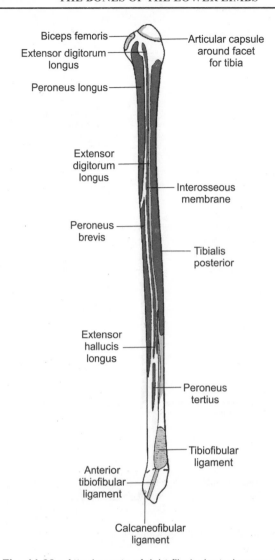

Fig. 11.28 : Attachments of right fibula (anterior aspect)

Posterior (Flexor) Surface (Fig. 11.31)

- **Medial are :** Origin of tibialis posterior muscle.
- **Medial crest :** Attachment of the intermuscular septum between the tibialis posterior (lying deep) and flexors digitorum and hallucis longus (lying superficial) muscles.
  Lateral area : (Fig. 11.29)
(a) Upper fourth : Origin of soleus muscle. The medial part of this origin shows a tubercle which gives attachment to the fibrous area of origin of the muscle.
(b) Lower three-fourths : Origin of flexor hallucis longus muscle.
- **Anterior border of triangular rough area :** Attachment of the anterior tibiofibular ligament.

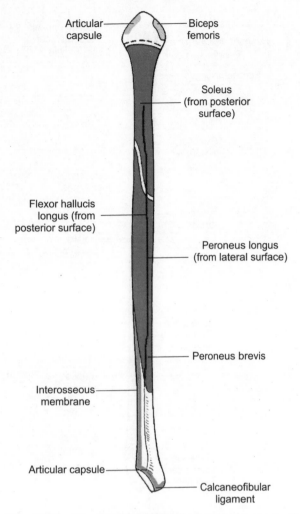

Fig. 11.29 : Attachments of right fibula (posterior aspect)

Labels for Fig. 11.29:
- Articular capsule
- Biceps femoris
- Soleus (from posterior surface)
- Flexor hallucis longus (from posterior surface)
- Peroneus longus (from lateral surface)
- Peroneus brevis
- Interosseous membrane
- Articular capsule
- Calcaneofibular ligament

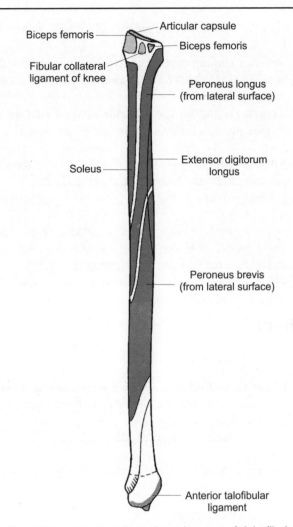

Fig. 11.30 : Attachments on lateral aspect of right fibula

Labels for Fig. 11.30:
- Biceps femoris
- Articular capsule
- Biceps femoris
- Fibular collateral ligament of knee
- Peroneus longus (from lateral surface)
- Soleus
- Extensor digitorum longus
- Peroneus brevis (from lateral surface)
- Anterior talofibular ligament

- **Posterior border of triangular rough area :** Attachment of the posterior-tibiofibular ligament.
- **Rough area between above two :** Attachment of interosseous tibiofibular ligament.
  Lateral (Peroneal) Surface (Fig. 11.28)
- Upper third and posterior part of middle third : Origin of peroneus longus muscle.
- Rest of the surface : Origin of peroneus brevis muscle.

TRIANGULAR FOURTH SURFACE

It is subcutaneous.

LOWER END

MEDIAL SURFACE (11.28) : It presents
- Triangular smooth area in front : Articulates with talus.
- A depression called malleolar fossa behind the above

(a) Its upper part : Attachment of the lower and deeper fibres of posterior (transverse) tibiofibular ligament.
(b) Its lower part : Attachment of posterior talofibular ligament.

LATERAL SURFACE : It is subcutaneous and easily palpable.

ANTERIOR SURFACE : Rounded and gives attachment to the anterior talofibular ligament.

POSTERIOR SURFACE : It presents a groove which has a prominent lateral border.
- **Groove :** Lodges the tendons of peroneus longus and brevis. The former is more superficial.
- **Lateral border of groove :** Gives attachment to superior peroneal retinaculum.

INFERIOR BORDER : It presents a notch to which is attached the calcaneofibular ligament.

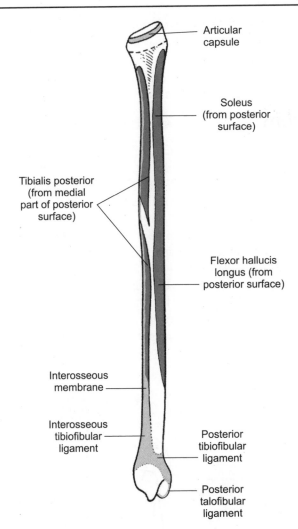

Fig. 11.31 : Attachments on medial aspect of right fibula

across the neck while that of the lower end runs above the malleolar facet. Both are therefore extracapsular.

NUTRIENT ARTERY

The nutrient artery is usually a branch of the peroneal artery. The foramen is directed downwards. Hence, the upper end of the bone is the growing end.

CLINICAL APPLICATION

- A fracture of the neck of the fibula may damage the common peroneal nerve.
- An excessive inversion of the foot causes an avulsion of the calcaneofibular ligament with a fracture of the tip of the lateral malleolus.
- An excessive eversion of the foot causes a transverse fracture of lateral malleolus above the facet for talus.

THE BONES OF THE FOOT

The bones of the foot can be subdivided into three groups, viz., (1) the tarsus, (2) the metatarsus and (3) the phalanges. The **tarsus** consists of seven bones named the calcaneus, talus, navicular, cuboid, and the three cuneiforms. (Fig. 11.32 & 11.33)

The **metatarsus** consists of five metatarsal bones.

The **phalanges** are fourteen in number. Each metatarsal bone carries three phalanges except the first which has one less.

OSSIFICATION

The fibula ossifies from three centres, one primary for the shaft and two secondary centres, one for each end.

Centre	Appearance	Fusion with shaft
1. Primary	8th week IUL	-
2. Upper end	4th year	1th year
3. Lower end	1st year	17th year

N.B. : The fibula violates one of the laws of ossification in the sense that the secondary centre appearing first is not the last to unite with the shaft.

EPIPHYSEAL LINE (Fig. 11.26)

The epiphyseal line of the upper end runs transversely

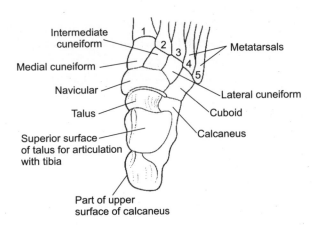

Fig. 11.32 : Tarsal bones : Dorsal aspect

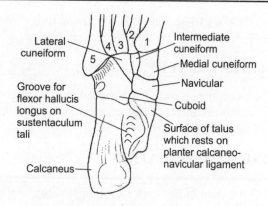

Fig. 11.33 : Tarsal bones : plantar aspect

THE TALUS

The talus articulates above and on the sides with the tibia and the fibula to form the ankle joint, below with the calcaneus to form the subtalar joint and in front with the navicular bone to form one of the midtarsal joints.

PARTS : It has a rounded head, a short neck and body which possesses a number of articular areas out of which a pulley shaped or trochlear surface and a triangular area are easily identified. (Figs. 11.34, 35, 36 & 11.37).

HEAD

It points anteriorly, slightly downwards and medially. It has anterior and plantar (inferior) surfaces.

ANTERIOR SURFACE : Oval, convex and smooth, it articulates with the navicular bone.

PLANTAR SURFACE : It exhibits three facets.
- Posteriormost facet : Largest and oval in shape, it rests on the upper surface of the sustentaculum tali of the calcaneus.
- Facet anterior and lateral to the above : It rests on the anteromedial part of the upper surface of the calcaneus.
- Facet medial to the above two : It lies in contact with the plantar calcaneonavicular (spring) ligament.

NECK

It is the connecting part between the head and the body and has upper and lower surfaces.

UPPER SURFACE : It provides the following attachments:
- **Anteriorly :** Dorsal talenavicular ligament.
- **Posteriorly :** Capsular ligament of the ankle joint.
- **Laterally :** Anterior talofibular ligament (also extends to the anterior border of the lateral surface).

LOWER SURFACE : It is grooved in the medial part which is known as the sulcus tali. In the articulated foot it forms a bony canal, the sinus tarsi, with the sulcus calcanei. The rough area of the neck provides attachments to the interosseous talocalcaneal and cervical ligaments.

BODY

It has five surfaces which are, dorsal, plantar (inferior), medial, lateral and posterior.

DORSAL SURFACE (FIG. 11.34) : It is completely occupied by the trochlear, surface which is convex anteroposteriorly and slightly concave from side to side and articulates with the inferior surface of the lower end of the tibia to form the ankle joint. The surface is narrow posteriorly. Hence, a certain amount of accessory movement is allowed in the joint during plantar flexion at the cost of stability. Posterolaterally, a triangular smooth impression on this surface comes in relation with the posterior tibiofibular ligament during dorsiflexion of the ankle joint.

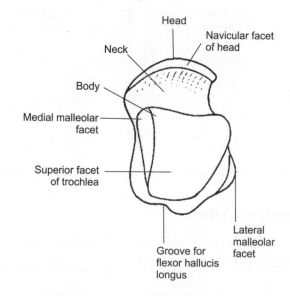

Fig. 11.34 : Right talus, dorsal aspect

PLANTAR SURFACE (Fig. 11.35) : Occupied by an oval concave facet, the entire surface articulates with the dorsal surface of the calcaneus.

MEDIAL SURFACE (Fig. 11.36) : It exhibits, (1) a comma-shaped facet superiorly for articulation with the medial malleolus of the tibia and (2) a rough ligamentous area below this for the attachment of the deep fibres of the deltoid ligament.

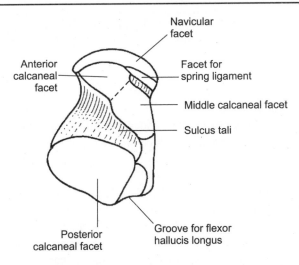

Fig. 11.35 : Right talus, plantar aspect

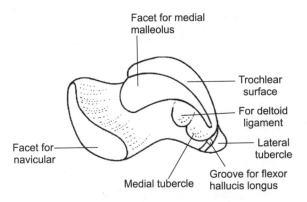

Fig. 11.36 : Right talus : Medial aspect

LATERAL SURFACE (Fig. 11.37) : It presents a triangular articular articular facet whose apex points downwards and is known as the lateral process.
- **Articular facet :** Articulates with the lateral malleolus of the fibula.
- **Anterior border :** Provides attachment to anterior talofibular ligament. (Fig. 11.38)

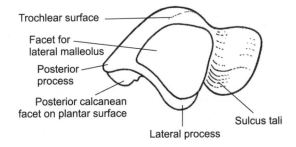

Fig. 11.37 : Right talus : Lateral aspect

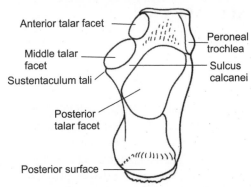

Fig. 11.38 : Right calcaneus, dorsal aspect

- **Lateral process :** Gives attachment to lateral talocalcanean ligament.
- **Posterior border of (1) :** The lateral talocalcanean ligament extends over here.

POSTERIOR SURFACE : Also known as the posterior process, it exhibits a groove flanked by a medial and a lateral tubercle.
- **Groove :** It lodges the tendon of flexor hallucis longus.
- **Medial tubercle :** It provides attachments to (a) superficial posterior fibres of the deltoid ligament above and (b) medial talocalcanean ligament below (a) (Fig. 11.39).

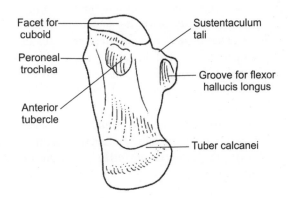

Fig. 11.39 : Right calcaneus, plantar aspect

- **Lateral tubercle :** It gives attachments to (a) posterior talofibular ligament above and (b) posterior talocalcanean ligament below, which extends to the posterior border of the lateral surface. (Fig. 11.40)

The talus does not have any muscular or tendinous attachments.

THE CALCANEUS

The calcaneus is the largest tarsal bone and articulates superiorly with the talus to form the subtalar joint and anteriorly with the cuboid to form one of the midtarsal joints.

SURFACES AND DETERMINATION OF SIDE : The bone has six surfaces, anterior, posterior, superior, plantar (inferior), lateral and medial. The upper surface bears a large facet while the plantar is rough and tuberculated. The medial surface possesses a shelf-like projection. The anterior surface has a concavoconvex facet and is thus distinguished from the posterior surface which is rough and nonarticular. Thus, the bone belongs to the side opposite to which the shelf-like projection points.

UPPER SURFACE (Fig. 11.38) : It is divisible into three areas :

- **Posterior one-third :** Rough and nonarticular, it is related to fibrofatty tissue interposed between the back of the ankle joint and the tendocalcaneus.
- **Middle one-third :** It possesses a facet for articulation with the posterior facet of the talus.
- **Anterior one-third :** It consists of articular and nonarticular areas.

(a) Nonarticular area : It is depressed and forms a groove medially. The groove is known as the sulcus calcanei and forms the sinus tarsi with the sulcus tali. The groove gives attachments to the (i) *interosseous talocalcanean ligament* (ii) *cervical ligament* and (iii) *inferior extensor retinaculum.* The rough area in front of the posterior facet of the talus gives attachments to (iv) extensor digitorum brevis muscle (origin), (v) stem of the bifurcated ligament, and (vi) inferior extensor retinaculum.

(b) Articular area : Situated anteromedially, it possesses two facets, named, middle and anterior, for the talus. The middle facet is actually situated on the sustentaculum tali.

PLANTAR SURFACE (Fig. 11.39) : This is the lower surface. Its posterior part is tuberculated and is known as the calcanean tuberosity which is further subdivided into a lateral and a medial process. In front of these is the anterior tubercle. A triangular area is enclosed between the process and the tubercle.

- **Medial process :** It provides attachments to (a) flexor retinaculum and (b) abductor hallucus (origin) medially and to (c) flexor digitorum brevis (origin) and (d) plantar aponeurosis lateral to (a) and (b).
- **Lateral process :** It gives origin to abductor digiti minimi muscle.
- **Triangular area :** It provides attachments to the (a) long plantar ligament over the whole area and (b) flexor digitorum accessorius muscle along its lateral margin.
- **Anterior tubercle :** The short plantar ligament is attached here.

ANTERIOR SURFACE (Fig. 11.40) : It is wholly articular and possesses a concavoconvex facet for articulation with the cuboid bone.

POSTERIOR SURFACE (Fig. 11.41) : It is divided into three areas, upper, middle and lower.

- **Upper area :** Related to a bursa and fatty tissue which lie between the bone and the tendocalcaneus.
- **Middle area :** It provides insertion to the tendocalcaneus over the whole area and to the plantaris medially.
- **Lower area :** It is subcutaneous and is separated from the skin by fibrofatty tissue.

LATERAL SURFACE (Fig. 11.41) : It exhibits a tubercle anteriorly, the peroneal tubercle, which separates two ill-defined grooves.

- **Peroneal tubercle :** It gives attachment to a slip of the inferior peroneal retinaculum.
- **Groove above and in front of (1) :** Related to the tendon of peroneus brevis.

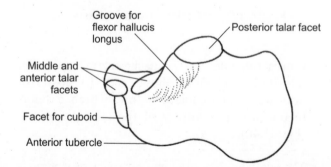

Fig. 11.40 : The right calcaneus : Medial aspect

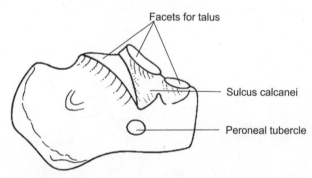

Fig. 11.41 : The right calcaneus : Lateral aspect

- **Groove below and behind (1) :** Related to the tendon of peroneus longus. The inferior margin of the groove gives attachment to the inferior peroneal retinaculum.
- **Elevation about 1 cm behind (1) :** Attachment of the calcaneofibular ligament.
- **Rest of the surface :** Subcutaneous.

MEDIAL SURFACE (Fig. 11.40) : It is concave and its anterior part shows a shelf-like projection, the sustentaculum tali.

Sustentaculum tali :
- **Its upper surface :** Articular and possesses the middle facet for talus.
- **Its inferior surface :** Possesses a groove which lodges the tendon of the flexor hallucis longus. The margins of the groove provide attachment to the slips of the flexor retinaculum.
- **Its medial surface :** Provides attachment to (i) plantar calcaneonavicular ligament, (ii) a slip of tibialis posterior (insertion), (iii) deltoid ligament, and (iv) medial talocalcanean ligament in that order anteroposteriorly. The lower part of the surface is sometimes grooved by the tendon of the flexor digitorum longus.

Rest of the surface : Gives origin to the medial head of the flexor digitorum accessorius muscle from a large area.

THE NAVICULAR BONE (FIGS. 11.32 & 11.33)

It is situated between the talus posteriorly and the three cuneiform bones anteriorly. It is shaped like a boat and possesses six surfaces.

ANTERIOR SURFACE : This surface is wholly articular and has three articular facets, each triangular in shape. The medialmost is the largest, its apex points medially and articulates with the medial cuneiform bone. Those for the other two cuneiforms are also triangular but their apices point inferiorly.

POSTERIOR SURFACE : It has a concave facet for articulation with the head of the talus.

DORSAL SURFACE : It is entirely ligamentous and gives attachments to the (1) dorsal talonavicular ligament posteriorly, (2) cuneionavicular ligaments anteriorly, and (3) cubonavicular ligament laterally.

PLANTAR SURFACE : It is rough and marked by a groove just lateral to the tuberosity of the medial surface.
- **Groove :** Lodges the tendon of the part of the tibialis posterior which proceeds forwards in the groove and is inserted in other tarsal and some of the metatarsal bones.

Surface lateral to the groove : Gives attachment to plantar calcaneonavicular (spring) ligament.

MEDIAL SURFACE : It presents the tuberosity of the navicular bone in its lower part which receives the insertion of the main part of the *tibialis posterior tendon*.

LATERAL SURFACE : It is usually nonarticular but may sometimes possess a facet for articulation with the cuboid bone. The rest of the surface gives attachment to the medial limb (calcaneonavicular part) of the bifurcated ligament.

THE CUBOID BONE (FIGS. 11.32 & 11.33)

The cuboid bone is situated between the calcaneus posteriorly and the fourth and fifth metatarsals anteriorly. On its medial side is the navicular bone. Like the other tarsals, it also has *six surfaces*.

ANTERIOR SURFACE : This surface provides articulation for the base of the lateral two metatarsals. That for the fourth is quadrangular and medial. The one for the fifth is triangular and lateral.

POSTERIOR SURFACE : It bears a triangular concavoconvex facet with a projecting inferomedial angle which articulates with the anterior surface of the calcaneus.

PLANTAR SURFACE : The plantar surface presents:
- A *groove* which lodges the tendon of the peroneus longus.
- **A ridge posterior to the groove :** Gives attachment to the long plantar ligament.
- **An area in front of the ridge :** Provides attachment to some fibres of the same ligament (long plantar).
- **Surface behind the ridge :** Gives attachment to the short plantar ligament.
- **Posteromedial projecting angle :** Receives insertion of a slip of the tibialis posterior tenbon.
- **Lateral end of the ridge :** Related to a sesamoid bone which is associated with the tendon of peroneus longus.

DORSAL SURFACE : It is entirely ligamentous and the ligaments attached here are, (1) dorsal calcaneocuboid posteriorly, (2) cubometatarsals anteriorly, (3) cubonavicular, and (4) cuneocuboid, both medially.

MEDIAL SURFACE : It has both articular and nonarticular areas.
- **Articular area :** It consists of one facet, occasionally two. The constant one articulates with the lateral

cuneiform bone. The other, when present, is behind the former and is meant for the navicular bone.

- **Nonarticular area :** It gives attachments to the (a) medial calcaneocuboid (lateral limb of bifurcated ligament), (b) cubonavicular, and (c) cuneocuboid ligaments.

LATERAL SURFACE : It is a narrow area and is nonarticular and nonligamentous. The groove for the peroneus longus commences here.

THE CUNEIFORM BONES (FIGS. 11.32 & 33)

These are three wedge-shaped bones, the medial, intermediate and lateral, which articulate with the navicular bone posteriorly and the three medial metatarsals anteriorly.

IDENTIFICATION : The medial cuneiform is the largest. Of the articular surfaces, one is bean-shaped and another is F-shaped. The *intermediate cuneiform* is the smallest. One of its articular surfaces is F-shaped. The lateral cuneiform is intermediate in size. None of its articular surfaces are either bean-shaped or F-shaped.

SURFACES, ARTICULATIONS AND ATTACH-MENTS : Each cuneiform bone has six surfaces. These are plantar, dorsal, anterior, posterior, medial and lateral. Each bone provides attachments to a few muscles and a large number of interosseous ligaments which bind it to the adjacent articulating bones.

MEDIAL CUNEIFORM

- It is the largest of the three cuneiform bones.
- Base of the wedge is plantar but in the other two it is dorsal.
- Lower surface is broader than its upper one.
- It presents articular surfaces for the navicular, the first and second metatarsals and the intermediate cuneiform.

INTERMEDIATE CUNEIFORM

- It is the smallest of the three cuneiforms.
- It has broader dorsal surface and however plantar surface.
- It has articular surfaces for the navicular, the second metatarsal, and the medial and lateral cuneiforms.

LATERAL CUNEIFORM

- Base of the wedge is dorsal, so this surface is broad.
- It articulates mostly with the navicular, the intermediate

cuneiform, the cuboid, and the 3rd metatarsal and to a small extent with the 2nd and 4th metatarsals.

THE METATARSUS (FIG. 11.42)

The metatarsus consists of five metatarsal bones situated between the tarsus and the phalanges and are numbered from the medial to the lateral side. Metatarsals are miniature long bones, each possessing a base, a head and a shaft connecting the two.

The bases are proximal and their principal articulations are with the corresponding tarsal bones. In addition, they articulate with the neighbouring metatarsal bones. It is convenient to remember that the second metatarsal bone projects a little more posteriorly than the rest. Hence, it articulates with the adjacent tarsal bones as well.

The shafts are concave on their plantar aspects. The plantar surface of a metatarsal bone will not touch the surface of a table when it is made to rest on the table on its plantar aspect.

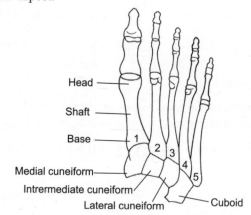

Fig. 11.42 : Metatarsus and phalanges

Meta-tarsal	Posterior articulat-ion.	Articulation with adjacent metatarsals	Articulation with adjacent tarsals
I.	Medial cuneiform	2nd metatarsal (contact only)	—
II.	Intermediate cuneiform	1st metatarsal (contact only)	Medial and lateral cun-eiform.
III.	Lateral cuneiform	2nd metatarsal 4th metatarsal	—
IV.	Cuboid	3rd metatarsal 5th metatarsal	Lateral cuneiform (occasional).
V.	Cuboid	4th metatarsal	—

The heads are round and are meant for articulation with the proximal phalanges. The articular surface is more extensive on the plantar aspect.

ATTACHMENTS : Two groups of structures, muscles and ligaments find attachment on the metatarsal bones.

Muscular attachments : These belong to two groups, the intrinsic muscles of the foot (interossei flexor digiti minimi brevis and adductor hallucis) and the tendons of some of the muscles of the leg.

- *Interossei :* These are seven in number in the foot, of which four are dorsal and three plantar.

The *dorsal interossei* arise by two heads from the adjacent metatarsal bones. Hence, the medial and lateral surfaces of the shafts of all the bones excluding the medial surface of the first metatarsal and the lateral surface of the fifth give origin to the dorsal interossei which encroach on the dorsal surfaces as well.

The *plantar interossei* take origin from the ventral aspects of the medial, fourth and fifth metatarsals only.

- *Flexor digiti minimi brevis* takes origin from the medial part of the plantar surface of the fifth metatarsal bone.
- *Adductor hallucis (oblique head)* arises from the plantar aspect of the bases of the second, third and fourth metatarsals but most of the attachment is on the plantar ligament of the tarsometatarsal joints.
- *Tibialis anterior* gives a slip of insertion to the plantar aspect of the medial surface of the first metatarsal.
- *Peroneus longus* also gives a slip of insertion to the first metatarsal, on the plantar aspect of the lateral surface of its base.
- *Peroneus brevis* and *Peroneus tertius* are inserted into the base of the fifth metatarsal bone, the former on the dorsal surface of its styloid process and the latter on the medial aspect of its dorsal surface
- *Tibialis posterior* finds insertion through small slips on the plantar aspect of the base of the second, third and fourth metatarsals but they are attached on ligaments and not directly on bone.

Ligaments : These are numerous and extend between each metatarsal and bones adjacent to it.

OSSIFICATION

Tarsal bones : Each tarsal bone is ossified from a single centre, except the calcaneus which has an additional centre for its posterior surface and the talus, the posterior process of which may also sometimes ossify from a separate centre. The order and the approximate age of their appearance are as follows:

Calcaneus : 5th month of intrauterine life (additional centre for posterior surface appears between 6th and 8th year and fuses by 16th year).

Talus : 6th month of intrauterine life. The posterior process, sometimes, may ossify from a separate centre and remain separate forming the ostrigonum.

Cuboid—9th month of intrauterine life.

Lateral cuneiform—1st year.

Medial cuneiform—2nd year.

Intermediate cuneiform—3rd year.

Navicular—3rd year.

Metatarsal bones : Each metatarsal bone ossifies from two centres, one primary and one secondary. The primary centre appears in the middle of the shaft between the 9th and 10th week of intrauterine life. The secondary centres appear in the 3rd year in the base of the 1st metatarsal bone and in the heads of the rest and fuse with the shaft between the 18th and 20th year.

Note particularly the following features in the skeleton of the foot.

- The plantar surface of the calcaneus with its three named prominences and at a higher level the plantar aspect of the sustentaculum tali.
- The deep groove and prominent ridge on the plantar surface of the cuboid.
- The tuberosity of the navicular at the junction of the medial and plantar aspect of the bone.
- The plantar calcaneonavicular (spring) ligament in the gap between the sustentaculum tali and navicular.
- The sagittal grooves, separated by a ridge, on the plantar aspect of the articular surface on the first metatarsal head.
- The tuberosity extending backwards and laterally from the base of the fifth metatarsal.
- No muscles insert on the dorsal aspect of any tarsal bone.
- The peroneus longus and tibialis anterior tendons are attached to the lateral and medial sides respectively of the inferior surface of the medial cuneiform bone adjacent to its articulation with the first metatarsal bone.
- The tibialis posterior is attached to all the cuneiform bones, to the cuboid and to the lateral of our metatarsal bones.

12

Lower Limb—Front of Thigh

INTRODUCTION

Parts and Regions of the Lower Limb

- The **thigh** which can be divided into three compartments—anterior or extensor, medial or adductor and posterior or flexor.
- The **gluteal region** is made up of hip and buttock and overlies the side and back of pelvis, above the posterior compartment of thigh.
- The **knee** is divisible into a posterior region, the popliteal fossa and an anterior or patellar region.
- The **leg** extends from the knee joint to the ankle joint. It also has three compartments—anterior or extensor, lateral or peroneal and posterior or flexor.
- The **foot** extends from the point of the heel to the roots of the toes. It has a dorsum or upper surface and a sole or plantar surface.

The lower limb is built for support and propulsion. It is constructed on the same fundamental plan as the upper limb. Assumption of erect posture by man has freed the upper limb from weight bearing and it has become specialized in that direction. Due to erect posture the burden upon the lower limb has become greater. It is specialized more in the direction of stability at the expense of some freedom of movement. In view of their function the bones of lower limb are larger than the corresponding bones of the upper limb. In order to prevent dislocation due to the forces to which they are subjected, the lower limb joints are more stable due to shape of joint surfaces and the number and strength of the ligaments.

BONY FRAMEWORK (FIG. 12.1)

Parts of the anterior aspect of hip bone and femur form the bony framework of the front of thigh.

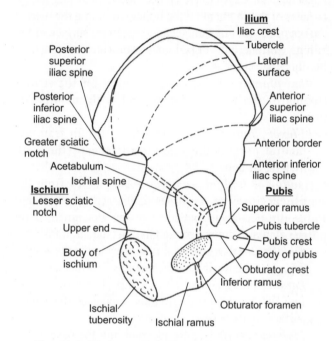

Fig. 12.1: Hip bone: Dorsal aspect of right hip bone.

The Hip Bone

The hip bone is a large flat bone of irregular shape which articulates with the sacrum and with its fellow of the opposite side to form the bony pelvis. It also articulates with the femur. It has three parts, the ilium, pubis and ischium which meet at the acetabular cavity. The **ilium** forms the upper part of the acetabulum and the fan-shaped bone above it. The **pubis** constitutes the anterior part of the acetabulum and the part of the bone associated with it. The rest of the bone forms the **ischium**. The pubis and ischium are also united medial to the obturator foramen to form the **ischiopubic ramus**.

The **ilium** possesses two ends which are upper and lower; three borders which are anterior, posterior and medial and two surfaces named lateral or gluteal and medial. The latter is subdivided into the iliac fossa and sacropelvic surface by a medial border.

The upper end is the expanded end and is limited anteriorly by a projection named the **anterior superior iliac spine**. The lower end forms a part of the acetabulum.

The anterior border extends between the anterior superior iliac spine and the acetabulum. Just above the latter it is marked by a rough projection, the **anterior inferior iliac spine**.

The **pubis** constitutes the anterior part of the hip bone. It possesses a body, which articulates with the pubis of the opposite side to form the **pubic symphysis**, a **superior ramus** which is directed upwards and backwards to meet the ilium and ischium at the acetabulum, and an inferior ramus which runs backward, downward and laterally (forming the medial boundary of the **obturator foramen**) to meet the ramus of the ischium and constitute the **ischiopubic ramus**.

The body of pubis is flattened anteroposteriorly and forms the anterior wall of the true pelvis. It has three surfaces which are anterior, posterior and medial or symphyseal and an upper border termed the pubic crest. **Pubic crest** ends laterally in a blunt projection termed the **pubic tubercle**. The crest has anterior and posterior borders which enclose a surface and meet at the pubic tubercle.

The superior ramus extends upward, backward and laterally from the upper lateral part of the body to the acetabulum. It has three surfaces, pectineal, pelvic and obturator enclosed between three borders viz., the pectineal line (pecten pubis), obturator crest and inferior border. **Pectineal line** is the sharpest of the three borders and extends from the pubic tubercle to the **arcuate line**. Together with the pubic crest it forms the pubic part of the arcuate line which is the boundary line between the false and the true pelvis. Medial border of ilium forms the iliac part of the arcuate line. The **obturator crest** is rounded and situated anterior to the pectineal line, it extends from the pubic tubercle to the acetabulum. The inferior border forms the anterior margin of the **obturator foramen**. The pectineal surface is limited by the pectineal line behind and the obturator crest in front. Pelvic surface is bounded above by the pectineal line and below by the inferior border. The obturator surface is bounded by the obturator crest in front and the inferior border behind.

The **inferior ramus** arises from the lower and lateral part of the pubis and runs downward, backward and slightly laterally forming the inferior boundary of the **obturator foramen**. It joins the ramus of the ischium and they are known together as the **ischiopubic ramus**.

The **ischium** constitutes the lower and posterior part of the hip bone and consists of a body and a ramus. The latter extends upward, forwards and medially from the lower part of the body, forms the lower boundary of the obturator foramen and meets the inferior ramus of the pubis to form the ischiopubic ramus.

The body has two ends, upper and lower, three borders (viz., dorsal or posterior, lateral and the margin of the obturator foramen) and three surfaces. The upper end forms a part of the acetabulum. The lower end is free and forms the **ischial tuberosity**. Femoral surface is the lateral surface of the body and is limited anteriorly by the margin of the obturator foramen and posteriorly by the lateral border. Dorsal surface is a continuation downwards of the gluteal surface of ilium. Pelvic surface is bounded in front by the margin of the obturator foramen and behind by the posterior border.

The **ischiopubic ramus** has external and internal surfaces and lateral and medial borders. The lateral border forms the margin of the obturator foramen.

The Femur (Fig. 12.12)

The femur is the skeleton of the thigh and is the longest and strongest bone of the body. It has two ends, upper and lower, joined by a shaft.

The **upper end** consists of a **head** joined to the rest of the bone by a **neck**. At the junction of the neck with the shaft are two projections, the **greater and lesser trochanters**. A rounded ridge called the intertrochanteric line extends between the two trochanters.

The **lower end** of the bone is expanded and is partly separated to form the **lateral and medial condyles**.

The **shaft** is narrow in the middle but expanded at the two ends. Its long axis inclines medially about 10° from the vertical axis. The middle third presents three surfaces, anterior, medial and lateral bounded by three borders, lateral, medial and posterior. The former two are indistinct but the posterior border is very prominent and is termed the **linea aspera**. The upper and lower third of the shaft present a fourth surface each bounded by the bifurcation of the lips of linea aspera.

At the lower end of femur, the anterior surface of both the condyles possess an articular surface for the patella which is a continuous area slightly grooved in the middle and concave from side to side. It extends higher on the lateral condyle.

The Patella (Fig. 12.12)

The **patella** is a sesamoid bone (the largest in the body) which has developed in the tendon of the quadriceps femoris and lies in front of the knee joint. It is a rounded triangle presenting anterior and posterior surfaces, superior (base), lateral and medial borders and an apex which is directed inferiorly.

THE FASCIA

The Superficial Fascia (Fig. 12.2)

The superficial fascia of the thigh presents two layers :

- A **superficial fatty layer** continuous with the superficial fatty layer of superficial fascia of the anterior abdominal wall (Camper's fascia).

- A **deep membranous layer** continuous with the deep membranous layer of superficial fascia of the anterior abdominal wall (Scarpa's fascia). It is loosely attached to the deep fascia of thigh except near the inguinal ligament where there is a linear, fairly from attachment to the deep fascia along a horizontal line from the pubic tubercle towards the lateral aspect of thigh.

The superficial fascia contains blood vessels, lymph nodes and lymph channels as well as cutaneous nerves supplying the skin.

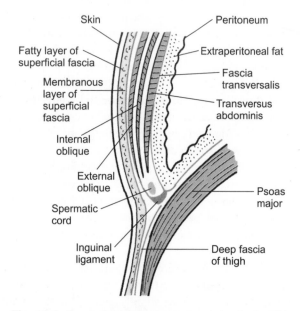

Fig. 12.2: Front of thigh and anterior abdominal wall in sagittal section to show the disposition of superficial and deep fascia of front of thigh

CLINICAL APPLICATION

In rupture of male urethra the urine passes into the anterior part of perineum. Its further course is determined by the disposition of fascia in the thigh. It cannot pass into the medial side of the thigh because of the attachment of the membranous layer of the superficial fascia to the side of the pubic arch and to the front of the pubis, but it ascends to the anterior abdominal wall between the membranous layer and the deep fascia. From the abdominal wall it cannot descend into the front of the thigh because of the connection between the membranous layer and the deep fascia of the thigh (Fig. 12.3).

THE DEEP FASCIA (FIG. 12.3)

The deep fascia of the thigh covers the entire thigh and is known as **fascia lata (Latus = Broad, *Latin*)**. It is attached on the front to the iliac crest, the inguinal ligament and the pubis and is especially thickened on the lateral side where it forms the **iliotibial tract** which is attached superiorly to the ilium along the outer border of its crest and there encloses the **tensor fascia lata**. About the distal two-thirds of thigh, the fascia lata sends medial, posterior and lateral intermuscular septa to the linea aspera of femur. The fascia lata is attached below to the patella, the tibial condyles and head of fibula. The inguinal ligament is convex downwards due to the attachment of the deep fascia.

Saphenous opening is an oval aperture in the deep fascia of the thigh 3 cm long and 1.5 cm wide with its centre lying 3 to 4 cm below and lateral to the pubic tubercle. It is covered by a thinner fascia called the **cribriform fascia,** perforated by certain vessels. Saphenous opening has a sharp lateral and inferior margins called the **falciform margin**. The upper margin goes upto the inguinal ligament and pubic tubercle and the lower margin turns medially to become continuous with the fascia covering the pectineus muscle and is called the **pectineal fascia**. The pectineal fascia slopes deeper laterally behind the femoral sheath. **Great saphenous vein** ascends from the medial side of the thigh and inclines anteriorly through the thigh to the saphenous opening, where it pierces the cribriform fascia and the femoral sheath to enter the femoral vein.

Three small branches of the femoral artery pierce the cribriform fascia. The superficial external pudendal radiates medially, the **superficial epigastric** upward and the **superficial circumflex iliac** laterally. They supply the skin

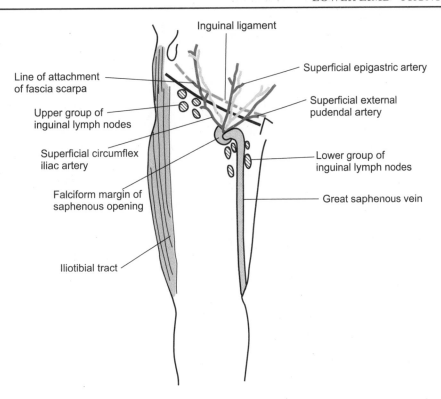

Fig. 12.3: The front of thigh : Deep fascia, superficial vessels and lymph nodes (dotted lines indicate the line of fusion of the membranous layer of superficial fascia with the deep fascia of thigh)

of the external genital organs, of the groin and of the lower part of the anterior abdominal wall and the inguinal lymph nodes.

The upper group of large **superficial inguinal nodes** lie spread out below the line of fusion of the membranous layer of superficial fascia with the deep fascia of the thigh. The lower group of large superficial inguinal nodes lie along both sides of the upper part of the great saphenous vein.

CLINICAL APPLICATION

Full relaxation of the abdominal wall for palpation of the abdominal viscera can be achieved by flexing the thighs. This eliminates the pull of the fascia lata on the inguinal ligament to which it is attached.

Cutaneous Nerves (Fig. 12.4)

(a) From the Lumbar Plexus in the Abdomen

- **The ilioinguinal nerve (L_1):** It is the second and lower branch of first lumbar nerve. It becomes superficial after passing through the superficial inguinal ring. It accompanies the structures of the spermatic cord and

supplies the skin of the thigh over the proximal and medial part of thigh. Most of its branches go to skin of superior part of scrotum, root and dorsum of penis in male and mons pubis and labium majus in female.

- **The femoral branch of the genitofemoral nerves (L_1 and L_2):** It issues out after piercing the femoral sheath and pierces the deep fascia 2 cm below the inguinal ligament, a little lateral to the saphenous opening. It supplies the skin of the upper part of thigh just below the inguinal ligament.

- **The cutaneous branch of the anterior division of obturator** is a fine twig which becomes cutaneous to supply the distal third of the medial side of thigh.

- **The lateral cutaneous nerves of thigh (L_2 and L_3)** leave the abdomen close to the anterior superior iliac spine, behind the inguinal ligament. It supplies the skin of the lateral side and front of thigh.

(b) From the Femoral Nerve

- **The intermedial cutaneous nerve of the thigh.** It pierces the deep fascia of thigh near the midline and extends upto the knee. It usually appears as two branches.

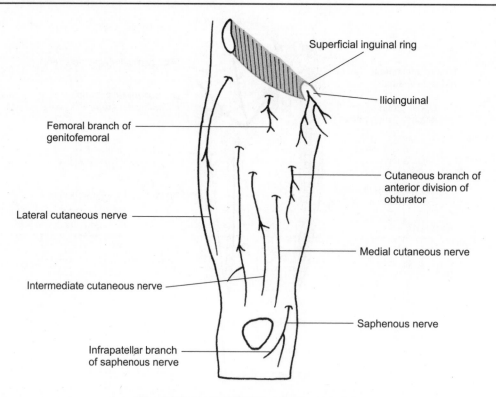

Fig. 12.4: Front of thigh: cutaneous nerves

- **The medial cutaneous nerve of the thigh.** It pierces the deep fascia on the medial side of the thigh and descends upto the knee.
- The **saphenous nerve** becomes subcutaneous on the medial side of knee and lies in front of the great saphenous vein. It gives off an **infrapatellar branch** before piercing the fascia.

THE FEMORAL TRIANGLE

A great part of the upper third of thigh is occupied by a hollow. The anterior aspect of this hollow is named femoral triangle.

Boundaries (Fig. 12.5)

Base

- Inguinal ligament.

Lateral Boundary

- The medial border of the sartorius.

Medial Boundary

- The medial border of the adductor longus.

Apex

- Meeting point of the medial borders of the above two muscles.

Floor (Fig. 12.5)

From medial to lateral side the floor is formed by adductor longus, pectineus, psoas major and iliacus. Adductor brevis may show up between the adductor longus and pectineus.

Contents (Fig. 12.6)

The area between the inguinal ligament and the superior pubic ramus is divided into two compartments:

(a) The muscular compartment which contains from lateral to medial side:
- The lateral cutaneous nerve of thigh.
- The iliopsoas.
- The femoral nerve.

(b) The vascular compartment which contains from lateral to medial side:
- The femoral artery with the femoral branch of genitofemoral nerve.

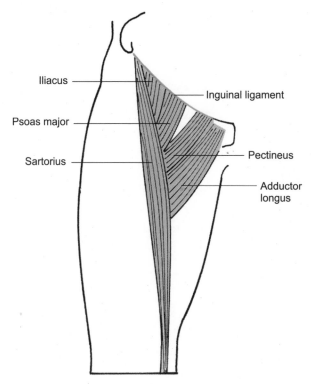

Fig. 12.5: Front of thigh : The femoral triangle—boundaries and floor

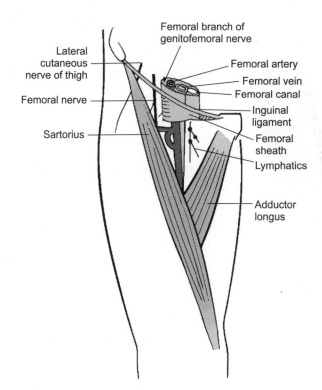

Fig. 12.6: The femoral triangle: Contents

- The femoral vein.
- The femoral ring containing lymphatics.
- The lacunar ligament.

The **femoral vessels traverse** the triangle from base to apex. The vein changes its relation with the artery from medial aspect at the base to the posterior aspect at the apex of the triangle. The **deep external pudendal** is a small artery arising from the medial side of the femoral artery near the base of the triangle. It is distributed to the scrotum in the male and the labium majus in the female.

The **profunda femoris** springs from the lateral side of the femoral artery 5 cm below the inguinal ligament. It soon passes deep to the artery and disappears behind adductor longus. The **profunda vein** is in front of its artery and ends in the femoral vein. Two large arteries spring from the profunda femoris near its origin. The **lateral circumflex** artery runs laterally and leaves the triangle behind the sartorius. The **medial circumflex artery** passes backward and disappears through the floor of the triangle between the psoas and the pectineus. The **circumflex veins** end in the femoral.

The **femoral branch of genitofemoral nerve** runs close to the artery on its lateral side and within the femoral sheath (Fig. 12.7).

The **femoral nerve** lies lateral to the femoral artery and outside the femoral sheath.

The **lateral cutaneous nerve of thigh** crosses the lateral angle of the triangle.

FEMORAL SHEATH (FIGS. 12.7 AND 12.8)

In the osteoligamentous pelvis there is a wide firm aperture which is bounded by the anterior border of the pelvis posteriorly and the inguinal ligament anteriorly. This aperture is situated at the junction of the abdomen and the thigh and unless it is fully packed, structures from abdomen may herniate into the thigh. This aperture is packed, by iliopsoas, pectineus, femoral vessels, femoral nerve, lateral cutaneous nerve of thigh and deep lymphatics. The iliopsoas which forms the posterior wall of abdomen is covered by **fascia iliac** which fuses with **fascia transversalis** which lines the anterior abdominal wall. The fusion of the two fasciae opposite the inguinal ligament along its lateral half seals off the abdominal cavity from the thigh. The external iliac vessels which become the femoral vessels in the thigh are situated within the fascial box of abdomen and thus when the vessels reach the inguinal ligament they are met by fascia iliaca behind and the fascia transversalis in front and the two fasciae are continued down into the thigh along

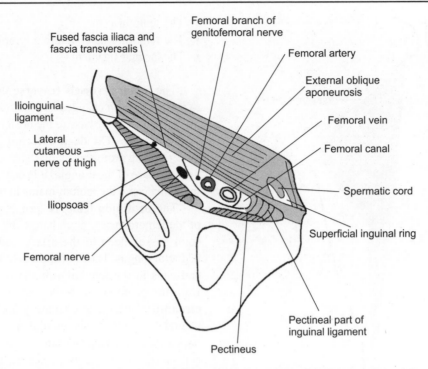

Fig. 12.7: Femoral sheath : Structures passing through the osteoligamentous gap of the pelvis

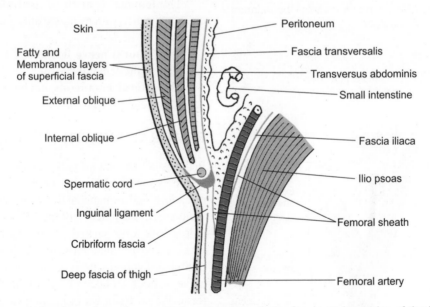

Fig. 12.8: Femoral sheath as shown in a sagittal section through the fascia and muscles of the inguinal region

the vessels and fuse over them. Thus, the fascial abdominal box is closed along the inguinal ligament in its lateral half and it is prolonged down in the thigh opposite the medial half of the ligament in the shape of a fascial pouch which is designated as the **femoral sheath**. Its various walls are related as follows:

- **Anterior wall** is covered by fascia lata in which is the fossa ovalis.
- **Posterior wall** lies on the psoas and pectineus.
- **Outer wall** is straight.
- **Inner wall** is oblique and shorter than the outer wall.

Femoral sheath has three compartments:

- **Lateral** occupied by the femoral artery and the femoral branch of genitofemoral nerve.
- **Intermediate** occupied by the femoral vein.
- **Medial** called the **'femoral canal'** occupied by fat, a lymph node and some loose areolar tissue.

FEMORAL CANAL (FIGS. 12.7 AND 12.9)

Femoral canal is 1.2 cm long and 1.2 cm wide. It lies under cover of the **cribriform fascia** which covers the saphenous opening. It contains fat and a lymph node belonging to the deep subinguinal group. The **femoral ring** is the mouth of the canal.

Boundaries

Anteriorly

The **inguinal ligament (Poupart's),** which is the inferior border of the external oblique aponeurosis between the anterior superior iliac spine and the pubic tubercle.

Posteriorly

The **pectineus** and the **pectineal ligament (Cooper's),** which is an extension of the **lacunar ligament (Gimbernat's)** along the pectineal line of the superior pubic ramus.

Laterally

- The femoral vein.

Medially

The **lacunar ligament (Gimbernat's),** which is a reflection of the inguinal ligament posteriorly to the pectinate line of the superior pubic ramus.

Contents

- A fat pad plugging the ring and known as **femoral septum**.
- A lymph node belonging to the deep inguinal group **(Cloquet's gland).**

CLINICAL APPLICATION

The femoral canal is a potential point of weakness in the abdominal wall through which a hernia can occur. The femoral hernia is more common in females due to a broader pelvis. The hernia passes through the femoral ring into the femoral canal and presents a bulge in the upper medial part of the thigh with the neck of the hernial sac below and lateral to the pubic tubercle. Its position easily differentiates it from the indirect hernia which comes through the inguinal canal and whose sac extends above and medial to the pubic tubercle as it comes out of the superficial inguinal ring.

After descending down the femoral canal the hernia passes forward through the saphenous opening then turns upwards along the course presented by the superficial epigastric and superficial circumflex iliac vessels, so it may come to project above the inguinal ligament. The course of the hernia is to be kept in mind, while reducing it. It is reduced first downwards, then backwards and finally upwards.

Irreducibility and strangulation of the hernia commonly occur at the neck of the femoral canal, which is very narrow and has the sharp lateral border of the lacunar ligament as its medial relation. To relieve pressure on the strangulated hernia the opening of the canal is enlarged by dividing the lacunar ligament. In 10% of persons an **abnormal obturator artery,** a branch of inferior epigastric artery, passes down along the edge of the lacunar ligament (Fig. 12.10). In such cases great care is to be exercised in cutting the ligament as serious haemorrhage follows division of the artery.

A femoral hernia has following coverings (Fig. 12.9):
- Femoral septum.
- Anterior wall of femoral sheath.
- Cribriform fascia.

COMPARTMENTS OF THIGH (FIG. 12.11)

Three intermuscular septa divide the muscles of the thigh into four compartments:
- The **anterior** containing leg extensors which are supplied by **femoral nerve**.
- The **medial** containing thigh adductors supplied by **obturator nerve**.
- The **posterior** containing the leg flexors supplied by the **tibial component of sciatic**.

A lateral compartment, containing thigh abductors mainly, is represented by gluteus minimus, the anterior part of gluteus medius and tensor fascia lata, is supplied by inferior gluteal nerve. Below the greater trochanter, it is represented only by the iliotibial tract.

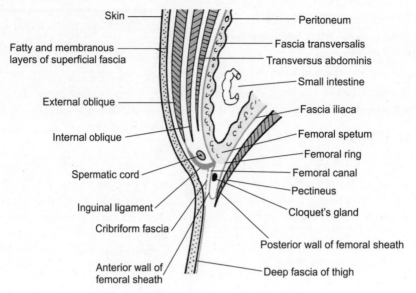

Fig. 12.9: Femoral canal in sagittal section

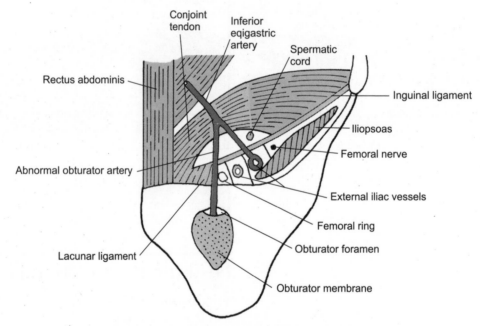

Fig. 12.10: Posterior surface of the lower part of anterior abdominal wall showing the course of an abnormal obturator artery

THE ANTERIOR COMPARTMENT OF THIGH

Bony Framework

This is already described (Fig. 12.1).

Muscles

Sartorius (Fig. 12.13)

This is an unipennate muscle with very long fibres. The upper third of the muscle forms the lateral boundary of the femoral triangle while the middle third forms the roof of the adductor canal.

Origin (Fig. 12.12)

• The lower half of the anterior superior iliac spine.

Insertion (Fig. 12.12)

It runs downward and medially, descends behind the medial

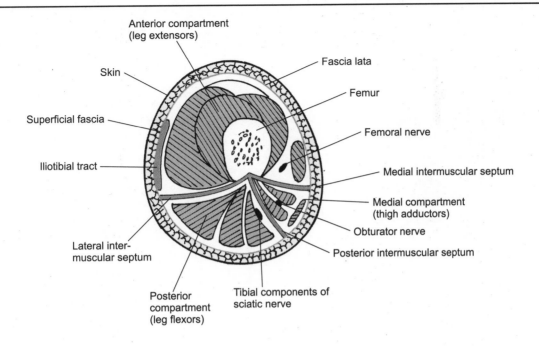

Fig. 12.11: Compartments of thigh

side of the knee joint and ends in a tendon which comes forward to get inserted into the upper part of the medial surface of tibia along with gracilis and semitendinosus.

Nerve Supply

- Femoral nerve.

Action

Abduction, flexion and lateral rotation of thigh at the hip and flexion and medial rotation of the leg at the knee.

Its action is said to produce the position of the lower limb associated with the tailor who sits sewing on a table (**Sartor = Tailor,** *Latin*).

Quadriceps Femoris (Fig. 12.13)

Quadriceps femoris consists of four parts viz., the rectus femoris, vastus medialis, vastus intermedius and vastus lateralis which form a massive muscle covering the anterior, medial and lateral aspects of the femoral shaft from the intertrochanteric line to the knee joint.

Rectus Femoris

Origin

- It is by two heads:
- **Straight head:** Upper half of anterior inferior iliac spine (Fig. 12.12).

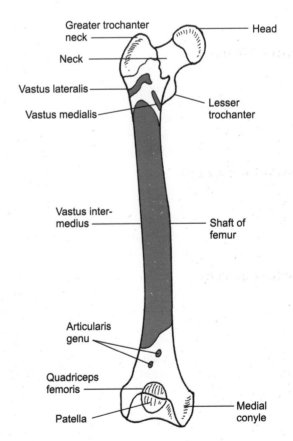

Fig. 12.12: Attachment of the muscles of anterior compartment

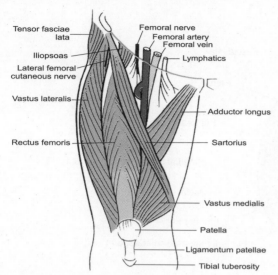

Fig. 12.13: Muscles of anterior (extensor) compartment of thigh. Tensor fascia lata belongs to the lateral (abductor) compartment

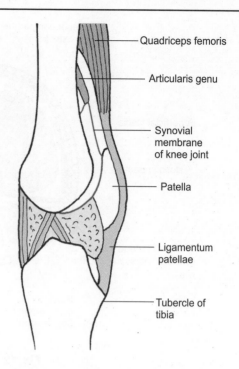

12.14: Insertion of quadriceps femoris

- **Reflected head:** The groove just above the acetabulum.

The two heads unite at an acute angle and form a powerful, fusiform bipennate muscle. The fibres have a pattern of an inverted V.

Vastus Medialis

Origin (Fig. 12.12)

Lower part of the trochanteric line, base of lesser trochanter, spiral line, medial lip of linea aspera and the upper part of the medial supracondylar ridge of femur.

Vastus Intermedius

Origin (Fig. 12.12)

- The proximal two-thirds of the anterior and lateral surface of femur.

Vastus Lateralis

Origin (Fig. 12.12)

The upper part of trochanteric line, base of greater trochanter, lateral lip of gluteal tuberosity and upper part of lateral lip of linea aspera and upper part of the lateral supracondylar ridge.

Insertion (Figs. 12.13 and 12.14)

The quadriceps femoris gives rise to a common tendon which is inserted into the tubercle of the tibia via the **ligamentum patellae**. The tendon has two laminae. A superficial lamina formed by the rectus femoris and a deep lamina formed by the three vasti. The superficial lamina is the main tendon and is attached to upper edge of patella. Its deep surface is joined by the membranous tendons of three vasti.

The medial and lateral vasti are attached also to the corresponding edges of the patella, and to the upper edge and vastus intermedius is attached to the lateral edge, by means of membranous expansions which blend with the capsule of the knee joint. Fascia lata blends with these expansions on each side forming the **medial** and **lateral patellar retinacula** which gain attachment to the medial and lateral tibial condyles.

The **patella** is a sesamoid bone in the tendon of the quadriceps. **Ligamentum patellae** represents the continuation of the tendon to the tibial tuberosity.

Nerve Supply

- Femoral nerve.

Action

- Principal extensor of knee joint.
- Strong flexor of the hip joint through rectus femoris. The above two movements are essential in kicking.

Articularis Genu

It is a small muscle lying deep to lower part of vastus intermedius and often considered a part of it.

Origin (Fig. 12.12)

- Lower part of front of femur 5 cm above the patellar surface.

Insertion (Fig. 12.14)

- Into synovial membrane of knee joint.

Nerve Supply

- Femoral nerve.

Action

- During extension of the knee joint it lifts up the synovial membrane of the knee joint to prevent its injury between the articular ends.

Tensor Fascia Lata (Fig. 12.13)

This muscle does not belong to the anterior group of thigh muscles which are supplied by the femoral nerve. It belongs to a lateral or abductor group. It has migrated anteriorly to become a flexor and medial rotator of thigh. It is enclosed between two layers of thickened fascia lata, which fuse below to form the iliotibial tract.

THE MEDIAL COMPARTMENT OF THE THIGH

Bony Framework (Fig. 12.15)

Pubis and Ischium

The osteology has already been described (Fig. 12.1).

Femur

The middle of the shaft of femur has three surfaces and three borders. The borders are lateral, medial and posterior. The former two are indistinct but the posterior border is very prominent and is termed the **linea aspera** which consists of a central rough part lineated on either side by medial and lateral lips. The upper and lower third of shaft possess a fourth surface each bounded by the bifurcation of the lips of the linea aspera. The fourth surface of the upper part, known as the posterior surface, is triangular and limited by the **gluteal tuberosity** laterally and the spiral

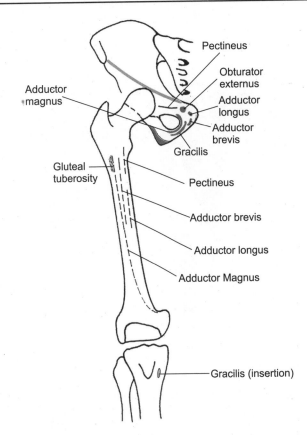

Fig. 12.15: Attachment of muscles of the medial compartment to hip bone and femur (Insertions in dotted are on the back of femur)

line medially. That in the lower part, named the popliteal surface, is also triangular and is bounded by the **medial and lateral supracondylar lines,** which are the continuation downward of the medial and the lateral lips respectively of the linea aspera. The medial supracondylar ridge terminates in the **adductor tubercle.**

MUSCLES OF THE MEDIAL COMPARTMENT

The group of adductor muscles on the medial side of the thigh is arranged in three layers. These are supplied by obturator nerve. Profunda femoris is the artery for this compartment.

FIRST LAYER (FIG. 12.16)

The first layer or the anterior layer has **pectineus, adductor longus** and **gracilis** which lie in the same plane. The adjacent borders of pectineus and adductor longus touch

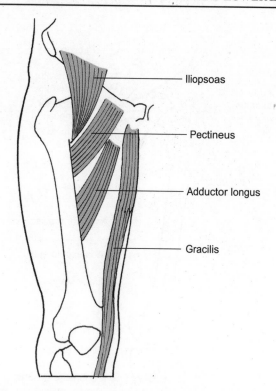

Fig. 12.16: Muscles of medial compartment. First layer (Pectineus, adductor longus and gracilis)

each other, but near the femur they are separated by a small interval.

The iliopsoas descends over the front of the hip joint and then passes backward inferior to it to get inserted into the lesser trochanter of the femur.

Pectineus

It is placed between the adductor longus and the psoas major muscles.

Origin

- Pecten pubis and the pectineal surface in front of it.

Insertion

- Pectineal line of the femur which descends from the lesser trochanter halfway to linea aspera.

Nerve Supply

- Femoral nerve.
- Sometimes additionally by obturator nerve.

Action

- Adduction of thigh.
- Flexion of thigh at the hip.

Adductor Longus

It is placed on the medial side of the pectineus. It is triangular in shape, being narrow at its origin and expanded at its insertion.

Origin

- Front of the body of pubis by a flat narrow tendon.

Insertion

- Middle one-third of the linea aspera.

Nerve Supply

- Anterior division of the obturator nerve.

Action

- Adductor of thigh.

Gracilis

It is a long slender muscle which rounds off the free, medial edges of the three adductors. In the distal third of thigh it narrows to form a slender cylindrical tendon.

Origin

- Medial margin of the lower half of the body of pubis.
- Whole length of the inferior ramus of pubis.

Insertion

Into a vertical line on the medial surface of tibia below the medial condyle between the insertions of sartorius and semitendinosus.

Nerve Supply

- Anterior division of the obturator nerve.

Action

- Adduction of thigh.
- Flexion the knee and medial rotation of the flexed leg.

SECOND LAYER (FIG. 12.17)

The second or the middle layer is formed by the **adductor brevis** alone and is behind the pectineus and the adductor longus. As it descends, it inclines backward.

Adductor Brevis

Origin

Anterior surface of the body and the outer surface of the inferior ramus of pubis, in the interval between gracilis and obturator externus.

Insertion

Along the line leading from the lesser trochanter to the linea aspera immediately behind the pectineus and the upper part of the adductor longus.

Nerve Supply

- Anterior division of the obturator nerve.
- Occasionally by posterior division of obturator.

Action

- Adduction of thigh.
- Lateral rotation of thigh.

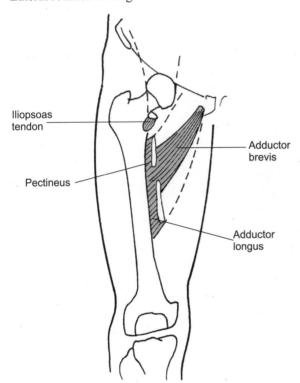

Fig. 12.17: Muscles of medial compartment : Second layer (Adductor brevis)

THIRD LAYER (FIG. 12.18)

The third or the posterior layer is formed by the **adductor magnus** and the **obturator externus**.

Adductor Magnus

It is the second largest muscle in the body, the largest being the gluteus maximus.

Origin

It is a composite muscle having two parts:
- An **adductor part** which arises from the outer surface of the combined ischiopubic ramus encroaching only slightly on the inferior ramus of pubis. The bundles arising anteriorly pass in a horizontal direction; the more posterior the origin, the more oblique the direction taken.
- A **hamstring part** arising from the lower and lateral parts of the ischial tuberosity just lateral to the part on which one sits.

Insertion

- Pubic fibres from inferior ramus of pubis into the medial lip of the gluteal tuberosity. These fibres are sometimes separate, on a more anterior plane than the rest of the muscle and then constitute **adductor minimus**.

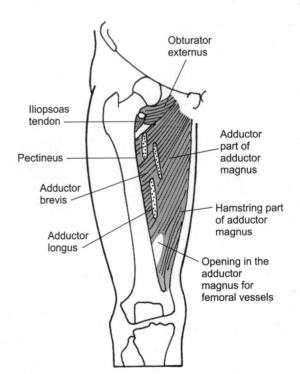

Fig. 12.18: Muscles of medial compartment : Third layer (Adductor magnus and obturator externus).

- Fibres from the ramus of ischium insert into linea aspera and the medial supracondylar ridge of the femur.
- Fibres from ischial tuberosity pass vertically downwards, end in a strong palpable tendon in the distal third of the thigh and get inserted into the adductor tubercle. The medial intermuscular septum attaches the tendon to the medial supracondylar ridge. This part constitutes the **hamstring part of adductor magnus**. The degenerated part of the hamstring part is the **tibial collateral ligament** of the knee joint.

There are five fibrous arches in the attachment of adductor magnus to the femur which allow passage to blood vessels. The upper four transmit perforating branches of profunda femoris artery. The lowest is a large aperture in the tendon of the muscle **(tendinous hiatus)** at the junction of the lower one-third and middle one-third of the thigh through which the femoral vessels pass to become the popliteal vessels.

Nerve Supply

- Posterior division of obturator supplies the fibres from the ischiopubic ramus (adductor part).
- Tibial component of the sciatic nerve supplies the fibres from the ischial tuberosity (hamstring part).

Action

- Adduction of thigh.
- Medial rotation of femur.
- Ischial fibres are weak extensors of the hip joint.

Obturator Externus

Origin

- Medial half of the obturator membrane.
- Medial and inferior margins of the obturator foramen over a wide strip.

Insertion

Trochanteric fossa of the femur, which is out of site from the front, by a narrow tendon.

The muscle passes posterolaterally, below the capsule of the hip joint and is closely applied to it.

Nerve Supply

- Posterior division of the obturator nerve.

Action

- Flexion and lateral rotation of thigh.

ADDUCTOR (SUBSARTORIAL) CANAL (FIG. 12.19)

It is also known as **Hunter's canal as John Hunter** was the first to ligate the femoral artery in this canal for **aneurysm** of the popliteal artery. It is an intermuscular space which occupies the middle third of the medial side of thigh.

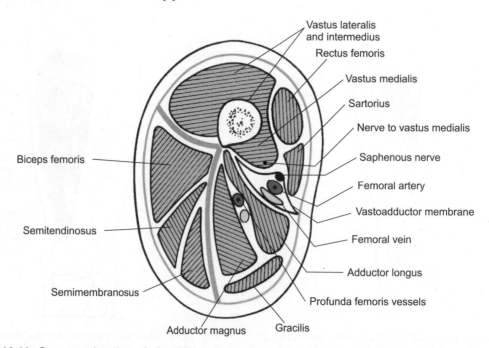

Fig. 12.19: Cross-section through the thigh in the region of the adductor or subsartorial canal of Hunter

Boundaries (Fig. 12.19)

Anterolaterally

• Vastus medialis.

Posteriorly

• Adductor longus.
• Adductor magnus.

Roof

• Sartorius.
• Vastoadductor membrane which is a fibrous sheath passing between adductor longus and the vastus medialis on which sartorius lies.

Contents

Entering the canal from above are:
• Femoral artery.
• Femoral vein behind the artery in the upper part and lateral to it in the lower part.
• Nerve to vastus medialis lies on the lateral side of the artery in the upper part then enters the muscle.
• Saphenous nerve lateral to the artery in the upper part. In the middle of the canal it crosses superficial to artery and then descends on its medial side in the lower part. It pierces the roof of the canal and becoming superficial continues distally along the medial side of the knee, leg and foot.

FEMORAL ARTERY (FIG. 12.20)

The femoral artery is the continuation of the external iliac artery and enters the thigh by passing behind the inguinal ligament midway between the anterior superior iliac spine and the symphysis pubis **(midinguinal point)**. It ends by passing through the tendinous hiatus in adductor magnus at the junction of middle and distal third of thigh to be continued as popliteal artery.

In the thigh the femoral artery traverses two regions viz., the femoral triangle and the adductor canal. The femoral artery bisects the formal triangle, thereby separating the motor territory of the obturator nerve from the motor territory of the femoral nerve.

Relations of the Artery in the Femoral Triangle

Anteriorly

• Skin, superficial fascia and fascia lata.

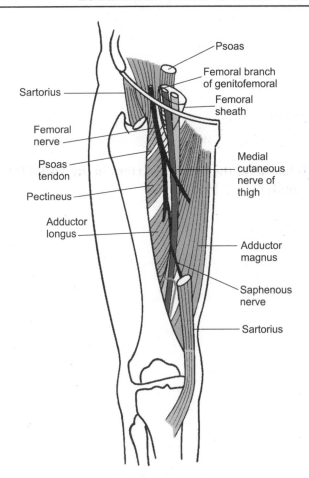

Fig. 12.20: Femoral artery and its relations

• Femoral sheath covering the upper 3.75 cm of the artery.
• Medial cutaneous nerve of the thigh crosses it at the apex of the femoral triangle.

Posteriorly from Above Downwards

• Psoas tendon behind which is the capsule of hip joint.
• Pectineus with profunda femoris vessels intervening.
• Adductor longus separated from the artery by the femoral vein.

At the apex of the femoral triangle, the femoral artery lies in front of the femoral vein which in turn lies in front of the profunda femoris vein and artery. Consequently, an injury to this region may serve all four vessels.
• Nerve to pectineus from the femoral nerve passes medially behind the upper part of the artery.

Laterally

- Femoral branch of the genitofemoral in the upper part as it lies in the lateral compartment of the femoral sheath.
- Femoral nerve and its branches.

Medially

- Femora vein in the upper part of the triangle.

Relations of the Femoral Artery in the Adductor Canal (Fig. 12.19)

Anteriorly

- Sartorius muscle.
- Fibrous roof with subsartorial plexus of nerves formed by branches from medial cutaneous nerve of thigh, saphenous nerve and anterior division of the obturator nerve.
- Saphenous nerve in front of the middle of the artery.

Posteriorly

- Femoral vein in the upper part of the canal.
- Adductor longus.
- Adductor magnus.

Laterally

- Nerve to vastus medialis in the upper part.
- Saphenous nerve in the upper half.
- Femoral vein in the lower part.

Medially

- Saphenous nerve in the lower part of the artery.

Branches (Fig. 12.21)

In the femoral triangle.

Superficial Branches (Fig. 12.3)

- Superficial circumflex iliac goes toward the anterior superior iliac spine and supplies the anterior abdominal wall.
- Superficial epigastric ascends upto supply the anterior abdominal wall.
- Superficial external pudendal supplies the external genitalia.

Deep Branches (Fig. 12.21)

- Deep external pudendal supplies the external genitalia.

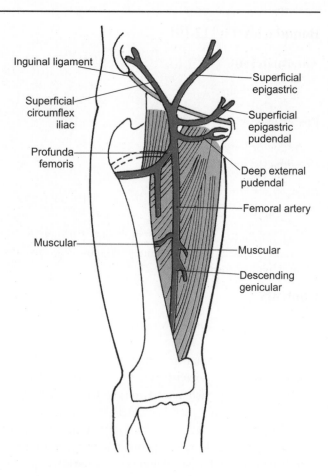

Fig. 12.21: The branches of the femoral artery

- Profunda femoris.
- Muscular.
- Descending genicular in the adductor canal. It divides into a superficial saphenous branch which accompanies the saphenous nerve and a deep muscular branch that enters the vastus medialis.
- Unnamed muscular branches.

Profunda Femoris Artery (Fig. 12.22)

The profunda femoris artery is the main source of blood supply to the muscles of the thigh. It is given off from the lateral side of the femoral artery in the femoral triangle and passes downward and medially to the apex of the femoral triangle, where femoral artery, femoral vein and profunda vein lies anterior to it. Next it descends deep into the adductor longus. Thus, from above downwards it lies on three muscles viz., the pectineus, the adductor brevis and the adductor magnus.

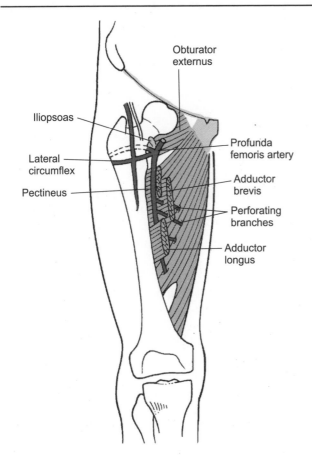

Fig. 12.22: The profunda femoris artery and its branches

The branches given off are:

(i) The **medial circumflex femoral** which passes backward and disappears through the floor of the femoral triangle between the psoas and the pectineus and then between the obturator externus and the adductor brevis to reach the back of thigh. It divides into ascending and transverse terminal branches.

(ii) The **lateral circumflex femoral** runs laterally amongst the branches of the femoral nerve and leaves the triangle behind the sartorius. It ends by dividing into ascending, transverse and descending branches.

(iii) The first three **perforating arteries**. They are so called because they perforate the deficiencies in the tendinous insertion of adductor magnus in the linea aspera.

The profunda femoris artery ends a little below the middle of the thigh as a fine terminal vessel called the fourth perforating artery, which passes backward through the adductor magnus.

(iv) A number of **muscular branches** supply the adductor muscles and some of them pierce the adductor magnus to reach the hamstring muscles.

Femoral Vein (Fig. 12.20)

The femoral vein is the continuation of the popliteal vein at the opening in the adductor magnus. It continues upwards through the adductor canal and femoral triangle at first posterior and then medial to the femoral artery. It lies in the middle compartment of the femoral sheath. At the inguinal ligament it becomes the external iliac vein.

Tributaries

- Profunda femoris which is the largest tributary and joins it 6 cm below the inguinal ligament.
- Great saphenous vein.
- Medial circumflex femoral vein.
- Lateral circumflex femoral vein.

Femoral Nerve (Fig. 12.23)

The femoral nerve arises from the dorsal divisions of anterior rami of L_2, L_3 and L_4 nerves. About 7.5 cm distal to the inguinal ligaments it divides into two sets of branches.

- Superficial set consisting of medial and intermediate cutaneous nerves of thigh and a muscular branch to sartorius (L_2).

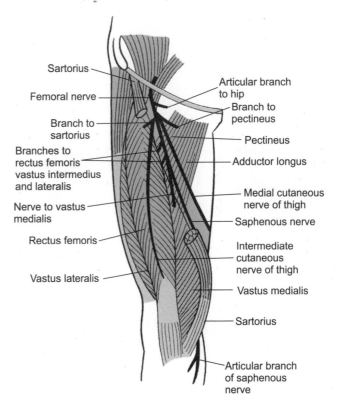

Fig. 12.23: The femoral nerve: Course and branches

- Deep set consisting of:
  - Muscular branches to:
  (a) Pectineus (L_2).
  (b) Quadriceps femoris (L_3 and L_4).
  - Articular branches to the hip and the knee joints via the branches to the rectus femoris and vasti respectively.
  - A cutaneous branch viz., the saphenous nerves (L_3 and L_4) which is continuation of femoral nerve and is the only part of the nerve to travel beyond the region of the thigh as it ends by supplying the skin of the leg and the medial border of the foot, but does not supply the medial side of the big toe.

Obturator Nerve (Fig. 12.24)

It is derived from the ventral divisions of anterior rami of L_2, L_3 and L_4 spinal nerves. It enters the thigh by passing through the obturator foramen (converted into a canal by the parietal pelvic fascia). It divides into anterior and posterior divisions.

The **anterior division** curves over the upper edge of obturator externus and lies in front of adductor brevis and behind the pectineus and adductor longus. It descends in the groove between the psoas and iliacus muscles to gain entry into the femoral triangle by passing posterior to the inguinal ligament. In the femoral triangle the nerve lies about 1 cm lateral to the femoral sheath. It breaks up into two sets of branches. It gives off:

- Articular twig to hip joint.
- Muscular branches to:
  - Adductor longus.
  - Adductor brevis.
  - Gracilis.
  - Pectineus (occasionally).
- Cutaneous branch to the medial side of thigh which joins the medial cutaneous nerve of thigh and a branch from the saphenous nerve to form the **subsartorial plexus** on the fibrous roof of the adductor canal.
- A terminal vascular twig to the walls of the femoral artery.

The **posterior division** pierces the obturator externus and descends behind the adductor brevis and superficial to adductor magnus. It gives the following branches:

- Muscular branches to:
  - Obturator externus.
  - Adductor part of adductor magnus.
  - Adductor brevis occasionally.
- Articular branch to knee joint called:
  - The genicular branch which perforates the lower part of adductor magnus to enter the back of the knee joint.

Accessory Obturator Nerve

It is present in 30% of the individuals. It arises from the lumbar plexus from the ventral division of the anterior primary **rami** of L_4 and L_3 nerves. It enters the thigh above the superior ramus of the pubis deep to the pectineus and not through the obturator canal. It supplies:

- Pectineus.
- Hip joint.
- A communicating branch to the anterior division of the obturator nerve.

CLINICAL APPLICATION

- Injury to femoral nerve results in loss of extension at the knee joint as the quadriceps femoris is paralysed. There is sensory loss on the area supplied by its saphenous branch i.e., medial side of the lower part of the leg and the medial border of the foot.
- Injury to obturator nerve, results in paralysis of all the adductors except the ischial part of adductor magnus, which is supplied by sciatic nerve.

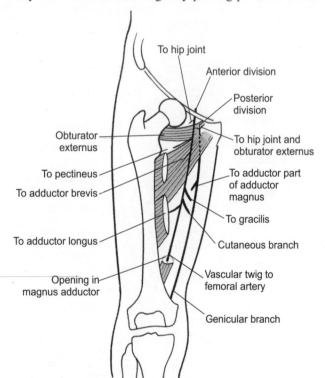

Fig. 12.24: The obturator nerve: Course and branches

- The clinical significance of the obturator nerve supplying both the hip and knee joint is that any pain arising from one joint may be referred to the other.
- To reduce the spasticity of adductor muscles without paralysing them completely the anterior division of the obturator nerve is divided. The inability to abduct the lower limb at the hip is thus improved.

Obturator Artery (Fig. 12.25)

The obturator artery is a branch of the anterior division of the internal iliac artery in the pelvis. It runs downward in the lateral wall of the pelvis to leave through the obturator canal. Just outside the obturator canal it divides into **anterior** and **posterior divisions,** which run anteriorly and posteriorly respectively on the outer surface of the obturator membrane, close to the obturator foramen and deep to the obturator externus muscle and anastomose with each other.

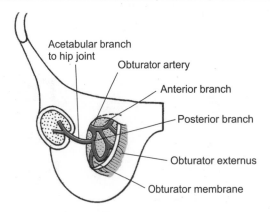

Fig. 12.25: The obturator artery

It supplies the muscles of the thigh. The posterior division sends an acetabular branch which passes through the acetabular notch to supply the hip joint. Branches are:

- Muscular from both branches.
- Articular to hip joint from the posterior branch. It enters the joint through the acetabular notch and runs along the ligamentum teres and supplies a small part of the head of femur.

13

The Gluteal Region, Back of the Thigh and the Popliteal Fossa

THE GLUTEAL REGION

The Osteoligamentous Framework of the Gluteal Region (Fig. 13.1)

The ilium forms most of the skeletal framework of the gluteal region. Its lateral or **gluteal surface** is divided into four areas by three ridges, the posterior, anterior and inferior gluteal lines.

- Area behind the posterior gluteal line gives:
  - Origin to **gluteus maximus** muscle from the upper rough part.
  - Attachment to **sacrotuberous ligament** below.
- Area between posterior and anterior gluteal lines:
  - Origin of gluteus medius muscle.

- Area between anterior and inferior gluteal lines:
  - Origin of gluteal minimus muscle.
- Area below the inferior gluteal lines:
  - **Groove above acetabulum:** Origin of reflected head of rectus femoris.
  - **Margin of acetabulum:** Attachment of capsular ligament of hip joint.

The upper end of the body of ischium forms a part of acetabulum. Its lower end forms the ischial tuberosity. The dorsal surface of the body also forms the skeletal framework of the gluteal region. It is a continuation downwards of the gluteal surface of ilium. The upper part of the surface is convex and smooth. This is followed by a grooved area. The lower part is continued into the ischial tuberosity. They relations are (Fig. 13.4):

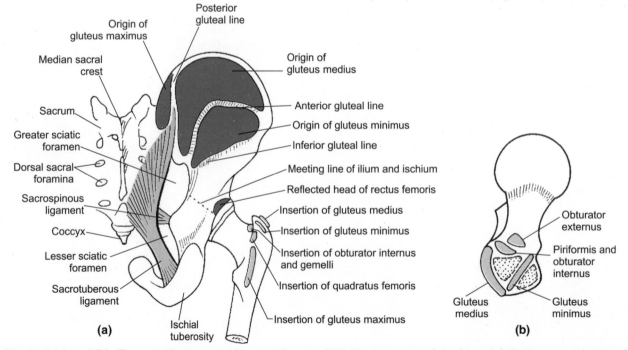

Fig. 13.1 (a) and (b): The osteoligamentous framework over which the structures of the gluteal region are superimposed

(i) *Convex part is related to:*
- Piriformis muscle.
- Sciatic nerve.
- Nerve to quadratus femoris.

(ii) *Grooved area is related to:*
- Obturator internus.
- Gemelli muscles.

(iii) *Ischial tuberosity.*
- Curved ridge on its medial margin gives attachment to:
  – Sacrotuberous ligament.

The posterior border of ischium is a continuation downwards of posterior border of the ilium. The two together from the **greater sciatic notch**. Posterior border of ischium has projection termed the **ischial spine** to the tip of which is attached the **sacrospinous ligament**. The greater sciatic notch is converted into the greater sciatic foramen by the sacrotuberous and sacrospinous ligaments. **Lesser sciatic notch** situated below the greater sciatic notch is converted into **lesser sciatic foramen** by the same two ligaments.

The dorsal surface of sacrum is also concerned with the gluteal region. In the midline it has **median sacral crest** representing spinous processes. On either side of the median sacral crest is the **intermediate sacral crest** representing fused articular processes. Lateral to the intermediate sacral crests are four pairs of **dorsal sacral foramina** representing dorsal parts of intervertebral foramina. Lateral to the dorsal foramina on each side is the **lateral sacral crest** which represents the fused transverse processes.

Skin and Fascia of the Gluteal Region

The skin is hairy, especially in males and presents a dimple opposite the posterior superior iliac spine. A line connecting the dimples of two sides pass through the spine of the second sacral vertebra. A horizontal fold, due to the attachment of the skin to the underlying fascia, marks the lower border of the buttock. This gluteal fold does not correspond with the lower border of the gluteus maximus which passes downward and laterally and is oblique and deep to the fold.

The superficial fascia is heavily laden with fat, particularly in the female, this being a secondary sex characteristic. The subcutaneous tissue is thickened over the ischial tuberosity and acts as a cushion for the bone in the sitting posture.

The Cutaneous Nerves of the Gluteal Region

In the figure the dotted line indicates the line of demarcation between the distribution of cutaneous nerves derived from the anterior and posterior primary rami (Fig. 13.2).

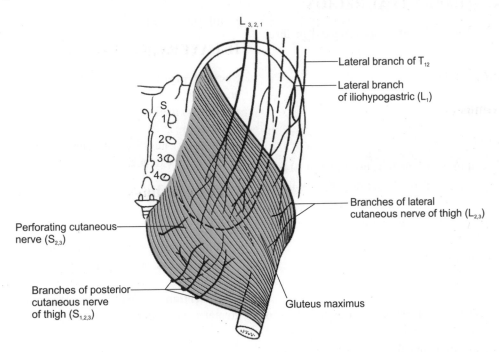

Fig. 13.2: Gluteal region: Cutaneous nerves. The dotted line indicates the line of demarcation between the nerves derived from the anterior and posterior rami

Branches from Anterior Rami

- **Lateral branch of subcostal (T_{12})**, descends anterior to tub of the iliac crest and descends upto the level of the greater trochanter.
- **Lateral branch of iliohypogastric (L_1)**, descends behind the tubercle of iliac crest and descends upto greater trochanter.
- **Lateral cutaneous nerve of thigh (L_2 and L_3).** Branches from its posterior division, supply the antero-inferior part of gluteal region.
- **Posterior cutaneous nerve of thigh (S_2 to S_3)**, two or three of its branches curl over the middle third of lower border of gluteus maximus and supply the skin of the postero-inferior part of gluteal region.
- **Perforating cutaneous nerve (S_2 and S_3)**, appears midway between the coccyx and the ischial tuberosity to supply the intermediate area of gluteal region.

Branches from Posterior Rami

- **Branches of L_1 to L_3** are long and descend across the iliac crest almost to the fold of the buttock.
- **Branches of S_1 to S_3** are short and emerge from the upper three posterior sacral foramina to supply the medial area.

MUSCLES OF THE GLUTEAL REGION

The muscles of the gluteal region are arranged in three layers:

I. LAYER (FIG. 13.3)

Gluteus Maximus

Origin (Fig. 13.1)

- Lateral surface of ilium behind the posterior gluteal line.
- Outer sloping surface of the dorsal one-third segment of iliac crest.
- Lower part of the lateral surface of sacrum and the adjoining coccyx.
- Sacrotuberous ligament.

Insertion

- Iliotibial tract has the insertion of upper half and superficial part of the lower half.
- Gluteal tuberosity of femur has the insertion of deep part of the lower half (Fig. 12.15).

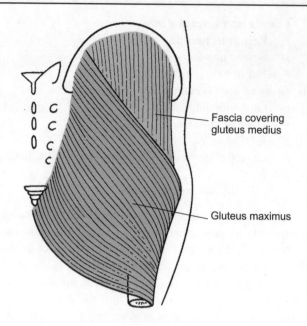

Fig. 13.3: Gluteal region: Muscle of first layer—the Gluteus maximus

Action

- Chief extensor of the hip.

Nerve Supply

- Inferior gluteal nerve.

II. LAYER (FIG. 13.4)

Second layer of muscles from above downwards are:
- Gluteus medius.
- Piriformis.
- Obturator internus-cum-gemelli.
- Quadratus femoris.

Gluteus Medius

Origin

- Gluteal surface of the ilium between the anterior and posterior gluteal lines (Fig. 13.1a).

Insertion on the oblique ridge on the lateral aspect of greater tronchanter of femur (Fig. 13.1b).

Action

- Abductor of hip joint.

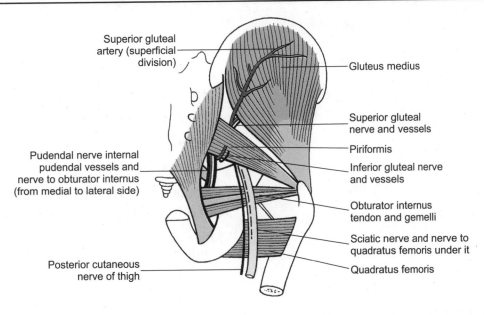

Fig. 13.4: Gluteal region: Muscles of second layer with nerves and vessels

Nerve Supply

- Superior gluteal nerve.

CLINICAL APPLICATION

Gluteus medius has a stabilising effect on the pelvis. During walking when one foot is supported by the ground the pelvis on the opposite side rises slightly and thus avoids the unsupported foot to sag downwards. This is because the gluteus medius of the supported foot acts from below and exerts a powerful pull on the hip bones and stabilises the opposite side of the pelvis. When the muscle is paralysed, this stabilising effect is lost and the pelvis on the unsupported limb sags. This is known as the **'Trendelenburg sign'**.

Piriformis

Origin

- The front of middle three pieces of sacrum mainly.
- Pelvic surface of ilium in front of preauricular surface gives origin to a few fibres.

Insertion

- By a round tendon into the superior border of the greater trochanter after passing through the greater sciatic notch (Fig. 13.1b).

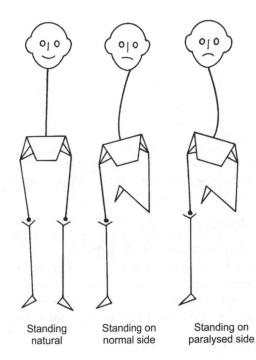

Fig. 13.5: Trendelenburg test: Dipping gait due to gluteus medius paralysis

Obturator Internus

Origin

- It is a fan-shaped muscle arising within the pelvis from

the inner surface of the obturator membrane and the surrounding bone.

Insertion

• Its tendon comes out of the lesser sciatic foramen to get inserted into the medial surface of the greater trochanter (Fig. 13.1b).

Gemelli

(a) **Gemellus superior** arises from the upper margin of the lesser sciatic notch and its fibres are inserted obliquely into the upper border of the tendon of obturator internus.

(b) **Gemellus inferior** arises from the lower margin of the lesser sciatic notch and its fibres are inserted into the lower border of the obturator tendon.

Quadratus Femoris

Origin

• Lateral border of the ischial tuberosity.

Insertion

• Quadrate tubercle situated below the middle of the intertrochanteric line and into the adjoining part of the shaft of the femur.

Action

• The piriformis, the obturator internus, the two gemelli, the quadratus femoris and the obturator externus are all small lateral rotator muscles of thigh.

Nerve Supply

• Piriformis—S_1 and S_2 in the pelvis.
• Obturator internus – Nerve to obturator internus.
• Gemellus superior – Nerve to obturator internus.
• Gemellus inferior – Nerve to quadratus femoris.
• Quadratus femoris – Nerve to quadratus femoris.

III. LAYER (FIG. 13.6)

Third layer of muscles comprise gluteus minimus only.

Gluteus Minimus

Origin

• From gluteal surface of ilium between anterior and inferior gluteal lines (Fig. 13.1 a).

Insertion

• Into the ridge on the lateral aspect of the anterior surface of the greater trochanter (Fig. 13.1 b).

Action

• Abductor of hip. The anterior fibres flex it.

Nerve Supply

• Superior gluteal nerve.

Immediate Coverings of the Capsule of Hip Joint (Fig. 13.6)

The immediate coverings of the capsular ligament are formed by piriformis, tricipital tendon (obturator internus and the two gemelli) and the obturator externus tendon. The obturator internus and the gemelli separate the sciatic nerve from the hip joint.

The capsule covers only the medial part of the neck and excludes the trochanteric fossa making only the medial half of the posterior surface intracapsular.

Structures under Cover of Gluteus Maximus (Fig. 13.4)

The key muscle after the reflection of gluteus maximus is

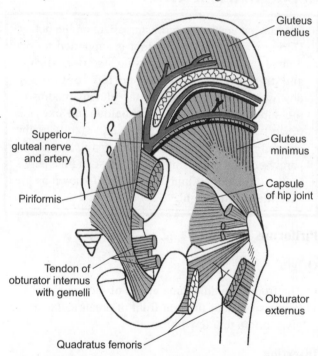

Fig. 13.6: Gluteal region: Muscles of third layer (Gluteus minimus and obturator externus) and superior gluteal nerve and artery. Muscles of the second layer are shown cut.

the piriformis which passes through the greater sciatic foramen. The deep relations of the gluteus maximus will be those that lie above and below the piriformis as they emerge from the greater sciatic foramen.

At the Upper Border of Piriformis

- The superior gluteal vessels.
- The superior gluteal nerve.

At the Lower Border of the Piriformis

- The sciatic nerve.
- The nerve to quadratus femoris deep to sciatic nerve.
- Inferior gluteal vessels.
- Inferior gluteal nerve.
- Posterior cutaneous nerve of thigh.

The following structures emerge from the greater sciatic foramen and then pass through the lesser sciatic foramen:
- Nerve to obturator internus lies on the base of the ischial spine.
- Internal pudendal vessels cross the tip of the spine.
- Pudendal nerve lies on the **sacrospinosis** ligament close to the ischial spine.

Besides the above structures, the following are also seen deep to the gluteus maximus:
- Greater trochanter of femur, ischial tuberosity and ischial spine.
- Sacrotuberous and sacrospinous ligaments.
- Trochanteric, ischial and gluteofemoral bursae of gluteus maximus lying on greater trochanter, lower and medial part of ischial tuberosity and tendon of vastus lateralis respectively.
- Gluteus medius muscle above and anterior to the piriformis.
- Tendon of obturator internus with the two gemelli.
- Upper border of adductor magnus.
- Gluteus minimus muscles.
- Quadratus femoris.
- Greater trochanter.
- Origin of the hamstring muscles.

The Superior Gluteal Nerve (L_4 and L_5, S_1) (Fig. 13.6)

It arises from the sacral plexus, enters the gluteal region through the greater sciatic foramen above the piriformis muscles. It accompanies the deep division of the superior gluteal artery and runs between the gluteus medius and minimus muscles and divides into upper and lower branches. The **upper branches** supply the gluteus medius.

The **lowest branch** crosses the middle of the gluteus minimus and supplies both the gluteus medius and minimus, it then passes between the anterior borders of these two muscles to supply the tensor fasciae latae from its deep surface.

The Superior Gluteal Artery (Figs. 13.4 and 13.6)

The superior gluteal artery is a branch of internal iliac artery and accompanies the superior gluteal nerve to enter the gluteal region where it immediately divides into superficial and deep divisions. The **superficial division** runs along the middle gluteal line and is distributed to the deep surface of the gluteus maximus. The **deep division** divides into a superior and an inferior branch. The superior branch follows the upper border of the gluteus minimus while the inferior branch accompanies the lowest branch of the superior gluteal nerve.

Sciatic Nerve (L_4 and L_5, S_1 to S_3) (Fig. 13.4)

It is a terminal branch of the sacral plexus and enters the gluteal region below the piriformis through the lower part of greater sciatic foramen. It traverses between the tuberosity of the ischium and the greater trochanter of femur before entering the back of the thigh. In the gluteal region it lies from above downwards on:
- Posterior surface of ischium with the nerve to quadratus femoris intervening.
- Gemellus superior, tendon of obturator internus and gemellus inferior.
- Quadratus femoris which separates the sciatic nerve from obturator externus and hip joint (Fig. 13.6).

Inferior Gluteal Artery (Fig. 13.4)

It is a branch of internal iliac artery and enters the gluteal region below the piriformis in accompaniment with the sciatic nerve. It is continued with the posterior cutaneous nerve to the back of thigh. Its branches are :
- Muscular branches to gluteus maximus.
- Cutaneous branches to the buttocks and the back of the thigh.
- Companion artery of the sciatic nerve which sinks into the substance of the nerve.

Inferior Gluteal Nerve (L_5; S_1 and S_2) (Fig. 13.4)

It is a branch of the sacral plexus. It enters the gluteal region below the piriformis through the lower part of the sciatic notch accompanied by the posterior cutaneous nerve of the thigh. It supplies the gluteus maximus muscle from its deep surface by breaking into several branches.

Internal Pudendal Artery, Pudendal Nerve and Nerve to Obturator Internus

As already mentioned they enter the gluteal region by emerging through the greater sciatic foramen and after a very small course enter the pelvis through the lesser sciatic foramen.

The Nerve to Quadratus Femoris

It enters the pelvis through the lower part of the greater sciatic foramen. It is deep to sciatic nerve and superficial to:
• Posterior surface of ischium.
• Capsule of hip joint.
• Obturator internus and the gemelli.

  It supplies:
• Quadratus femoris
• Hip joint.
• Inferior gemellus.

CLINICAL APPLICATION

• Paralysis of the superior gluteal nerve, results in **"abductor lurch",** a rolling (Trendelenburg) gait because of loss of stability of the pelvis due to the paralysis of gluteus medius. During normal walking the gluteus medius and minimus of both sides contract alternately first on one side and then on the other side. This permits the leg to be raised off the ground before taking a step forward. If these two glutei are paralysed, the pelvis sags down on the opposite side, when the foot of the sound side is raised off the ground. The patient has a dipping or lurching gait and this is known as a positive Trendelenburg's sign.
• Paralysis of the inferior gluteal nerve results in difficulty in rising from a seated position and in climbing stairs due to weakness of hip extension caused by the paralysis of gluteus maximus.
• The sciatic nerve is usually damaged in posterior dislocation of the hip since the femora head comes to lie either superior or inferior to the obturator internus tendon. The damage results in paralysis of the hamstrings and all muscles of the leg and foot, there is loss of joint sense and all movements in the lower limb below the knee joint with foot drop deformity.
• The pudendal nerve provides the principal

innervation of the perineum. In obstetric practice it can be blocked with local anaesthetic prior to forceps delivery.
• The upper and outer quadrant of the buttock is the standard site for intramuscular injection as there are the gluteus maximus medius and minimus in this region and there is no risk of injury to any nerve or blood vessel.

BACK OF THIGH

The Osseous Framework of the Back of the Thigh

Ischial tuberosity is the lower end of the body of the ischium. It is divided by a near transverse ridge into an upper quadrilateral area and a lower triangular area.

The upper quadrilateral area is further subdivided by a diagonal line into:

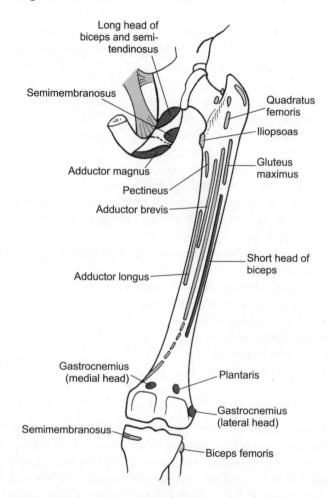

Fig. 13.7: Back of thigh: Osseous framework

- Upper lateral area from where **semimembranous muscle** arises.
- Lower medial area for the origin of the **long head of biceps** and **semitendinosus muscle**.

The lower triangular area is divided by a vertical line into:
- Lateral area for the origin of **ischial fibres of adductor magnus muscle**.
- Medial area which is related to fibrofatty tissue and the **ischial bursa of gluteus maximus**.

The **short head of biceps** arises from the lateral lip of linea aspera and the upper half of the lateral supracondylar ridge. The **semitendinosus** is inserted into the upper part of medial surface of tibia along with the tendon of **sartorius** and **gracilis**.

The **semimembranosus** is inserted into the floor of the groove on the back of medial condyle of the tibia.

The **biceps femoris** is inserted into the head of the fibula.

The **medial head of the gastrocnemius** arises from a rough, raised area on the popliteal surface of the femur above the medial condyle.

The **plantaris** arises from the popliteal surface above the lateral condyle.

The **lateral head of the gastrocnemius** arises from the lateral surface of the lateral condyle of the femur.

CUTANEOUS NERVES OF POSTERIOR COMPARTMENT (FIG. 13.8)

- Posterior cutaneous nerve of thigh issues out of the lower compartment of the greater sciatic foramen posterior to the sciatic nerve on which it frequently lies (Fig. 13.4). It continues down the midline of the back of the thigh supplying the skin of the back of thigh and the upper part of the leg. Just below the gluteal fold, it gives off a perineal branch which curves upwards and medially to supply the skin of the medial aspect of the upper thigh and the adjacent part of the perineum (Figs. 10.19 and 10.35).
- Anterior division of the obturator nerve gives cutaneous branches to the medial side of the thigh which extend to the back as well.
- Lateral cutaneous of thigh sends a few twigs to back of the thigh.

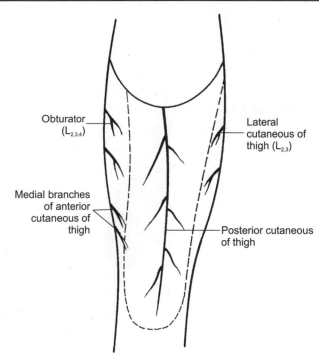

Fig. 13.8: Cutaneous nerves of back of thigh

MUSCLES OF POSTERIOR COMPARTMENT OF THIGH

Muscles of the back are arranged in three layers. The three layers from behind to forward are formed by biceps femoris, semitendinosus and semimembranosus. These are known as Hamstring muscles.

I. LAYER

Biceps Femoris

Origin (Fig. 13.7)

Long head: Lower medial part of the upper quadrilateral area of ischial tuberosity.

Short head: Lateral lip of linea aspera and the upper half of the lateral supracondylar ridge of femur (Fig. 13.10).

Insertion (Fig. 13.7)

Head of fibula: The tendon of insertion crosses the postero-lateral surface of the knee and then it is first grooved and then split by the fibular collateral ligament before getting inserted into the head of fibula.

Action

- Flexion of knee.
- Extension of the hip.

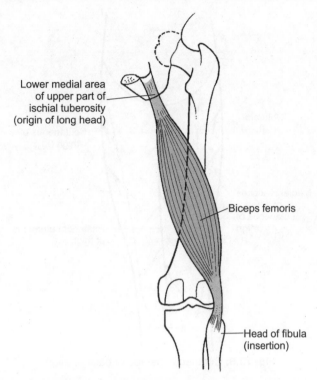

Fig. 13.9: Back of thigh: Muscle of first layer (Long head of biceps femoris)

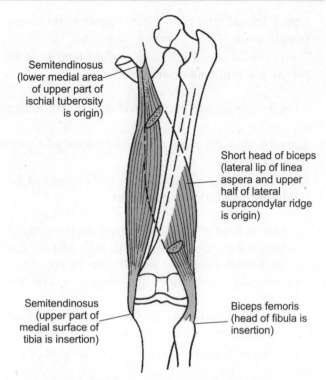

Fig. 13.10: Back of thigh: Muscles of second layer (short head of biceps and semitendinosus)

Nerve Supply

- Long head by the tibial part of sciatic nerve and short head by the common peroneal part of sciatic nerve.

II. LAYER (FIG. 13.10)

Short head of biceps and semitendinosus form this layer.

Semitendinosus

Origin (Fig. 13.7)

- Same as long head of biceps i.e., lower medial part of the upper quadrilateral area of ischial tuberosity.

Insertion (Fig. 13.7)

- Upper part of medial surface of tibia.
- The muscle lies on semimembranosus.

Action

- Flexor of the knee.
- Medial rotator of flexed knee.
- Extensor of the hip.
- The short head has been described above.

III. LAYER

Semimembranosus

Origin (Fig. 13.7)

- Upper lateral part of the upper quadrilateral area of the ischial tuberosity.

Insertion (Fig. 13.7)

- Floor of the groove on the back of the medial condyle of tibia. It sends extension which form.
- Oblique posterior ligament of knee and
- Fascia of the popliteus (Fig. 13.17).

Action

- Same as those of semitendinosus.

Nerve Supply

- Tibial part of sciatic nerve.

Adductor Magnus

The part of the adductor magnus inserted into the adductor tubercle is associated at its origin from the ischial tuberosity

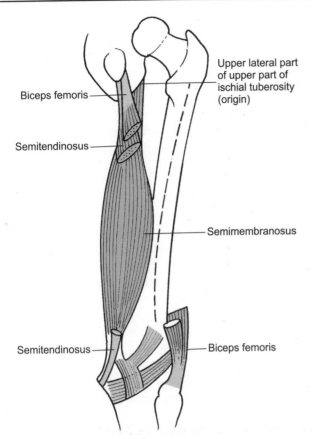

Fig. 13.11: Back of thigh: Muscle of third layer (Semimembranosus)

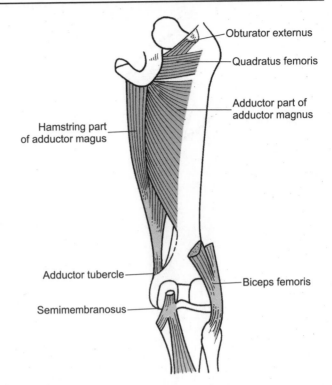

Fig. 13.12: Adductor magnus from behind. The three layers of the muscles of the back of thigh lie over it

with the hamstrings and belonging to the same flexor group is designated as its hamstring part. The degenerated part of the hamstring part is the tibial collateral ligament of the knee. The hamstring part is thus also supplied by the tibial part of sciatic nerve.

Relations of Adductor Magnus

Anterior (Figs. 12.21, 12.22 and 12.24)

- Adductor longus and brevis.
- Femoral and profunda vessels.
- Posterior division of obturator nerve.

Posterior (Fig. 13.13)

- Semitendinosus, semimembranosus and biceps femoris.
- Sciatic nerve.
  Between its upper border and quadratus femoris emerges the:
- Medial circumflex femoral artery.
  Through the tendinous arch in the linea aspera emerge the:

- Perforating arteries.
  Through the deficiency in its insertion in the medial supracondylar ridge pass to the popliteal fossa the:
- Femoral vessels.

SCIATIC NERVE (FIG. 13.13)

- Bed of sciatic nerve is formed:
  (a) In the gluteal region under cover of gluteus maximus by:
- Posterior surface by ischium.
- Obturator internus with the gemelli.
- Quadratus femoris.
  (b) In the back of the thigh deep to biceps femoris it lies on:
- Semimembranosus.
- Adductor magnus.

Branches of the Sciatic Nerve

Sciatic nerve usually ends halfway down the back of the thigh by dividing into two large branches known as the **common peroneal** and the **tibial nerves**.

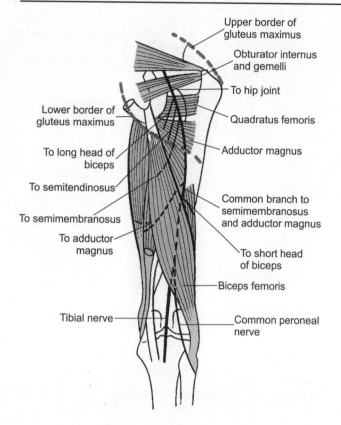

Fig. 13.13: Sciatic nerve : Muscles forming its bed and its branches

The nerves to the hamstrings arise from the medial side of the main trunk **(tibial part)** as the level of ischial tuberosity and a little lower down. These are:
- One branch to long head of biceps.
- Two branches to semitendinosus.
- One common branch for semimembranosus and the ischial part of adductor magnus.

The lateral side of the main trunk **(common peroneal part)** gives the following branches:
- One branch to short head of biceps.
- One articular twig to hip joint from the upper part of the nerve.

PROFUNDA FEMORIS ARTERY

It is a branch of the femoral artery given from its lateral side in the femoral triangle which it leaves by passing posteriorly between the pectineus and the adductor longus. It then descends behind the adductor longus. The artery lies on three muscles which from above downwards are pectineus, adductor brevis and adductor longus.

Branches

- **Medial circumflex femoral** arising in the femoral triangle ends near the upper border of the adductor magnus by dividing into:
  – Ascending branch and a
  – Transverse branch.
- **Lateral circumflex femoral,** also arises in femoral triangle and running laterally to the deep surface of rectus femoris divides into:
  – Ascending branch,
  – Transverse branch and a
  – Descending branch.
- **Muscular branches** are inconsistent.
- **Four perforating branches** so called because they perforate the deficiencies in the tendinous insertion of adductor magnus in the linea aspera. They pass backwards and laterally to end in the vastus lateralis.
- The first passes between the pectineus and adductor longus.
- The second pierces adductor brevis and adductor magnus.
- Third pierces the adductor magnus.
- Fourth is termination of profunda.

Anastomoses on the Back of Thigh

- Trochanteric anastomosis formed by:

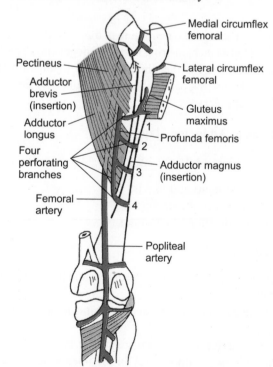

Fig. 13.14: Back of thigh: Arteries

- Superior gluteal artery.
- Inferior gluteal artery.
- Ascending branch of the medial circumflex femoral.
- Cruciate anastomosis:
  - Descending branch of inferior gluteal artery from above.
  - Transverse branch of lateral circumflex femoral from lateral side.
  - Transverse branch of medial circumflex femoral from medial side.
  - First perforating from below.
- Perforating arteries anastomose among themselves and through the first perforating link up with the cruciate anastomosis.
- Fourth perforating anastomoses below with the upper muscular branches of the popliteal artery to the hamstrings.

Thus, a longitudinal chain of anastomosis occurs in the back of the thigh from the gluteal region to the popliteal fossa linking the internal iliac, the femoral and the popliteal arteries.

THE POPLITEAL FOSSA

It is a diamond-shaped space behind the knee opposite the lower third of femur and upper part of tibia.

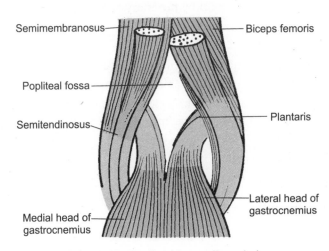

Fig. 13.15: Popliteal fossa: Boundaries

Boundaries

- Laterally and above.
  - Biceps femoris muscle.
- Medially and above.
  - Semitendinosus lying on the back of

- Semimembranosus
- Laterally and below.
  - Lateral head of gastrocnemius.
  - Plantaris.
- Medially and below.
  - Medial head of gastrocnemius.

Roof

The roof is formed by skin, superficial fascia and deep fascia and contains.
- Moderate amount of fat.
- Small saphenous vein.

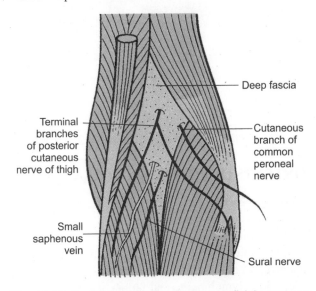

Fig. 13.16: Popliteal fossa: Roof and superficial structures

- Terminal part of posterior cutaneous nerve of thigh which is most superficial.
- Posterior branch of medial cutaneous nerve of thigh.
- Peroneal communicating nerve.

Floor

- The floor from above downwards is formed by:
  - Popliteal surface of the femur.
  - Capsule of the knee joint covered by oblique posterior ligament of the knee.
  - Popliteal fascia covering popliteus muscle.

The tendon of semimembranous is inserted into the floor of the grooves on the back of the medial condyle of the tibia. It sends extensions which form:
- Oblique popliteal ligament of the knee joint.
- Fascia of the popliteus, through which it is inserted into the soleal line of tibia.

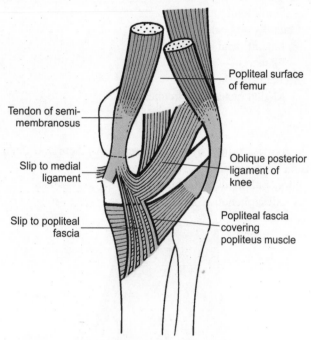

Fig. 13.17: Popliteal fossa: Floor

Labels in figure:
- Popliteal surface of femur
- Tendon of semimembranosus
- Slip to medial ligament
- Slip to popliteal fascia
- Oblique posterior ligament of knee
- Popliteal fascia covering popliteus muscle

CONTENTS OF POPLITEAL FOSSA

- Popliteal vessels.
- Tibial and common peroneal nerves.
- Termination of small saphenous vein.
- Lower end of the posterior femoral cutaneous nerve.
- Genicular branch of obturator nerve.
- Few small lymph nodes and fat.

Popliteal Artery

Popliteal artery is the continuation of the femoral artery. It enters the popliteal fossa through the opening in the adductor magnus and ends at the distal border of the popliteus muscle by dividing into the anterior and posterior tibial arteries.

Relations

Anterior

- As seen from the back, it lies from above downwards on:
  - Popliteal surface of femur.
  - Capsule of the knee joint and the oblique posterior ligament of the knee.
  - Fascia covering popliteus.

Posterior

- Semimembranous above.

- Gastrocnemius and plantaris below.
- Popliteal vein and tibial nerve in the middle. The vein separates the artery from the nerve.

Lateral

- In the upper part of the popliteal fossa:
  - Popliteal vein.
  - Tibial nerve.
  - Common peroneal nerve and biceps femoris.
  - Lateral condyle of femur.
- In the lower part of the popliteal fossa:
  - Plantaris.
  - Lateral head of gastrocnemius.

Medial

- In the upper part of the popliteal fossa:
  - Semimembranosus.
  - Medial condyle of femur.
- In the lower part of the popliteal fossa.
  - Popliteal vein.
  - Tibial vein.
  - Medial head of gastrocnemius.

Branches

The branches given off by the artery are:
- Muscular.
- Genicular.
  - Superior and inferior lateral genicular.
  - Superior and inferior medial genicular.
  - Middle genicular which pierces the oblique posterior ligament to supply the interior of the joint.
- Terminal.
  - Anterior tibial.
  - Posterior tibial.

Popliteal Vein

Its commencement is at the distal border of the popliteus muscle by the union of the vena comitantes of the anterior and posterior tibial arteries. It lies in the same fibrous sheath as the artery and crosses it superficially from medial to posterolateral side as it ascends upward. Its tributaries correspond to the branches of the popliteal artery and after passing through the opening in the adductor magnus it continues as femoral vein. For relations refer to popliteal artery.

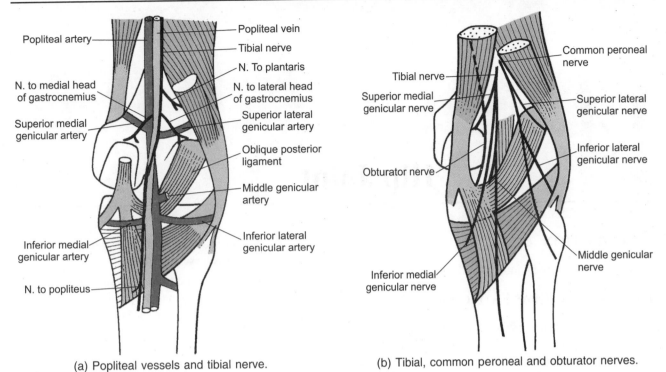

(a) Popliteal vessels and tibial nerve.

(b) Tibial, common peroneal and obturator nerves.

Fig. 13.18: Popliteal fossa: Contents

Tibial Nerve (L$_4$ and L$_5$; S$_1$ and S$_3$)

It is larger of the two terminal branches of the sciatic nerve and begins about the back of the middle of thigh. It enters the popliteal fossa at its upper angle emerging from under cover of the biceps femoris. It lies almost in the midline and crosses the popliteal vessel from lateral to medial sides as it courses downwards.

Branches

- Cutaneous:
  - Sural.
- Muscular to:
  - Plantaris.
  - Both heads of gastrocnemius.
  - Soleus.
  - Popliteus. The nerve to this muscle arises lower down than the others.
- Genicular branches are given off in the fossa and accompany the corresponding genicular arteries.
  - Superior medial genicular runs above the medial femoral condyle.
  - Middle genicular: Supplies the cruciate ligament.
  - Inferior medial genicular is larger than the other two.

Common Peroneal Nerve (L$_4$ and L$_5$; S$_1$ and S$_2$)

It is smaller of the two terminal branches of the sciatic nerve

and arises about the middle of the thigh. It passes along the upper lateral boundary of the popliteal fossa on the inner edge of the biceps femoris tendon. It lies next on plantaris and lateral head of gastrocnemius. Passing downwards between lateral head of gastrocnemius and biceps tendon, it divides into **deep** and **superficial peroneal nerves** under cover of peroneus longus muscle at the lateral side of neck of fibula, where it can be rolled under the finger.

Branches

- Cutaneous:
  - Peroneal communicating which joins the sural nerve.
  - Lateral cutaneous nerve of calf for the skin of the lateral and anterior surfaces of the upper part of leg.
- Genicular accompanying the corresponding arteries:
  - Superior lateral genicular.
  - Inferior lateral genicular.
  - Recurrent genicular from the termination of the common peroneal nerve.

Genicular Branch of the Obturator Nerve

It is a continuation of the posterior division of the obturator nerve. It pierces the distal part of adductor magnus to enter the popliteal fossa. It lies on the posterior surface of the popliteal artery before piercing the oblique popliteal ligament to enter the knee joint.

14

Hip Joint

INTRODUCTION

The hip joint is a synovial joint of ball and socket variety.

ARTICULAR SURFACES (FIG. 14.1)

(i) The **head of femur** is spherical, smooth and covered with articular cartilage. On the upper part of the head is a small pit **(fovea capitis)**.

(ii) The bony **acetabulum** which is a cup-shaped cavity on the lateral aspect of the hip bone and has a contribution from all the three components of the bone. It has:

• A projecting margin, the rim of the acetabulum, which gives attachment to the cartilaginous **acetabular labrum**.

• An **acetabular notch,** which is a deficiency in the rim situated inferiorly and giving attachment to the **transverse ligament**.

• A horseshoe-shaped articular surface occupying the anterior, superior and posterior parts of the cavity called the **lunate surface** which is covered by articular cartilage.

• An **acetabular fossa,** a rough nonarticular floor on the inferior aspect. It lodges a pad of fat **(Haversian gland)** ensheathed in synovial membrane.

The Capsule

The capsule is a loose thick fibrous sac enclosing the joint cavity.

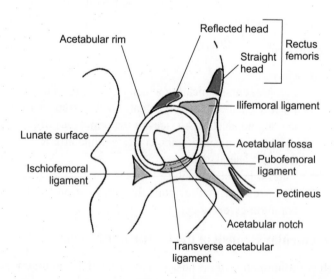

(A) Bony acetabulum.

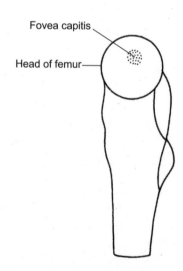

(B) Head of Femur.

Fig. 14.1: The hip joint: Articular surfaces

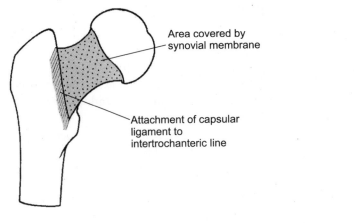

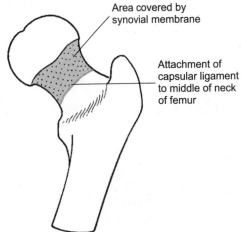

(A) Anterior aspect of upper end of femur

Area covered by synovial membrane

Attachment of capsular ligament to intertrochanteric line

(B) Posterior aspect of upper end of femur

Area covered by synovial membrane

Attachment of capsular ligament to middle of neck of femur

Fig. 14.2: Hip joint: Fibrous capsule

- Proximally it is attached to the margins of the acetabulum 5 or 6 cm away from the labrum acetabulare.
- Distally it is attached along the whole length of the intertrochanteric line anteriorly while posteriorly to the posterior surface of the neck just beyond its medial half. Therefore, only the medial half of the posterior surface is intracapsular, while the whole of anterior surface of neck is intracapsular (Fig.14.2).
- The fibres of the capsule travel distally in an increasingly spiral fashion to enclose the head and neck of the femur. This spiralling is most marked posteriorly and is thought to be due to the rotation of the limb during development and to assumption of erect posture in man.
- From attachment to the femur, the fibres of the capsule run upwards and medially along the neck of the femur to form **superior** and **inferior retinacula** which contain blood vessels to supply the neck and lower three-fourths of the head of femur. Some fibres run circumferentially about the neck and are known as **zona orbicularis**.

Ligaments (Figs. 14.3 and 14.4)

Three ligaments reinforce the capsule of the hip joint:
1. **The iliofemoral ligament ('Y'-shaped ligament of Bigelow):** The stem of 'Y' arises from the lower half of the anterior inferior iliac spine and the acetabular rim. The diverging limbs are attached to the upper and lower ends of the intertrochanteric line. It limits extension at the hip joint. The line of weight transmission, passes behind the hip joint and consequently there is a tendency for the trunk to roll backwards on the femoral head. This is counteracted

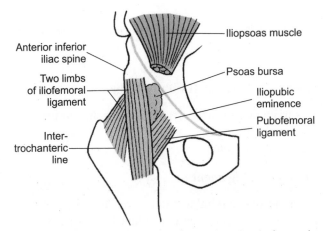

Fig. 14.3: The hip joint: The iliofemoral and pubofemoral ligaments

by the bracing action of the iliofemoral ligament which becomes taut in the standing position. It is the thickest and strongest of all ligaments.
2. **The pubofemoral ligament** is triangular and extends from the iliopubic eminence and obturator crest to the capsule on the inferior part of the neck of the femur. Between it and the medial band of iliofemoral ligament and deep to iliacus is the psoas bursa.
3. **The ischiofemoral ligament** is also triangular and is the weakest of the three. Arising from the postero-inferior margin of the acetabulum, its fibres spiral upward to form a band of fibres that run in the capsule transversely around the femoral neck. They form the zona orbicularis. Very few fibres reach the femur to get inserted into the base of the greater trochanter.

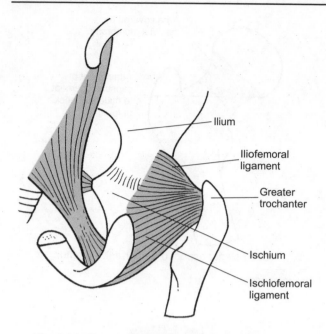

Fig. 14.4: The hip joint : The ischiofemoral ligament

Round Ligament of Head of Femur

It is triangular in shape. Its apex is attached to the pit on the femoral head. The base is attached to the margins of the acetabular notch.

Transverse Ligament

Margins of acetabular notch give attachment to the transverse ligament of the acetabulum. Converting the notch into the acetabular foramen.

The Synovial Membrane

It covers the inner surface of the capsule and the nonarticular surfaces of the joint and occasionally bulges out anteriorly to form a bursa beneath the psoas tendon.

Below the lunate articular surface of the acetabulum, is a nonarticular area filled with a pad of fat **(Haversian gland)** ensheathed in the synovial membrane.

Nerve Supply

- Following the **Hilton's law** the joint is supplied by the femoral, sciatic and obturator nerves.

Blood Supply

- Branches of the superior and inferior gluteal circumflex femoral and obturator arteries supply the joint.

Relations

Anteriorly there are three muscles which from lateral to medial side are:
- Straight head of rectus femoris.
- **Iliopsoas:** Femoral nerve lies in the groove between the iliacus and psoas major. Tendon of psoas major intervenes between the capsule of the joint and the femoral artery in the femoral sheath. Deep to psoas is a bursa which communicates with the joint.
- Pectineus separates the capsule of the joint from the femoral vein in the femoral sheath.

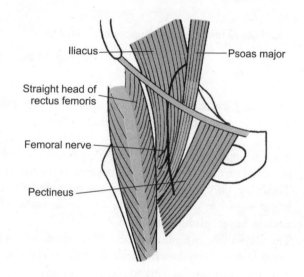

Fig. 14.5: The hip joint: Anterior relations

Posteriorly from Above Downwards

- Piriformis
- Tendon of obturator internus with the gemelli .
- Quadratus femoris.
- Sciatic nerve.
- Gluteus maximus more superficially.

Laterally

The relations are:
- Tendon fascia lata.
- Gluteus medius .
- Gluteus minimus.

Inferiorly

- Obturator externus winds posteriorly below the capsule and lies between the capsule and quadratus femoris (Fig. 13.6).

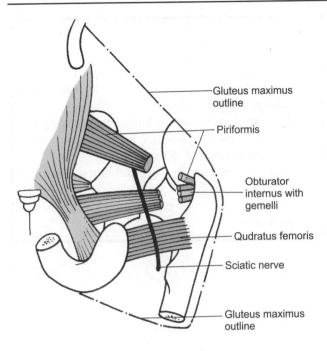

Fig. 14.6: The hip joint : Posterior relations

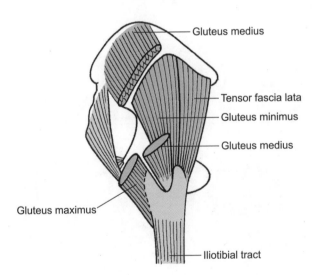

Fig. 14.7: The hip joint : Lateral relations

Superiorly

• Reflected head of rectus femoris lying in contact with the joint capsule.

Movements

• Flexion is free with the knee flexed. It is arrested only

by the anterior aspect of thigh being approximated to the anterior abdominal wall. It is carried out by:
– Iliopsoas: Main.
– Pectineus.
– Sartorius   Assist
– Rectus femoris (straight head).
• Extension is limited by iliofemoral ligament and is carried out by:
– Gluteus maximus: Main.
– Hamstring muscles: Assist.
• Abduction is restricted by pubofemoral ligament and is carried out by:
– Gluteus medius.   Main
– Gluteus minimus.
– Tensor fascia lata: Assist.
• Adduction:
– Adductor longus.
– Adductor brevis.   Main
– Adductor magnus (adductor part).
– Pectineus.   Assist
– Gracilis.
• Medial rotation:
– Gluteus medius et minimus (anterior fibres)   Main
– Iliopsoas.
• Lateral rotation:
– Gluteus maximus: Main.
– Obturator.
– Gemelli   Assist
– Quadratus femoris.

CLINICAL APPLICATION

• The retinacular fibres transmit arteries which supply the head and neck of femur. These may be torn in some cases of intracapsular fracture of neck of femur leading to avascular necrosis of the head of femur. This does not occur in the case of children as the artery passing along the ligamentum teres is capable of maintaining the nutrition of the head.
• Paralysis of gluteus medius and minimus which are powerful abductors of the thigh results in a **'dipping gait'**. During walking these muscles tilt the pelvis towards the side of the foot which is on the ground, so that the opposite foot can clear the ground. In case of paralysis of these

muscles the pelvis sinks on the unsupported side with an easily noticeable lowering of the gluteal fold. This is the basis of positive **Trendelenburg test** (Fig. 13.5).

- The hip joint is notable for its strength and is rarely dislocated. The weakest part of the joint is below and here the head leaves the capsule. It will then pass backward or forward depending on the line of force. In all dislocations the iliofemoral ligament remains intact.

- Flexion tends to unwind the ligaments, so that the hip is least stable in the flexed position. Posterior dislocation is thus more frequent, as and when the flexed thigh comes violently into contact with the dashboard during a car accident. The sciatic nerve, a close posterior relation of the hip, is in danger of damage in these injuries.

- The nerves supplying the hip joint also supply the knee joint and for this reason the pain of a diseased hip may be referred to the knee.

- Acute osteomyelitis of the upper femoral metaphysis involves the neck which is intracapsular and which, therefore, rapidly produces pus in the joint cavity.

15

Front of the Leg and the Dorsum of the Foot

INTRODUCTION

The leg is that part of the lower extremity that lies between the knee and ankle. The muscles and bones of the leg are enclosed within a cylindrical sheath of deep fascia. The space between this facial tube and the leg bones is divided into three compartments viz., anterior, lateral and posterior (Fig. 15.1).

Because the muscles of the leg act across the ankle joint as well as joints of the foot, the leg, the ankle and the foot are best studied as a functional unit.

ANTERIOR COMPARTMENT OF LEG AND DORSUM OF FOOT

BONY FRAMEWORK

The skeletal framework is provided lateral surface of the

tibia, medial surface of the fibula and the interosseous membrane (Fig. 15.1).

Tibia (Fig. 15.2)

The tibia is the medial and stronger bone of the leg.

The bone has a shaft connecting the upper and lower ends. The upper end is more massive and expanded to form the **medial** and **lateral condyles**. The lower end projects medially to form the **medial malleolus**. The most **conspicuous** feature of the shaft is its sharp anterior border. The shaft is triangular on section and possesses three borders viz., anterior, interosseous and medial, which enclose three surfaces, medial, lateral and posterior (Fig. 15.1).

The lateral surface is bounded by the anterior and interosseous borders, its upper two-thirds is hollowed out for the origin of **tibialis anterior muscle** (Fig. 15.6).

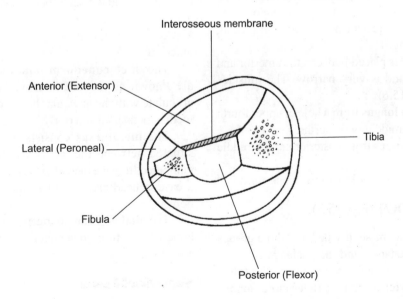

Fig. 15.1: The osteofascial compartments of leg

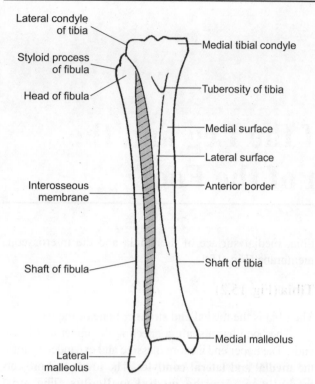

Fig. 15.2: Front of the leg: Bony framework

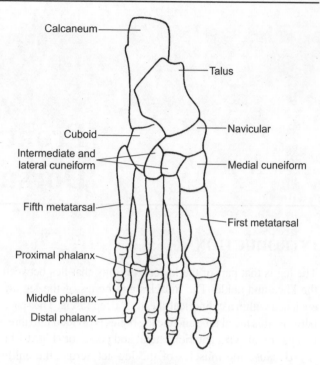

Fig. 15.3: Skeleton of foot

Fibula (Fig. 15.2)

The fibula is the lateral bone of the leg. It is slender and does not take any part in the transmission of body weight. It has two ends, the upper or the **head** and the lower or the **lateral malleolus,** connected by shaft. The upper end has a projection termed the **styloid process.** The shaft of the fibula has three borders viz., anterior, interosseous and posterior which enclose three surfaces which are medial, posterior and lateral (Fig. 15.1).

The medial surface is placed between the anterior and interosseous borders and is very narrow. The muscles taking origin are (Fig. 15.6):

- **Extensor digitorum longus** from whole of upper fourth and anterior part of middle two-fourths.
- **Extensor hallucis longus** from posterior part of middle two-fourths.
- **Peroneus terteus** from whole of lower one-fourth.

SKELETON OF FOOT (Fig. 15.3)

The bones of the foot can be subdivided into three groups viz., the tarsus, the metatarsus and the phalanges.

The **tarsus** consists of seven bones named the **talus, calcaneus, cuboid, navicular** and the **three cuneiforms**–medial, intermediate and lateral.

The **talus** articulates with the leg bones above and is the only bone of the foot having no muscular attachments. Below it articulates with calcaneus and in front with the navicular.

The **calcaneus** is the bone of the heel.

The **navicular** is shaped like boat. It is situated between the talus posteriorly and three cuneiform bones anteriorly.

The **cuboid** is situated between the calcaneus posteriorly and fourth and fifth metatarsals anteriorly. On its medial side is the navicular bone posteriorly and lateral cuneiform anteriorly.

The three **cuneiform bones** are wedge-shaped and are known as medial, intermediate and lateral which articulate with the navicular bone posteriorly and the three medial metatarsal anteriorly.

The **metatarsus** consists of five metatarsal bones situated between the tarsus and the phalanges and are numbered from the medial to the lateral side. Each possesses a base, a head and a shaft as they are miniature of long bones.

The **phalanges** are fourteen in number. Each metatarsal bone carries three phalanges except the first which has only two.

Superficial Fascia

The superficial fascia of the front medial and the lateral

side contains only a small amount of fat which contains the following cutaneous veins and nerves.

Cutaneous Veins

- **Dorsal digital veins:** There is a dorsal digital vein on each side of the dorsum of the toe. The ones on adjacent sides of two toes unite to form a common stem which ends in the dorsal venous arch. The dorsal digital veins on the medial side of the great toe and the lateral side of the little toe join the ends of the arch.
- **Dorsal venous arch** lies on the anterior parts of the metatarsal bones. Its medial end is continuous with the **great saphenous vein** which lies in front of the medial malleolus while its lateral end is continuous with the small saphenous vein which lies behind the lateral malleolus and then upwards on the back of the leg.
- **Great saphenous vein** passes obliquely across the distal third of tibia to reach its medial border along which it ascends. The two saphenous veins are connected by a profuse plexus of smaller veins so they have no exact drainage area. The small saphenous vein can be regarded as draining the lateral part of the foot and the posterior and lateral aspects of the leg, while the great saphenous vein drains the superficial fascia and skin of the rest of the lower limb.

CLINICAL APPLICATION

The great saphenous vein is used as a graft in surgery. The most important use is to bypass narrowed coronary arteries to improve the blood supply to the cardiac musculature. It is usually covered by a thin condensed layer of superficial fascia, which has to be incised to expose it.

Cutaneous Nerves

- **Saphenous nerves (L_3 and L_4)** supply the upper and medial parts of the front of the leg and medial side of the dorsum of foot.
- **Lateral cutaneous nerves of calf (L_5; S_1 and S_2),** given off by the common peroneal, are distributed to the skin between the infrapatellar region and the junction of the middle and distal third of the leg.
- **Cutaneous branch of the superficial peroneal nerve,** supplies the remainder of the front of the leg, their areas of distribution and segmental origin, the intermediate area of the dorsum of the foot and the toes not supplied by the sural nerve and deep peroneal nerve.
- **Sural nerve** supplies the lateral side of the dorsum of foot and lateral side of little toe.

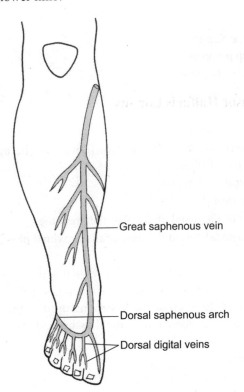

Fig. 15.4: Front of leg and dorsum of foot: Superficial veins

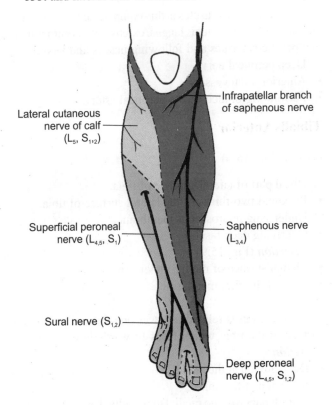

Lateral cutaneous nerve of calf (L_5, $S_{1,2}$)

Infrapatellar branch of saphenous nerve

Superficial peroneal nerve ($L_{4,5}$, S_1)

Saphenous nerve ($L_{3,4}$)

Sural nerve ($S_{1,2}$)

Deep peroneal nerve ($L_{4,5}$, $S_{1,2}$)

Fig. 15.5: Front of leg and dorsum of foot: Cutaneous nerves

- **Cutaneous branch of the deep peroneal nerve** supplies the adjacent sides of the first and second toes.

ANTERIOR COMPARTMENT OF LEG

Skeletal Framework

The skeletofascial frame is provided by lateral surface of the tibia, anterior surface of the fibula and the interosseous membrane (Fig. 15.1).

(i) **Lateral surface of the tibia:** It is bounded by the anterior and interosseous borders. Upper two-thirds hollowed out for the origin of **tibialis anterior muscle**.

(ii) **Medial surface of the fibula:** It is placed between the anterior and interosseous borders and is very narrow. The muscles taking origin are (Fig. 15.6):

- Whole of upper fourth and anterior part of middle two-fourths give origin to **extensor digitorum longus**. The muscles also arise from the anterior surface of the head of fibula.
- Posterior part of middle two-fourths gives origin to **extensor hallucis longus muscle**.
- Whole of lower one-fourth gives origin to **peroneus tertius muscle**.

There are four muscles in this compartment viz., tibialis anterior, extensor hallucis longus, extensor digitorum longus and peroneus tertues and following nerves and vessels:
- Deep peroneal nerve.
- Anterior tibial vessels.
- Perforating branch of the peroneal artery.

Tibialis Anterior

Origin (Fig. 15.6)

- Distal part of lateral condyle of tibia.
- Proximal two-thirds of the lateral surface of tibia.
- Underlying interosseous membrane.
- Overlying deep fascia.
Insertion (Fig. 15.9)
- Medial surface of medial cuneiform.
- Base of the first metatarsal.

The tendon is related to lower one-third of the lateral surface of the tibia which faces forwards lower down.
Action
- Dorsiflexion at the ankle.
- Inversion at the ankle.
- Maintenance of the medial longitudinal arch of the foot.

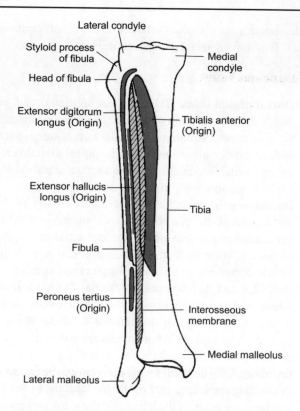

Fig. 15.6: Anterior compartment skeletal frame with muscle markings

Nerve Supply
- Deep peroneal.
- Recurrent genicular.

Extensor Hallucis Longus

Origin (Fig. 15.6)
- Posterior part of middle two-fourths of the anterior surface of fibula.
- Interosseous membrane.
Insertion (Fig. 15.9)
- Base of the distal phalanx of the great toe.
- Occasional slip to the base of the proximal phalanx.

It is a thin muscle hidden between the tibialis anterior and the extensor digitorum longus. It comes to the surface near the ankle to cross the lower one-third of the lateral surface of tibia where it lies lateral to the tendon of tibialis anterior.
Action
- Extension of the phalanges of the great toe.
- Dorsiflexion of the foot.

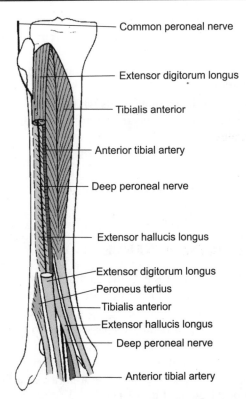

(a) The muscles of anterior compartment: The extensor digitorum has been cut to expose the extensor hallucis longus.

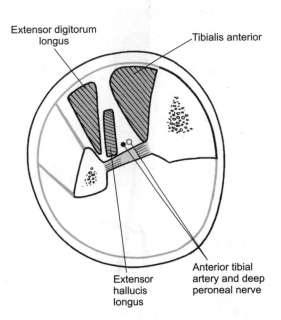

(b) Contents of anterior compartment in a transverse section.

Fig. 15.7: The anterior compartment of leg

Nerve Supply
- Deep peroneal nerve.

Extensor Digitorum Longus

Origin (Fig. 15.6)
- Whole of upper fourth and anterior part of middle two-fourths of the anterior surface of fibula.

Insertion (Fig. 15.9)
- Middle and distal phalanges of the lateral four toes.

The tendon lies on the lower part of the lateral surface of the tibia lateral to the tendon of **extensor hallucis longus**.

Action
- Extension of the interphalangeal and metatarsophalangeal joints of the lateral four toes.
- Dorsiflexion of the foot.

Nerve Supply
- Deep peroneal nerve.

Peroneus Tertius

Origin (Fig. 15.6)
- Lower one-fourth of the anterior surface of the fibula.
- Interosseous membrane.

It is continuous at its origin with the extensor digitorum longus of which it appears to be a separated part.

Insertion (Fig. 15.9)
- Dorsal surface of the base of the fifth metatarsal bone.

Action
- Dorsiflexion as the ankle.
- Eversion of the foot.

Nerve Supply
- Deep peroneal nerve.

Its tendon lies on the lower end of tibia lateral to the tendon of extensor digitorum longus.

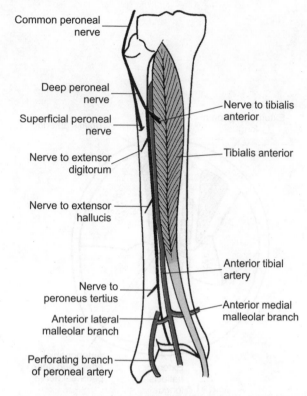

Common peroneal
nerve

Deep peroneal
nerve

Superficial peroneal
nerve

Nerve to extensor
digitorum

Nerve to extensor
hallucis

Nerve to
peroneus tertius

Anterior lateral
malleolar branch

Perforating branch
of peroneal artery

Nerve to tibialis
anterior

Tibialis anterior

Anterior tibial
artery

Anterior medial
malleolar branch

Fig. 15.8: Anterior compartment of leg: Deep peroneal
nerve and anterior tibial artery

ANTERIOR TIBIAL ARTERY

It is one of the two terminal branches of the popliteal artery
given at the distal border of the popliteal muscle in the
popliteal fossa. It enters the anterior compartment of the
leg by passing between the two heads of tibialis posterior
through an opening in the upper part of the interosseous
membrane.

Relations

Anteriorly
- Extensor digitorum longus in the upper two-thirds of
  the leg.
- Deep peroneal nerve in the middle one-third of the leg.
- Tendon of extensor hallucis longus crosses it from lateral
  to medial side in the lower one-third (Fig. 15.10).

Posteriorly
- Interosseous membrane in the upper two-thirds of the
  leg.
- Front of tibia and ankle in the lower one-third of the leg.

Laterally
- Extensor digitorum longus throughout its whole course.

- Deep peroneal nerve in the upper and lower one-third of
  the leg. The nerve is anterior to the artery only in the
  middle third of the leg.
- Peroneus tertius in the lower one-third of the leg.
  Medially
- Tibialis anterior throughout its whole course.
- Extensor hallucis longus tendon in front of the ankle.
  Branches
- Anterior recurrent running upwards through the tibialis
  anterior.
- Anterior medial and anterior lateral malleolar which ramify
  from the malleoli.
- Muscular branches.

DEEP PERONEAL NERVE

It is the terminal division of the common peroneal nerve
given off at the level of the neck of fibula. It enters the
anterior compartment of the leg by piercing the anterior
intermuscular septum and then passes deep to or through
the extensor digitorum longus. It courses downward and
after passing through the superior and inferior extensor
retinacula ends by dividing into a lateral and a medial branche
in front of the ankle (Fig. 15.11).

Relations

Medially
- Tibialis anterior throughout.
- Extensor hallucis longus in the lower third of the leg as
  its tendon crosses the nerve from lateral to medial side
  (Fig. 15.10)
  Laterally
- Extensor digitorum longus throughout the leg.
- Extensor hallucis longus in the middle one-third of the leg.
- Peroneus tertius in the lower one-third of the leg.

The deep peroneal nerve lies lateral to the artery in the
upper one-third of the leg. In the middle one-third it is in
front of the artery, **'hesitates'** to cross the medial side of
the artery, but goes back to the lateral side of the artery in
the lower one-third of the leg. Hence, it is referred to as
"nervous hesitans".
Branches (Fig. 15.8)
- Muscular branches to all the four muscles of anterior
  compartment.
- Articular branch to the ankle joint.
- Terminal branches (Fig. 15.11)
  (i) Medial terminal supplies the first dorsal
      interosseous muscle and the skin of the adjacent
      sides of first and second toes.

(ii) Lateral terminal ends in a pseudoganglion under extensor digitorum brevis supplying it and the tarsal and metatarsal joints of lateral side of foot.

Perforating Branch of the Peroneal Artery

Appears in the anterior compartment by perforating the interosseous membrane above the lateral malleolus.

DORSUM OF THE FOOT

Skeleton of Foot-Dorsal Surface

The bones of the foot consist proximally of seven short tarsal bones (the talus, calcaneus, cuboid, navicular and the three cuneiforms) collectively, known as the tarsus. They articulate with each other and distally with the five metatarsal bones (the metatarsus), each of which carries the phalanges of the corresponding toe.

Extensor digitorum brevis takes origin from the upper surface of calcaneus in front of the posterior facet. The **dorsal interossei** arise by two heads from the adjacent metatarsal bones. Hence, the medial and lateral surfaces of the shafts of all the bones excluding the medial surface of the first metatarsal and the lateral surface of the fifth give

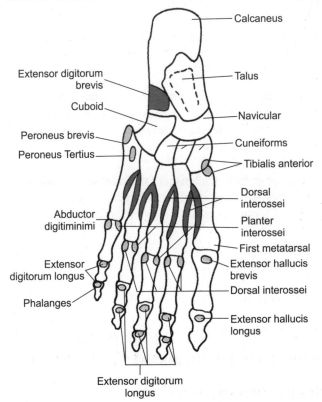

Fig. 15.9: Dorsum of foot: Skeletal framework with muscle markings

origin to the dorsal interossei which encroaches on the dorsal surface as well.

Peroneus brevis is inserted on the dorsal surface of the styloid process of the fifth metatarsal bone. **Peroneus tertius** is inserted on the medial aspect of the base of the fifth metatarsal.

The four tendons of extensor digitorum longus expand into dorsal digital extension, which divide distally into three slips. The middle slip inserts near the base of the middle phalanx, while the two lateral slips unite and insert near the base of the distal phalanx.

The tendon of **extensor digitorum brevis** to the great toe is inserted directly into base of the proximal phalanx. The tendon of **extensor hallucis longus** is inserted into the base of the distal phalanx of the great toe.

Deep Fascia

Retinacula around the ankle are thickenings of deep fascia which help in keeping the tendons in position as they pass deep into them.

The Superior Extensor Retinaculum

Attachments

• Lower ends of the anterior margins of the tibia and fibula.
   It splits at its medial end to enclose the tibialis anterior tendon.

Relations (Fig. 15.10)

Deep to the retinaculum from medial to lateral side are:
• Tendon of tibialis anterior with its own synovial sheath.
• Tendon of extensor hallucis longus.
• Anterior tibial artery.
• Deep peroneal nerve.
• Tendon of extensor digitorum longus with asynovial sheath which also enclose the tendon of peroneus tertius.

The Inferior Extensor Retinaculum

It is a Y-shaped structure antero-inferior to the ankle joint (Fig. 15.10).

Attachments

• The stem of the Y is lateral and is attached to the upper surface of the calcaneus and to the floor of sinus tarsi.
• The upper limb of the Y passes obliquely upwards to be attached to the anterior margin of medial malleolus.
• The lower limb of the Y passes medially to merge with the deep fascia of the sole.

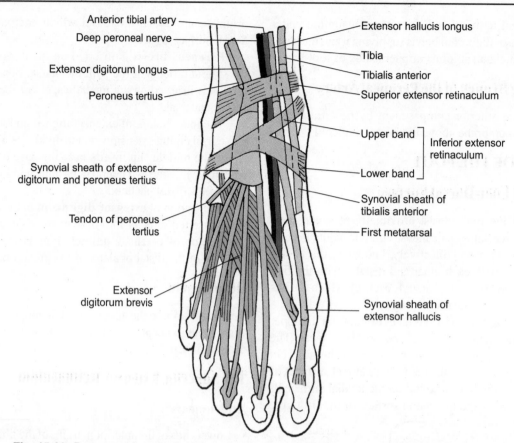

Anterior tibial artery
Deep peroneal nerve
Extensor digitorum longus
Peroneus tertius
Synovial sheath of extensor digitorum and peroneus tertius
Tendon of peroneus tertius
Extensor digitorum brevis

Extensor hallucis longus
Tibia
Tibialis anterior
Superior extensor retinaculum
Upper band
Inferior extensor retinaculum
Lower band
Synovial sheath of tibialis anterior
First metatarsal
Synovial sheath of extensor hallucis

Fig. 15.10: Dorsum of foot: Retinacula, tendons, synovial sheaths and extensor digitorum brevis

Synovial Sheaths on the Front of the Ankle (Fig. 15.10)

- The tendon of tibialis anterior has its own synovial sheath, extending from just above the superior extensor retinaculum almost to the medial cuneiform.
- The synovial sheath of the tendon of extensor hallucis longus begins between the retinacula and extends to the proximal of the big toe.
- The synovial sheath enclosing the tendons of the extensor digitorum longus and peroneus tertius extends from the lower border of the superior retinaculum for about 2.5.cm in front of the stem of the Y.

MUSCLE

Extensor Digitorum Brevis (Fig. 15.11)

It is the only muscle on the dorsum of the foot and forms a fleshy swelling in front of the lateral malleolus.

Origin (Fig. 15.9)

- Dorsum of the calcaneus medial to the attachment of the inferior extensor retinaculum.

Insertion

- By means of four tendons into the medial four toes. The tendon to the big toe crosses the dorsalis pedis artery and is attached independently to the base of the proximal phalanx. This part of the muscle is known as **extensor hallucis brevis**.
- The other three tendons join the extensor expansions of the second, third and fourth digits.
- The fifth toe lacks a short extensor tendon.

Action

- Extension of the toes.

Nerve Supply

- Deep peroneal nerve.

NERVE ON THE DORSUM OF THE FOOT

Deep peroneal nerve (15.11)

On the dorsum of the foot it emerges between the tendous of the extensor hallucis longus and the extensor digitorum

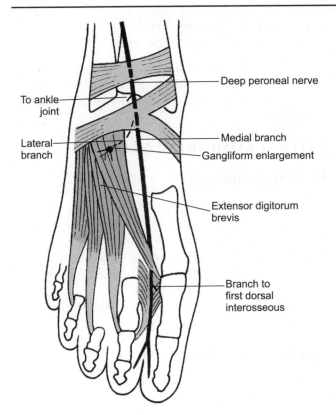

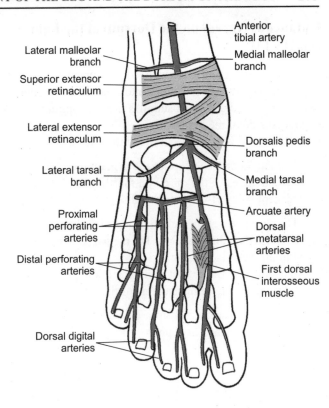

Fig. 15.11: Dorsum of foot : Extensor digitorum brevis and deep peroneal nerve

Fig. 15.12: Dorsum of foot: Dorsalis pedis artery and its branches

longus (Fig. 15.10). It divides into a medial and lateral branch.

- The medial branch continues forward supplies first dorsal interosseous and divides into dorsal digital nerves for the lateral side of the hallux and the medial side of the second toe.
- The lateral branch passes deep to extensor digitorum brevis and becomes enlarged into a pseudoganglion which supplies the muscle and torsal and metatorsophalangeal joints.

Arteries on the Dorsum of the Foot (Fig. 15.12)

Dorsalis pedis artery, begins in front of the ankle joint as continuation of the anterior tibial artery. It terminates by entering the sole between the two heads of the first dorsal interosseous muscle. In the sole of the foot it unites with the **lateral plantar artery** to form the **plantar arch.** Its successive deep relations on the dorsum of the foot are:

- Interosseous membrane.
- Lower third of lateral surface of tibia.
- Talus

- Navicular
- Intermediate cuneiform
- Capsules of the intervening joints.

It lies between the deep peroneal nerve laterally and the extensor hallucis longus tendon medially.

Branches

- **Lateral tarsal artery,** arising opposite the navicular.
- **Medial tarsal artery.**
- **Arcuate artery,** arises near the base of the second metatarsal. It runs laterally, with a slight anterior convexity, toward the lateral edge of the foot. It gives :
- Three **dorsal metatarsal arteries,** each of which divides into two dorsal digital arteries for contiguous sides of the lateral four toes. The lateral one sends a twig to the lateral side of the little toe.
- First dorsal metatarsal divide into dorsal digital branches for medial side of the big toe and the adjacent sides of the big toe and second toe.

Cutaneous Nerves on the Dorsum of the Foot
(Fig. 15.13)

The superficial peroneal nerve becomes superficial in the distal third of the foot. It divides into a medial and a lateral branch. The medial branch supplies the skin on the:
- Medial side of the big toe.
- Adjacent sides of the second and third toes.

The lateral branch supplies the skin on the:
- Adjacent sides of the third and fourth toes.
- Adjacent sides of the fourth and fifth toes.

The deep peroneal nerve at the level of the ankle divides into lateral and medial branches. The medial branch supplies the skin on the (Fig. 15.11):
- Adjacent sides of the first digital cleft and gives:
  – Articular twig to medial side of the foot.

The lateral branch ends in a gangliform enlargement which sends branches to supply:

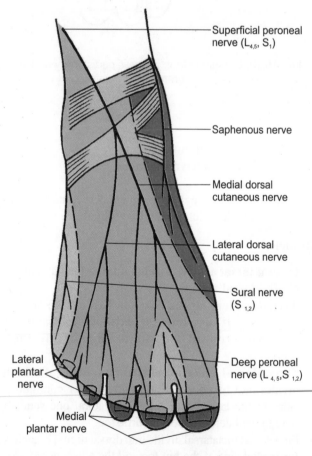

Fig. 15.13: Dorsum of right foot: Cutaneous nerves. Their areas of distribution and segmental origins

- The **extensor digitorum brevis**.
- Joints of the lateral side of the foot.

The nail beds and the tips of toes of the medial three and one-half toes are supplied by the medial plantar nerve and those of the lateral one and one-half toes by the lateral plantar nerve.

LATERAL COMPARTMENT OF LEG

The Bony Framework

Lateral (peroneal) surface of fibula is enclosed between the anterior and posterior borders, its lower fourth inclines posteriorly and its terminal part becomes continuous with the groove on the posterior surface of the lateral malleolus.
- Upper third and posterior part of middle third gives origin to **peroneus longus muscle**.
- Rest of the surface gives origin to **peroneus brevis muscle**.

Muscles of the Lateral Compartment

This compartment has two muscles, peroneus longus and peroneus brevis.

Peroneus Longus

Origin (Fig. 15.14)

- Upper two-thirds of the lateral surface of the shaft of fibula.
- Deep fascia overlying it.
- Anterior and posterior intermuscular septa.

Insertion (Fig. 15.9)

- Base of first metatarsal.
- Adjoining part of medial **cuneiform**.

The tendon of peroneus longus passes behind the lateral malleolus, where it is superficial to peroneus brevis tendon. It passes deep to superior peroneal retinaculum, lying in a common synovial sheath with brevis. Passing deep to the inferior peroneal retinaculum and below the peroneal tubercle on the lateral side of calcaneum, it has its own synovial sheath. The tendon then enters the fourth layer of the sole to reach its insertions.

Action

- Evertor of foot.
- Plantar flexor of the anckle joint.
- Maintenance of the longitudinal arch of the foot.

Nerve Supply

- Superficial peroneal nerve.

Peroneus Brevis

Origin (Fig. 15.14)

- Lower two-thirds of the lateral surface of the shaft of fibula.
- Anterior and posterior intermuscular septa.

Insertion (Fig. 15.9)

- Tuberosity on the base of the fifth metatarsal bone. Its tendon passes behind the lateral malleolus and lies in front of the tendon of peroneus longus in a common synovial sheath. The two tendons pass deep into superior and inferior peroneal retinacula to reach the lateral surface of calcaneum. The tendon of peroneus brevis passes above the peroneal tubercle enclosed in a separate synovial sheath.

Nerve Supply

- Superficial peroneal nerve.

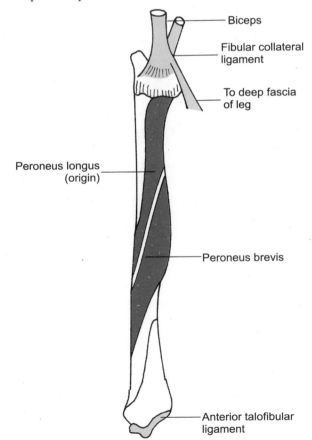

Fig. 15.14: Peroneal or lateral compartment bony framework

SUPERFICIAL PERONEAL NERVE

The common peroneal nerve lies on the neck of the fibula undercovers the origin of the peroneus longus muscle and it is here that it divides into three branches:

- Recurrent genicular.

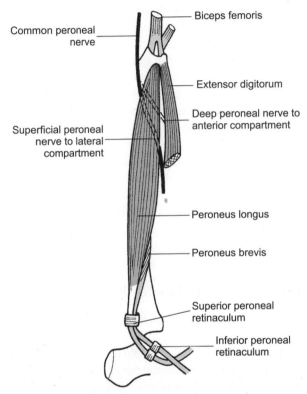

(a) Peroneus longus muscle and peroneal nerves

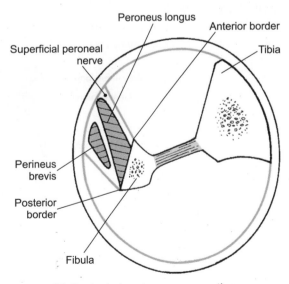

(b) Contents in a transverse section

Fig. 15.15: Lateral compartment of leg

- Deep peroneal.
- Superficial peroneal.

Recurrent genicular pierces the extensor digitorum longus, accompanies the anterior tibial recurrent through the upper part of tibialis anterior to reach the knee joint and the superior tibiofibular joint which it supplies.

Deep peroneal nerve, pierces the extensor digitorum longus to reach the anterior compartment of leg, where it has been studied (Fig. 15.15).

Superficial peroneal nerve passes downward between the peronei and extensor digitorum longus.

It pierces the deep fascia of the leg in the lower one-third of the leg and divides into a medial and a lateral branch which reach the dorsum of the foot (Fig. 15.13).

- *Branches*
- Muscular to peroneus longus and peroneus brevis.
- Cutaneous to the skin of the lower part of the front of the leg.
- Skin of the dorsum of the foot excluding the medial and lateral borders.
- Medial border of the big toe.
- Adjacent sides of second, third and fourth toes.

Lateral Aspect of Ankle (Fig. 15.17)

The **superior peroneal retinaculum** is firmly attached between:

- The back of the arterial malleolus.
- The lateral surface of the calcaneus.

It retains the tendons of peroneus longus and brevis along with their common synovial sheath in the hollow behind the lateral malleolus.

The **inferior peroneal retinaculum** is attached to the anterior part of the upper surface of calcaneous where

it is continuous with the stem of the inferior extensor retinaculum to be attached to:

- The peroneal trochlea midway.
- The lateral surface of calcaneus below.

It forms an osseofibrous canal above for the tendon of peroneus brevis and another below for the tendon of peroneus longus. Each canal has a separate synovial sheath.

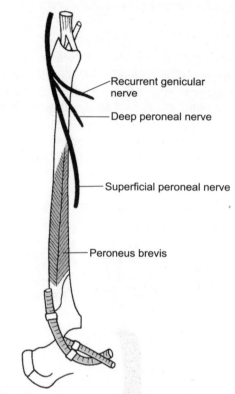

Fig. 15.16: Lateral compartment of leg: Peroneus brevis muscle

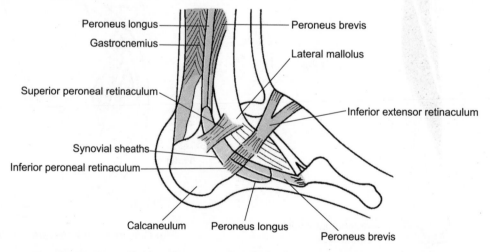

Fig. 15.17: The peroneal retinacula and the synovial sheaths of peroneal tendons

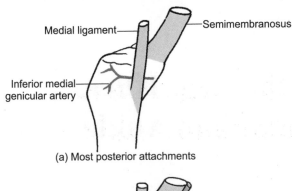

(a) Most posterior attachments

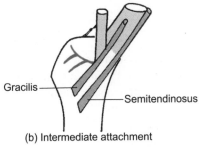

(b) Intermediate attachment

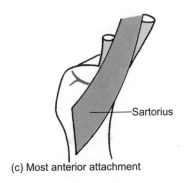

(c) Most anterior attachment

Fig. 15.18: Attachment of tendons and medial ligament of the knee to the upper part of medial surface of tibia from deep to superficial layers

The **common synovial sheath** is deep to the superior peroneal retinaculum. The sheath of peroneus brevis reaches almost to the fifth metatarsal, that of peroneus longus may extend across the sole to the attachment of the tendon.

Medial Side of Leg

This region is composed of the medial surface of the tibia covered over by periosteum, superficial fascia and skin.

The surface is enclosed by the anterior and medial borders and is mostly subcutaneous.

Upper Part

Anteriorly gives insertion from before backward to:
• Sartorius.
• Gracilis.
• Semitendinosus.

The insertion of sartorius is inverted J-shaped and the hook overlooks the insertion of the other two muscles. The insertions are separated by a bursa known as **bursa anserina**.

More posteriorly, the surface gives attachment to:
• Anterior fibres of the tibial collateral (medial) ligament of the knee joint for which there is an elongated impression.
• Insertion to an expansion of semimembranosus muscle.
• The tibial collateral ligament of the knee partly covers the insertion of the semimembranosus into the tibial condyle. The inferior genicular artery passes deep to it.
• The tendons of sartorius, gracilis and semitendinosis superficial to the medial ligament of the knee joint

Lower Part

It is related to:
• Great saphenous vein.

16 Back of the Leg, Knee, Tibiofibular and Ankle Joints

POSTERIOR COMPARTMENT

SKELETAL FRAMEWORK

Skeletal framework of the posterior compartment is provided by the posterior surface of tibia and fibula and of the talus, calcaneum and the interosseous membrane.

Posterior surface of tibia is bounded by the medial and interosseous borders. Soleal line running from above downwards and medially divides it into upper and lower

areas. The lower area is further subdivided by a vertical line in its upper three-fourths into medial and lateral areas (Fig. 16.1 a). The attachments on the areas are as follows (Fig. 16.1 b):

- *Upper (Triangular) Area*
- Insertion of **popliteus**.
- *Soleal Line from above Downwards*
- **Fascia covering popliteus**.
- **Fascia covering soleus**.
- Origin of **soleus**.

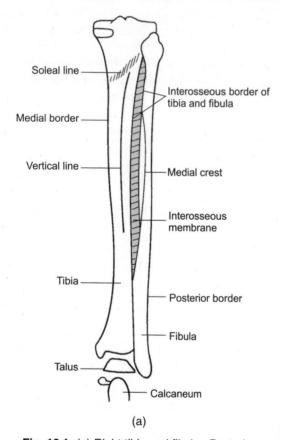

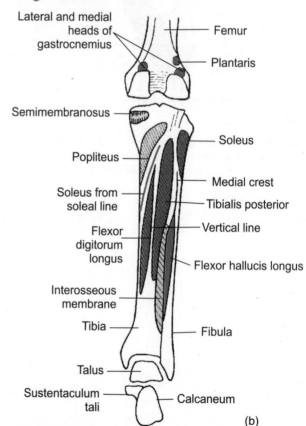

Fig. 16.1: (a) Right tibia and fibula : Posterior aspect bony features. (b) Posterior aspect with muscle markings

- **Fascia covering the deep muscles of the back of the leg.**

The upper lateral end of the line gives attachment to the medial end of the tendinous arch of origin of the soleus muscle.

- *Vertical Line*
  - Fascia covering the **tibialis posterior**.
- *Medial Area below Soleal Line*
  - Origin of **flexor digitorum longus**.
- *Lateral Area below Soleal Line*
  - Origin of **tibialis posterior**.

Posterior surface of fibula is bounded by the interosseous and posterior borders. Medial crest, which runs at first downwards and then inclines forward to meet the interosseous border, divides the upper two-thirds of the posterior surface of fibula into a lateral and a medial area. The attachments on these areas are as follows:

- *Medial Area*
  - Origin of the **tibialis posterior**.
- *Medial Crest*
  - Intermuscular septum between tibialis posterior lying deeply and flexor digitorum longus and flexor hallucis longus lying superficially.
- *Lateral Area*
  - Origin of **soleus** from the upper fourth part. The medial part of this origin shows a tubercle which gives attachment to the fibrous arch of origin of the muscle.
  - Origin of **flexor hallucis longus** from the lower three-fourths part of the area.

SUPERFICIAL FASCIA

The superficial fascia of the back of the leg has no special features.

Superficial Vein (Fig. 16.2)

The **short saphenous vein** begins at the lateral end of the dorsal venous arch. It ascends through the superficial fascia of the calf, pierces the lower part of the popliteal fascia and ascends through the fossa to join the upper part of the **popliteal vein**. The long and short saphenous veins are connected to the deep veins by communicating vessels known as **perforators,** which pierce the deep fascia. These perforators are most numerous in the posterior compartment and have valves which direct the blood flow from the superficial to the deep veins.

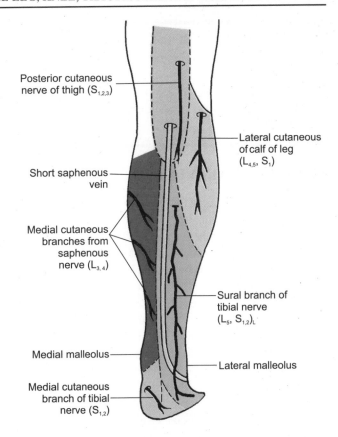

Posterior cutaneous nerve of thigh ($S_{1,2,3}$)

Lateral cutaneous of calf of leg ($L_{4,5}$, S_1)

Short saphenous vein

Medial cutaneous branches from saphenous nerve ($L_{3,4}$)

Sural branch of tibial nerve (L_5, $S_{1,2}$)

Medial malleolus

Lateral malleolus

Medial cutaneous branch of tibial nerve ($S_{1,2}$)

Fig. 16.2: Posterior aspect of right leg: Superficial vein and cutaneous nerves and their areas of distribution and segmental origin

CLINICAL APPLICATION

- The venous return through both the superficial and deep veins has to operate against a considerable hydrostatic pressure in the erect posture. The force which overcomes this pressure is different in the superficial and deep veins.
  In deep veins the pressure on the walls of the veins originates from the contraction of muscles, which are in a rigid osteofascial compartment.
  In superficial veins the joint movements create tension in the overlying skin which squeezes the vessels against the underlying deep fascia.
  In walking both forces operate, while in static standing little force is exerted on the superficial veins.
- Veins of the lower limb are prone to dilation and consequent valvular incompetence, since they have

to withstand high pressures. This results in the formation of **varicose veins** because the incompetency of the communicating vessels allow the blood to leak in the wrong direction from deep to superficial vessels particularly during standing.

CUTANEOUS NERVES (FIG. 16.2)

The cutaneous nerves are derived partly from the femoral nerve but mostly from the tibial and common peroneal nerves and their branches.

- **The posterior cutaneous nerves of thigh (S₁ to S₃),** continues downwards below the knee to supply a strip along the midline of the calf as much as half or two-thirds the length of the leg.
- **The saphenous nerves (L₃ and L₄),** from the femoral as it runs downwards with the great saphenous vein on the anterior aspect of the leg, give off a series of **medial cutaneous branches** to the back of the leg.
- **The sural nerves (L₅, S₁ and S₂),** arise from the tibial nerve and pierces the deep fascia about half way down the calf. In the superficial fascia it follows the short saphenous vein downwards and passes behind and below the lateral mallous to run along the lateral border of the foot.
- The lateral cutaneous of calf of leg (L₄, and S₅; S₁) is

given off in the popliteal fossa. It supplies the upper lateral part of the back of leg.

BOUNDARIES (FIG. 16.3)

Anteriorly

- Tibia.
- Interosseous membrane.
- Fibula.
- Posterior intermuscular septum.

Posteriorly

- Deep fascia extending from the medial border of the tibia to the posterior intermuscular septum. It covers the superficial muscles.

The compartment is subdivided into three by two strong fascial septa.

First septum from medial border of the tibia to the posterior border of fibula. It covers the:

- Flexor digitorum longus.
- Flexor hallucis longus.
- Posterior tibial vessels.

Second septum is attached medially to the proximal part of soleal line of the tibia and the vertical ridge on the posterior surface of the tibia and laterally to the medial crest of fibula.

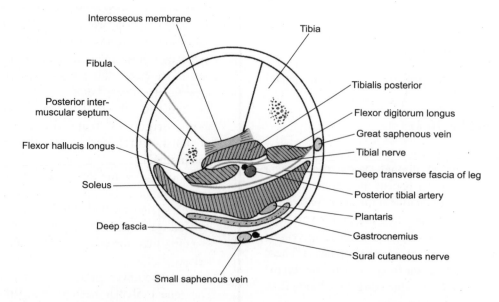

Fig. 16.3: Posterior compartment of leg: Boundaries and contents

MUSCLES

The muscles of the posterior compartment are arranged in four layers:

Layer I: Gastrocnemius.
Layer II: Plantaris and soleus.
Layer III: Flexor digitorum longus and flexor hallucis longus.
Layer IV: Tibialis posterior and popliteus.

Layer I (Fig. 16.4)

• **Gastrocnemius**

Origin

From distal end of femur by two heads (Fig. 16.1 b):
• Lateral head from lateral surface of lateral condyle.

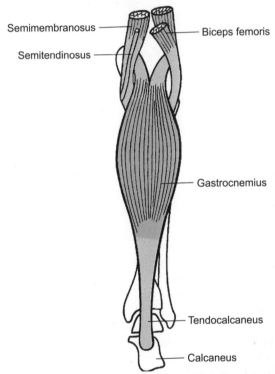

Fig. 16.4: Posterior compartment of leg: First layer muscle (Gastrocnemius)

It often contains a small sesamoid bone known as **'fabella'**.
• Medial head from popliteal surface of femur above the medial condyle.

Each head arises by a tendon which forms two fleshy bellies. Near the middle of the leg they end in a thin, aponeurotic tendon which joins the tendon of the soleus to form the tendocalcaneus, a short distance below the middle of the leg.

Insertion

• Middle portion of the posterior surface of the calcaneus.

Action

• Plantar flexion at the ankle.

Nerve Supply

• Tibial nerve.

Layer II

• **Plantaris**

It is a small muscle which lies partly hidden by the medial side of the lateral head of gastrocnemius.

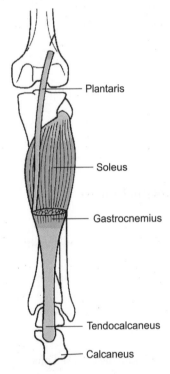

Fig. 16.5: Posterior compartment of leg: Second layer muscles (Plantaris and soleus)

Origin (Fig. 16.1 b)

• Popliteal surface of femur above the lateral condyle.

Insertion

• Middle portion of posterior surface of calcaneus medial to the insertion of tendoncalcaneus independently or blended with it.

Nerve Supply

• Tibial nerve.

Soleus

It is a flat, thick muscles

Origin (Fig. 16.1 b)

- Back of the head and upper third of the posterior surface of the shaft of the fibula.
- Soleal line.
- Middle of the medial border of the tibia.
- Tendinous arch between the lateral end of soleal line and the fibular origin of soleus.

Insertion

- Middle portion of posterior surface of calcaneus through tendocalcaneus which is its combined tendon with gastrocnemius.

Action

- Plantar flexion at ankle.
- Stabilization of the ankle joint on standing.

Nerve Supply

- Tibial nerve.

Layer III

Flexor Digitorum Longus

Origin (Fig. 16.1 b)

- Posterior surface of tibia below the soleal line, medial to the vertical ridge.

  It crosses superficial to the lower part of tibialis posterior. The tendon becomes lateral to the tendon of tibialis posterior to enter the sole of the foot.

Insertion (Fig. 17.1)

- By four tendons into the terminal phalanges of the lateral four toes.

Action

- Flexion of interphalangeal and metatarsophalangeal joints.
- Plantar flexion.
- Inversion of the foot.

Flexor Hallucis Longus

Origin (Fig. 16.1 b)

- Lower three-fourths of the lateral area of the posterior surface of fibula below the medial crest.

  Its tendon occupies grooves on the posterior surface of talus and the sustentaculum tali before entering the sole.

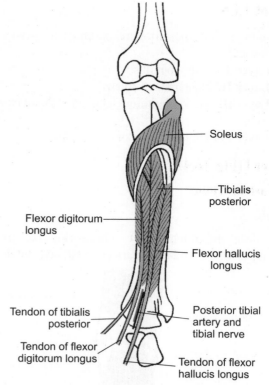

Fig. 16.6: Posterior compartment of leg: Third layer muscles (Flexor digitorum longus and flexor hallucis longus)

Insertion (Fig. 17.1)

- Terminal phalanx of the big toe.

Action

- Flexion of interphalangeal and the metatarsophalangeal joints of the big toe.
- Plantar flexion at ankle.
- Inversion of the foot.

Layer IV

Tibialis Posterior

Origin (Fig. 16.1 b)

- Area of the posterior surface of tibia below the soleal line and lateral to vertical line.
- Area of the posterior surface of fibula above the medial crest.
- Interosseous membrane.

  The upper end of the muscle is bifid for the passage of anterior tibial vessels. Its tendon inclines medially under the flexor digitorum longus, grooves on the back of medial malleolus before entering the sole.

Insertion (Fig. 17.1)

- Tuberosity of navicular.
- Medial cuneiform bone.
- All the other tarsal bones except the talus.
- Middle three metatarsals.

Action

- Plantar flexion at ankle.
- Inversion of the foot.

Popliteus

Origin (Fig. 16.10 c)

- Anterior part of the popliteal groove of the femur. Origin is intracapsular but extrasynovial.

Insertion (Fig. 16.1 b)

- Triangular area of the posterior surface of tibia above the soleal line.
- Popliteal fascia covering it.

Action

- Flexion of the knee.
- Medial rotation of leg at the beginning of flexion.

Nerve Supply

- Tibial nerve. The nerve to popliteus hooks arround the distal margin to reach its deep surface.

POSTERIOR TIBIAL ARTERY

It is the larger of the two terminal branches of the popliteal artery which divides at the distal border of popliteus muscle.

Relations

Superficial

- Upper part:
  - Gastrocnemius.
  - Soleus.
- Lower part:
  - Flexor retinaculum.
  - Abductor hallucis.

Deep

- From above downwards the artery lies on:
  - Tibialis posterior.
  - Flexor digitorum longus.
  - Back of tibia.
  - Back of ankle joint.

Branches

- **Circumflex fibular** runs laterally around the neck of fibula. May arise from anterior tibial.
- **Peroneal** is the first branch. It runs downward and laterally on the tibialis posterior deep to the flexor hallucis longus. After emerging from undercover of this muscle, it pierces the deep fascia and ends by dividing into lateral calcaneal arteries. The branches are:
  - Muscular.
  - Nutrient to fibula.
  - Perforating.
  - Lateral calcaneal.
- **Nutrient artery to tibia.**
- **Muscular.**
- **Communicating branch to peroneal artery.**
- **Medial calcaneal branches.**
- **Terminal medial** and **lateral plantar arteries** in the sole.

ANTERIOR TIBIAL ARTERY (FIG. 16.7)

Only a small part of the artery is seen in the posterior compartment. It passes through the interosseous membrane to the anterior compartment of the leg.

TIBIAL NERVES (L_4 AND L_5; S_1 TO S_3)

It is larger of two terminal branches of the sciatic and begins about the middle of the back of thigh. It then enters the popliteal fossa where it has been studied.

In the upper two-thirds of the posterior compartment of leg, its relations are:
- Superficial:
  - Gastrocnemius.
  - Soleus.
- Deep:
  - Tibialis posterior.
  - Flexor digitorum longus.

In the lower third of the leg relations are:
- Superficial:
  - Deep fascia.
- Deep:
  - Posterior surface of tibia.
  - Posterior surface of ankle.

In the leg, first the nerve is medial to the artery, then it crosses posterior to the artery from medial to lateral side (Fig. 16.7).

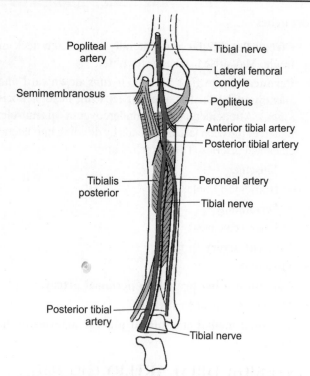

Fig. 16.7: Posterior compartment of leg: Fourth layer muscles, tibialis posterior and popliteus and posterior tibial artery and nerve

Branches

- **Muscular to:**
  - Tibialis posterior.
  - Flexor hallucis longus.
  - Flexor digitorum longus.
  - Deep part of soleus.
- **Cutaneous:**
  - Medial calcaneal nerves.
- **Articular:**
  - To ankle.

MEDIAL ASPECT OF ANKLE

Flexor retinaculum is attached between (Fig. 16.8):
- The medial margin of the groove on the back of the medial malleolus and;
- The medial process of the calcaneus.

Septa pass from its deep surface to form four osseofacial compartments which from medial to lateral side contain:
- The tendon of tibialis posterior.
- The tendon of flexor digitorum longus.
- The posterior tibial vessels and tibial nerve.
- The tendon of flexor hallucis longus.

The tendons are covered by synovial sheaths. Each extends about 2.5 cm above the tip of the medial malleolus. Distally the extent is:
- Tibialis posterior almost to the navicular.
- Flexor digitorum longus a little more anteriorly.
- Flexor hallucis longus still more, to about the middle of the first metatarsal.

KNEE JOINT

The knee joint is a complex synovial joint of a modified hinge variety.

Articular Surfaces

The articular surfaces are provided by the femur, patella and tibia. There are in fact two joints viz.:
- The tibiofemoral and;
- The patellofemoral.

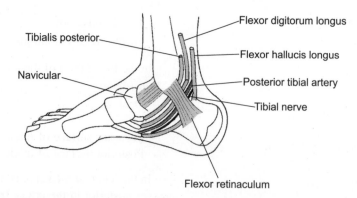

Fig. 16.8: Medial aspect of ankle: Flexor retinaculum with structures passing under it and the related synovial sheaths

Femoral Articular Surface (Fig. 16.9 a)

The lower end of femur is widely expanded more in the transverse axis; further it projects posteriorly. It consists of two condyles which are united anteriorly and are continuous with the shaft as one mass. Posteriorly they are independently continuous with the shaft being separated from each other by the intercondylar notch.

Patellar articular surface occupies the anterior surfaces of both the condyles and forms a continuous area, which is slightly grooved in the middle and is concave from side to side. It extends higher on the lateral condyle and is separated from the tibial articular surfaces by two grooves. Each groove is related to the respective meniscus during full extension of the knee.

Tibial articular surfaces are meant for articulation with the condyles of the tibia. They are limited anteriorly by the grooves for the menisci and are separated from each other by the intercondylar fossa. Each surface is convex from side to side as well as anteroposteriorly. The antero-posterior curve is:

- More sharp posteriorly in both condyles.
- Longer in the medial condyle.
- More gentle in the lateral condyle.

These features have important bearings on the movement and stability of the knee joint.

Tibial Articular Surface (Fig. 16.9 c)

The upper surfaces of two condyles are separated by non-articular intercondylar area. It is marked by an intercondylar eminence in the middle formed by the medial and lateral intercondylar tubercles which divide the area into anterior and posterior parts. Each condylar facet is slightly concave in the centre and flattened at the periphery.

The Patellar Articular Surface (Fig. 16.9 b)

Posterior surface of patella has an upper oval articular area and a lower rough area. Oval articular area has the following features:

- A vertical ridge dividing the area into a large lateral and a smaller medial facet. The ridge fits into the groove on the patellar area of the femur.
- The medial part of the media facet forms an elongated strip which comes in contact with the femur during extreme flexion.
- The rest of the medial surface is indistinctly divided into an upper and al lower area. The former remains in

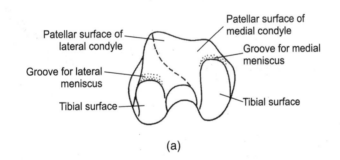

(a)

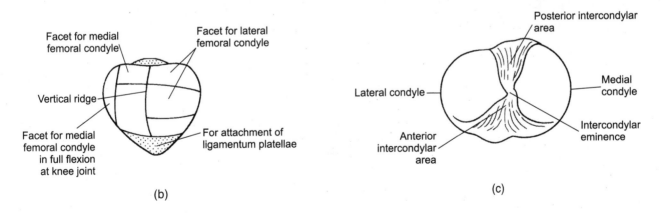

(b)

(c)

Fig. 16.9: Knee joint: Articular surfaces (a) Femoral. (b) Patellar. (c) Tibial

contact with the femur in moderate flexion and the latter in extension.

- The lateral articular area is larger and is indistinctly divisible into three areas from above downwards. The upper and middle areas are in contact with the femur, the former during moderate flexion and the latter during extension the lowermost area is related to fat.

THE FIBROUS CAPSULE (FIG. 16.10)

It is a sac which covers the joint except anteriorly. Its attachments are as follows on the femur:

- Posteriorly to the upper margins of the medial and lateral femoral condylar surfaces and the whole of the intercondylar line (Fig. 16.10 b).
- Medially along a line about 1 cm away from the articular margin of the medial condyle (Fig. 16.11).
- Laterally along a line about 1 cm away from the articular margin of the lateral condyle passing above the popliteal groove (Fig. 16.10 c).
- Anteriorly there is no capsule and the deficiency is covered by (Fig. 16.10 a):

- The broad **tendon of the quadriceps femoris,** muscle which descends from the thigh. It contains a very large sesamoid bone, the patella.
- **Medial** and **lateral patellar retinacula,** which are expansions of the aponeurosis for the vastus medialis and lateralis muscles.
- **Ligamentum patellae,** which is attached to the upper smooth part of the tibial tuberosity below and to the apex of patella above.

Extracapsular Ligaments

The **collateral ligaments** are strong and extracapsular. On the lateral side, ligament and capsule are separate. On the medial side, they are structurally continuous.

Medial Collateral Ligament (Tibial Collateral)

Medial ligament (Fig. 16.11) is attached above to the medial epicondyle of femur above the adductor tubercle and below to the medial condyle and medial surface of the shaft of the tibia. It has a superficial and a deep part.

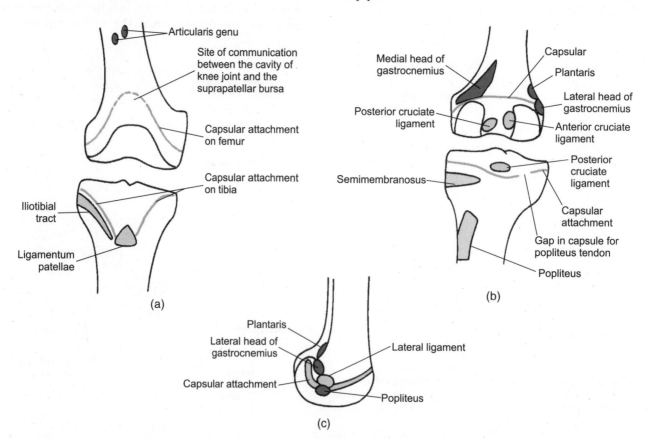

Fig. 16.10: Knee joint: Attachment of fibrous capsule (a) On anterior aspects of femur and tibia. (b) On posterior aspects of femur and tibia. (c) On lateral aspect of lateral condyle of femur

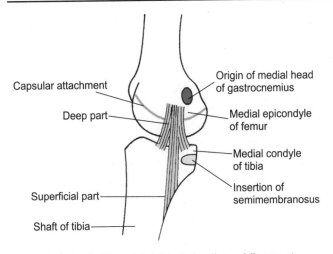

Fig. 16.11: Knee joint: Medial collateral ligament

The superficial part is attached to medial condyle and medial surface of the shaft of tibia far about 3.5 cm. The deep part is attached to the tibia above the groove for the insertion of semimembranous muscle. At the sides, the ligament fuses with the capsule of the joint and the medial meniscus making the meniscus immobile.

Lateral Collateral Ligament (Fibular Collateral)

Lateral ligament (Fig. 16.12) is cord-like and is attached superiorly to lateral epicondyle of femur above the origin of popliteus and inferiorly to the head of the fibula. Superficially the tendon of the biceps overlaps it and is said to be split by the ligament.

Oblique Posterior Ligament (Fig. 16.13)

It is an expansion from the tendon of insertion of

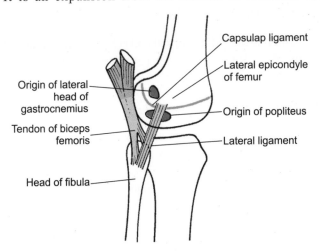

Fig. 16.12: Knee joint: Lateral collateral ligament

semimembranous on the back of medial tibia condyle. Passing upwards and laterally it is attached to the intercondylar line and the lateral condyle thereby strengthening the capsule on the back of the knee. It forms the floor of middle of popliteal fossa. It is pierced by the middle genicular artery and the genicular branch of the obturator nerve.

Arcuate Popliteal Ligament (Fig. 16.13)

The capsule of the knee joint presents a defect, below and laterally, through which the tendon of popliteus leaves its position from inside the capsule to run to its insertion on the tibia. A thickening at the upper edge of this defect is known as the arcuate ligament. Its fibres are attached below to the head of the fibula but spread out above in an upward and medial direction.

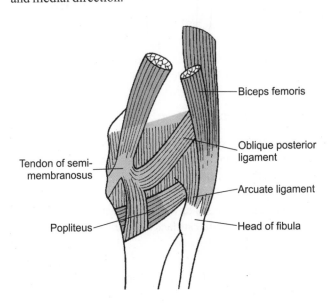

Fig. 16.13: Knee joint: Oblique posterior ligament and arcuate ligament

Ligamentum Patellae (Fig. 16.14)

It is a continuation of the insertion of quadriceps tendon to the tibia and is attached above to the apex of the patella and below to the upper half of the tuberosity of the tibia.

INTRACAPSULAR STRUCTURES

Cruciate Ligaments

These are two in number, their names refer to their attachments to the tibia and the fact that they cross each other like letter X.

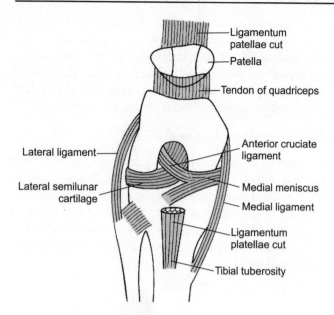

Fig. 16.14: Knee joint: Anterior cruciate ligament in anterior view with knee joint opened up

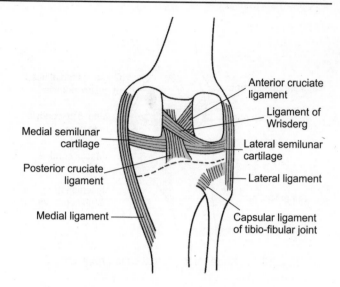

Fig. 16.15: Knee joint: Posterior cruciate ligament in posterior view with knee joint opened up

Anterior Cruciate Ligament

- **Inferiorly,** it is attached to the anterior upper surface of tibia in front of the intercondylar eminence and between the anterior horns of medial and lateral semilunar cartilages (Fig. 16.16).
- **Superiorly,** it passes upward, backward and laterally to be attached to medial surface of lateral condyle of femur (Figs. 16.10 and 16.14).

Anterior cruciate ligament is longer than the posterior cruciate ligament.

Posterior Cruciate Ligament

- Inferiorly, it is attached to the posterior part of upper surface of tibia behind the semilunar cartilages and between the condyles (Fig. 16.16).
- Superiorly, it passes upward and forward, medial to the anterior cruciate ligament, to be attached to the lateral surface of medial femoral condyle (Figs. 16.10 and 16.15).

The cruciate ligaments are essential to the antero-posterior stability of the knee joint, especially in the flexed position. In full extension the anterior cruciate is tough and the posterior cruciate ligament is slightly lax. In full flexion the posterior cruciate ligament is tough, while the anterior ligament is lax.

Semilunar Cartilages or Menisci

These are two—a medial and a lateral. They lie on the upper surface of tibial condyles and articulate with respective femoral condyles. Their outer convex margins are thick and the inner concave margins are thin. Their upper femoral surface is concave and the inferior tibial surface is flat. Their ends are thickened to form the anterior and posterior horns. Their anterior margins are bound together by the transverse ligament. Structurally, they consist of more fibrous tissue and less of cartilage. Their peripheral parts are fed by capillaries from capsule and most of the inner parts are avascular.

Medial Meniscus (Fig. 16.16)

It is comma-shaped, the broad end is behind. It is attached to the deep surface of the capsule and tibial collateral ligament.

Lateral Meniscus (Fig. 16.16)

It is more or less circular and so is more rounded. Its anterior and posterior **horns** lie within the horns of the medial meniscus which is more crescentic. Posteriorly it is separated from the fibular collateral ligament by the tendon of the popliteus which is attached to the meniscus.

The cruciate ligaments and the menisci are attached to the tibial intercondylar area in the following manner from front to backward (Fig. 16.16):

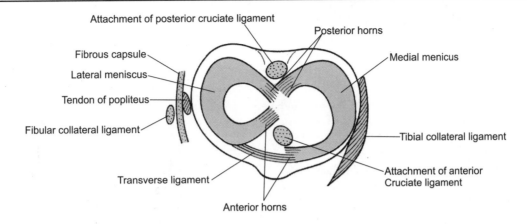

Fig. 16.16: Knee joint: Semilunar cartilages

- Anterior horn of medial meniscus.
- Lower end of anterior cruciate ligament.
- Anterior horn of lateral meniscus.
- Posterior horn of lateral meniscus behind the lateral intercondylar tubercle.
- Posterior horn of medial meniscus behind the medial intercondylar tubercle.
- Lower end of posterior cruciate ligament on the posterior most sloping area.

Transverse Ligament (Fig. 16.16)

It connects the anterior horns of the medial and lateral menisci.

Coronary Ligaments (Fig. 16.17)

These are short ligamentous fibers which connect the peripheral portions of the menisci to the peripheral margins of the tibial condyles. They merge with the lower part of the fibrous capsule of the knee joint.

Meniscofemoral Ligaments (Fig. 16.18)

These arise from the posterior surface of the lateral meniscus as two ligamentous slips, one runs along the anterior aspect of the posterior cruciate ligament **(ligament**

of Humphry) and the other on its posterior aspect **(ligament of Wrisberg)**. They are attached to the medial condyle of femur.

Origin of Popliteus

The popliteus arises from the anterior part of the groove on the lateral surface of lateral condyle of femur. The tendon comes out of the knee joint through an opening on the posterolateral aspect of the capsule and so becomes extracapsular. Its origin is intracapsular but extrasynovial.

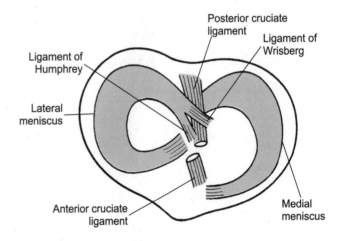

Fig. 16.18: Knee joint: Meniscofemoral ligaments

SYNOVIAL MEMBRANE (FIGS. 16.19 AND 16.20)

- The synovial membrane lines the fibrous capsule and covers those intracapsular bone surfaces which are not covered by articular cartilage.

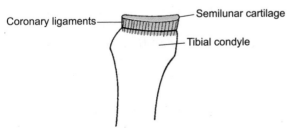

Fig. 16.17: Knee joint: Coronary ligament

- Posteriorly, the membrane is invaginated forward by the cruciate ligaments. Thus, the posterior aspects of these ligaments have no synovial covering i.e., they are intracapsular but extrasynovial.
- On either side, the membrane is invaginated by the menisci. Due to compression between the femoral and tibial condyles, it disappears from the central parts of their upper and lower surfaces and is present only on the peripheral parts of these surfaces.
- Anteriorly above the patella, the synovial membrane forms a pouch, which extends up beneath the quadriceps femoris muscle for a short distance forming the **suprapatellar bursa**. The articularis genu is inserted into it.
- Anteriorly below the patella, the wedge-shaped space between the ligamentum patellae and the anterior aspects of the tibial condyles is occupied by the **infrapatellar pad of fat**. The synovial membrane runs backward over the upper surface of this fat pad from the lower margin of the articular surface of the patella to the intercondylar area of the tibia forming the **infrapatellar fold**. The apex of this fold is attached to the anterior edge of the intercondylar notch of the femur. The infrapatellar fold is continued laterally on either side as the **alar folds**. The free lateral margins of these folds project backward from the sides of the patella. These folds are produced by extrasynovial fat pad and they adopt their shape to the contours of the bones in different positions of the

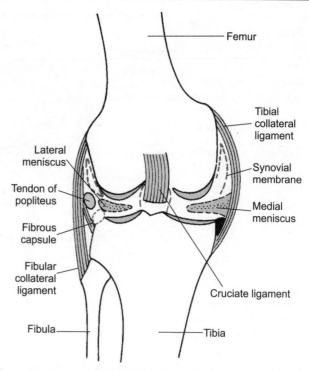

Fig. 16.20: Knee joint: Synovial membrane in a frontal section

knee. By keeping the synovial membrane in contact with the articular surfaces of the femoral condyles, they act as **Haversian fat pads** whose function is to occupy spaces where bony surfaces are incongruous.

Bursae Around the Knee

There is a large number of bursae related to the knee joint. The following are important:

Anterior Bursae (Fig. 16.21)

- **Suprapatellar bursa,** lies between the anterior surface of the lower part of femur and the deep surface of the quadriceps. It extends for about three finger-breadths above the upper border of patella, when the limb is at rest in extension. It always communicates with the synovial cavity of the knee joint.
- **Prepatellar bursa,** lies in front of the lower half of the patella and the upper half of the ligamentum patellae.
- **Superficial infrapatellar bursa,** lies in the subcutaneous tissue between the skin and the front of the lower part of the ligamentum patellae and the lower part of the tibial tuberosity.
- **Deep infrapatellar bursa,** lies between the ligamentum patellae and the tibia.

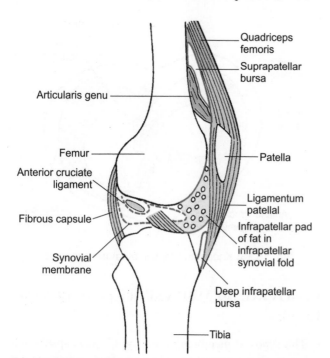

Fig. 16.19: Knee joint: Synovial membrane in sagittal section

Posterior Bursae (Fig. 16.21)

- **Semimembranosus bursa,** lies between the medial head of gastrocnemius and the capsule. It usually communicates with the joint cavity.
- **Bursa between lateral head of gastrocnemius and the capsule.**

Medial Bursae (Fig. 16.22)

- **Tibial intertendinous bursa (bursa anserina),** separates the tendons of gracilis, sartorius and semitendinosus from the tibial collateral ligament.

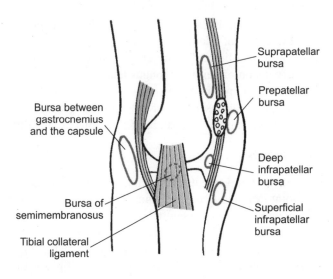

Fig. 16.21: Knee joint: Anterior and posterior bursae

- **Bursa separating the tendon of semimembranosus from the tibial collateral ligament medially and the head of tibia laterally.**

Lateral Bursae (Fig. 16.22)

- **Bursa between the biceps femoris tendon and the fibular collateral ligament.**
- **Bursa between the fibular collateral ligament and the tendon of popliteus.**
- **Popliteal bursa** between the popliteus tendon and the lateral condyle of femur.

Relations of the Knee Joint

Anteriorly

- Quadriceps tendon.
- Patella.
- Ligamentum patellae.

Anterolaterally

- Lateral patellar retinaculum derived from the vastus lateralis.

Posterolaterally

- Tendon of popliteus (intracapsular).
- Tendon of biceps femoris (extracapsular).
- Fibular collateral ligament deep to biceps.
- Common peroneal nerve running along the medial margin of biceps tendon.

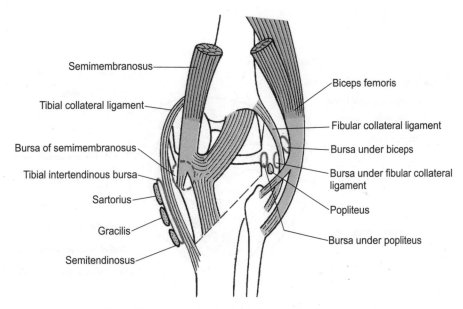

Fig. 16.22: Knee joint: Medial and lateral bursae

Posteriorly

- Popliteal vessels.
- Tibial nerve.
- Medial and lateral heads of gastrocnemius overlapping the popliteal vessels.
- Plantaris deep to the lateral head of gastrocnemius.

Posteromedially

- Semimembranosus lies medial to medial head of gastrocnemius and separates the tendon of semitendinosus from the capsule.
- Tendon of sartorius and gracilis.
- Great saphenous vein accompanied by saphenous nerve.

Anteromedially

- Medial patellar retinaculum derived from the vastus medialis.

Nerve Supply

- Articular branches of the femoral nerve.
- Genicular branches from the tibial and common peroneal nerves.
- Descending genicular branch from the posterior division of the obturator nerve.

Blood Supply

- Branches from femoral, lateral circumflex femoral, popliteal and anterior and posterior tibial arteries supply the joint.

Stability of the Knee Joint

In spite of the lack of congruency of its articular surfaces, the knee joint is one of the most stable of all joints. The stability is provided by the following:

- **Expansions from muscles,** which surround the joint from all sides viz.:
  - Patellar retinacula from medial and lateral vasti on either sides.
  - Iliotibial tract on the lateral side having the attachments of tensor fascia lata and gluteus maximus.
  - Oblique popliteal ligament, an expansion from the tendon of semimembranosus, at the back.
  - Medial collateral ligament considered to be an expansion of adductor magnus.
  - Lateral collateral ligament considered to be an expansion of peroneus longus tendon.
- **Muscular support** by origins of the gastrocnemius posteriorly, the insertions of the sartorius gracilis and semitendinosus medially and that of the biceps laterally.

Movements

The principal movements are flexion and extension as the knee joint is a modified hinge joint. The movement of the tibia on femur occurs in a sagittal plane around a transverse axis passing through the two femoral condyles.

- **Flexion** is a backward movement of the leg on the thigh and is associated with medial rotation of the tibia on the femur in the beginning. The main flexors are the hamstring muscles viz.:

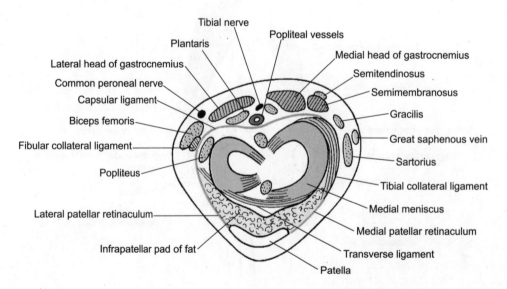

Fig. 16.23: Knee joint: Relations as seen in a horizontal section through the right knee joint above the menisci

- Semimembranosus.
- Semitendinosus.
- Biceps femoris.

These are supplied by the sciatic nerves (L_4 and L_5; S_1 and S_2). The sartorius, gracilis and popliteus may assist in this movement and the gastrocnemius is involved in a resisted flexion movement at the knee joint.

- **Extension** is a forward movement with the restoration of the flexed leg to the neutral position with lateral rotation of the tibia on femur at the end. The quadriceps femoris is the muscle, which extends the knee and is supplied by the femoral nerves (L_2 to L_4).
- **Rotation** occurs about a longitudinal axis and is the other normal movement at the joint. Active rotation is possible only in a flexed knee. Description of such movement as medial or lateral rotation must always indicate which bone is being regarded as the fixed element and which the moving element. Thus, medial rotation of the femur on the grounded tibia is the same movement as lateral rotation of the free tibia on the femur such axial rotations are possible only when the knee joint is flexed. The media rotators are:
  - Semimembranosus.
  - Semitendinosus.
  - Gracilis.
  - Sartorius.
  - Popliteus.

  The lateral rotators are:
  - Biceps femoris.

Locking Mechanism of the Knee

- The final limit of extension occurs at a sagittal **angulation** of about 190° between femur and tibia. This final limitation is brought about by a very complex looking mechanism, which operates over the last 5° or so of the movement and results in the ligaments getting taut especially the anterior cruciate, fibular and tibial collateral and oblique popliteal ligaments.
- In the locking mechanism the features of the articular surfaces are operative. On the lateral side, the articular surface of the lateral tibial condyle is shorter anteroposteriorly as compared to the medial condyle. Consequently the lateral meniscus and the articular surface of the lateral femoral condyle are also short. The medial femoral condyle has a longer and more curved articular surface than the lateral femoral condyle.
- As the joint passes from full flexion to extension, the

shorter lateral femoral condyle exhausts its forward roll faster than does the longer articular surface of the medial condyle. The extra-articular surface on the medial condyle which is still not used up allows for the final passive medial rotation of the femur on the tibia (**screw home movement**) to complete the process of extension. The rotation is around an arc of a circle whose centre is situated about the middle of the lateral condyle with the anterior cruciate ligament acting as a pivot. Quadriceps femoris is the muscle, which extends and locks the knee and is supplied by the femoral nerves (L_2 to L_4). The lowest fibres of vastus medialis, which are attached at right angles to the medial side of patella, are of great importance in obtaining the final degrees of complete extension.

- **Unlocking** is performed by the popliteus, supplied by the tibial nerves (L_4 and L_5; S_1) which rotates the femur laterally at the commencement of flexion. The popliteus also pulls the posterior end of the lateral meniscus backwards.

CLINICAL APPLICATION

- The collateral ligaments are taut in full extension of the knee and are, therefore, only liable to injury in this position.
- The anterior cruciate ligament, which is taut in extension, is torn by violent hyperextension of the knee or in anterior dislocation of the **tibia** on femur. This results in increased forward mobility with the leg not locking upon full extension.
- The posterior cruciate ligament, which is a key stabilizer of the knee joint, is torn in a posterior dislocation causing increased backward mobility.
- The medial meniscus gets split, if the knee is forcibly abducted and externally rotated (footballers injuries). A bucket handle tear, which is longitudinal, occurs as the more internal fibres are fixed and the force acts on the periphery of the meniscus. The medial meniscus is fixed at one point by the tibial collateral ligament. If its anterior part is subjected to any strain which tries to elongate the meniscus, it may tear away for this part causing a transverse tear. This meniscus is more vulnerable to injury because of its firm attachment to medial ligament.
- The lateral meniscus is torn if there is severe adduction and internal rotation. The injury of this meniscus is not common as the popliteus draws it backward from the 'harms way'.
- The prepatellar bursa is affected by prolonged

kneeling forwards, as in scrubbing floors (**housemaid's knee** or prepatellar bursitis).

- The bursa over the ligamentum patellae is involved by years of kneeling in a more erect posture as in praying (**clergyman's knee or infrapatellar bursitis**).
- Bursitis of the popliteal bursa may be caused by abnormal stress or strain. When distended it is called **'Baker's cyst'**. It may disappear during flexion of the knee because of its communication with the joint cavity.
- Synovitis of the knee results in fluid collecting in the knee joint. This gives rise to swelling above and at the sides of the patella due to the distension of the suprapatellar bursa.
- The prominent articular surface of the lateral femoral condyle and the medial pull of the longermost fibres of vastus medialis which insert almost horizontally along the medial margin of patella resist the dislocation of patella. Recurrent dislocation of patella may occur, if the lateral femoral condyle is underdeveloped as in knock knee deformity (**genu valgum**).

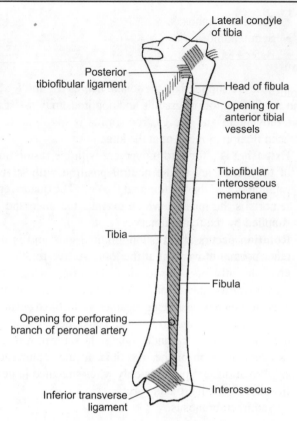

Fig. 16.24: Tibiofibular joints

TIBIOFIBULAR JOINTS

Superior Tibiofibular Joint (Fig. 16.24)

It is a synovial joint of the plane type.

Articular Surfaces

- Head of fibula.
- Facet on the postero-inferior aspect of the lateral condyle of tibia.

Fibrous Capsule

It is a weak capsule with thickening anteriorly and posteriorly.

Synovial Membrane

The membrane lines the capsule. If the fibrous capsule is deficient posteriorly, then the synovial membrane becomes continuous with that of the knee joint.

Movements

- Slight gliding movements are possible.

Nerve Supply

- Recurrent genicular branch of common peroneal.
- Nerve to popliteus.

Middle Tibiofibular Joint (Fig. 16.24)

It is a fibrous type of joint.

Articular Ends

- Interosseous borders of tibia and fibula.

Ligament

It is constituted by the interosseous membrane which attaches the interosseous border of the shafts of tibia and fibula. The fibres of the membrane pass downwards and laterally from the tibia to the fibula. Above there is an opening through which the anterior tibial vessels enter the anterior compartment of the leg. Inferiorly the membrane is continuous with the interosseous ligament of the inferior tibiofibular joint. Several muscles of the anterior and posterior compartments of leg are attached to the surfaces of the membrane.

Nerve Supply

- Nerve to popliteus.

Function

Holds the shafts to the bones of the leg together.

Inferior Tibiofibular Joint (Fig. 16.24)

It is a fibrous joint being a classical example of syndesmosis.

Articular Surfaces

- Rough triangular area above the articular facet on the medial side of the lower end of the fibula.
- Concave fibular notch on the lateral side of the lower end of the tibia.

Ligaments

- **Interosseous ligament** joins the articular surfaces and is continuous superiorly with the interosseous membrane.
- **Anterior tibiofibular** connects the anterior margins of the articular surfaces. The fibres are directed downward and laterally.
- **Posterior tibiofibular** connects the posterior margins of the articular surfaces. Its fibres are also directed downward and laterally (Fig. 16.28).
- **Inferior transverse tibiofibular** is formed by the lower and deep fibres of the posterior tibiofibular ligament. It forms a strong band passing transversely from the upper part of the malleolar fossa of the fibula to the posterior border of the articular surface of the tibia almost as far as the medial malleolus (Fig. 16.28). The deep surface of the ligament forms part of the articular socket for the talus at the ankle joint.

Nerve Supply

- Deep peroneal nerve.

Movements

- Small amount of gliding in association with movements occurring at the ankle joint.
- The joint contributes to the rigid mortise in which talus moves at the ankle joint.

THE ANKLE JOINT

- Ankle joint is a modified hinge joint.

Articular Surfaces (Fig. 16.25)

Superiorly, a socket formed by:
- The inferior articular surfaces of the tibia and fibula.
- The articular surfaces of the medial and lateral malleoli.
- The transverse tibiofibular ligament.

Inferiorly, the articular surface is provided by:
- The trochlear surface of the talus. The superior articular surface of the talus is wider anteriorly.

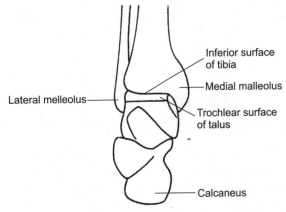

Fig. 16.25: Ankle joint: Articulating bones—anterior aspect

Capsular Ligament

The capsule surrounds the joint and is thin and weak in front and behind.

Ligaments

- **Medial ligament,** (Fig. 16.26) also known as **deltoid ligament** is triangular in shape. It has the following attachments and is exceptionally strong. Its apex is attached above to the lower border of medial malleolus. The base of the ligament is attached from front to backward to the:
  - Tuberosity of navicular.
  - Medial side of the neck of talus (anterior talotibial).
  - Medial margin of plantar calcaneonavicular ligament.
  - Medial edge of the sustentaculum tali of the calcaneum (calcaneotibial).
  - Medial side of the body of the talus below the posterior end of the comma-shaped articular surface (posterior talotibial).

Relations

Superficially the ligament is related to the tendons of the tibialis posterior and the flexor digitorum longus.

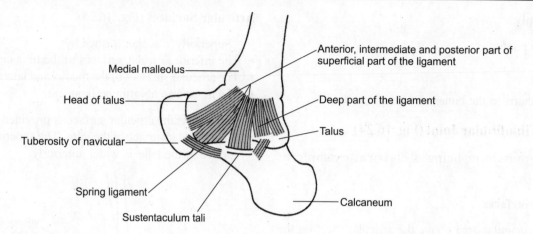

Fig. 16.26: Ankle joint: Medial ligament

Lateral Ligament (Fig. 16.27)

- It is attached above to the lateral malleolus and comprises three parts having the following attachments:
  - One part connects the anterior margin of the lateral malleolus to the lateral side of the neck of the talus is known as **anterior talofibular ligament**.
  - Second part connects the tip of lateral malleolus to the peroneal tubercle on the lateral side of **calcaneus** and is known as **calcaneofibular ligament**.
  - Third part attached to the malleolar fossa of the fibula proximally and to the posterior tubercle of talus distally is known as **posterior talofibular ligament**.

The strong parts of the medial and lateral ligaments are directed downwards and backwards, although the posterior talofibular ligament is almost horizontal.

Synovial Membrane

The **synovial membrane lines** the fibrous capsule and extends for a short distance between the tibia and the fibula.

Nerve Supply

- The deep peroneal nerve.
- The tibial nerve.

Blood Supply

- The anterior tibial artery.
- The peroneal artery.

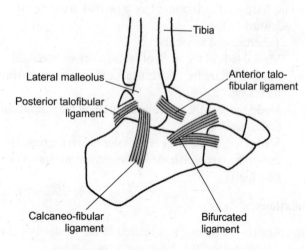

Fig. 16.27: Ankle joint: Lateral ligament

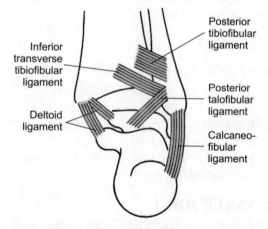

Fig. 16.28: Ankle joint: Posterior talofibular and calcaneo-fibular ligaments

Relations (Figs. 16.29 and 16.30)

Anteriorly structures are passing under the extensor retinaculum. These are from medial to lateral side.
- Tendon of tibialis anterior.
- Tendon of extensor hallucis longus.
- Anterior tibial artery.
- Deep peroneal nerve.
- Tendon of extensor digitorum longus.
- Tendon of peroneus tertius.

Posteromedially structures are passing under the flexor retinaculum. These are from medial to lateral side.
- Tendon of tibialis posterior.
- Tendon of flexor digitorum longus.
- Posterior tibial artery and vein.
- Tibial nerve.
- Tendon of flexor hallucis longus.

Posterolaterally structures are passing under the peroneal retinacula. These are:
- Tendon of peroneus longus.
- Tendon of peroneus brevis.

Posteriorly the joint is some distance from the surface, because of the presence of:
- Tendocalcaneus.
- Pad of fat.

Movements

- Dorsiflexion in which foot is raised upwards and the angle between the foot and leg is decreased. It is performed by:
  - Tibialis anterior.
  - Extensor digitorum longus.
  - Extensor hallucis longus.
  - Peroneus tertius.
- Plantar flexion, which causes the sole of the foot to bend down, so that the angle between the dorsum of the foot and leg is increased. The muscles involved are:
  - Gastrocnemius and soleus which are inserted in the tendocalcaneous.
  - Peroneus longus.
  - Peroneus brevis.
  - Flexor digitorum longus.
  - Flexor hallucis longus.

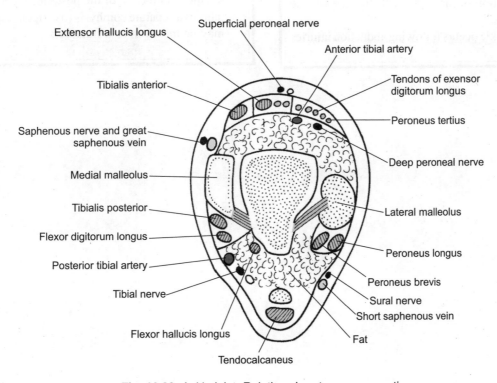

Fig. 16.29: Ankle joint: Relations in a transverse section

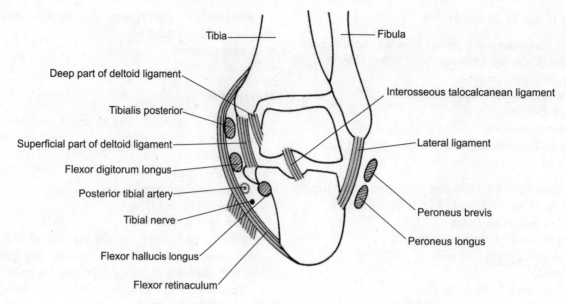

Fig. 16.30: Ankle joint: Relations in a coronal section

CLINICAL APPLICATION

- The strong tibiofibular socket is deepened by the transverse tibiofibular ligament and thus makes the ankle a very stable joint. Pure dislocation is rare and dislocation occurs only with fracture of one of the malleoli.
- Sprained ankle occurs following abduction injuries and in this avulsion of the medial malleous occurs as the deltoid ligament is very strong. The sprains of the lateral ligament are more common.
- In children the X-ray of the ankle region may show the medial tubercle of the posterior process of the talus as a separate epiphysis (os-trigonum) and this may be mistaken as a fracture.

17

Sole of the Foot, Joints and Arches of Foot

SKELETON OF FOOT

Plantar aspect

Muscular attachments (Fig. 17.1)

Calcaneum: The posterior part of its plantar surface is known as **calcaneal tuberosity,** which is further subdivided into a lateral process and a medial process.
- **Abductor hallucis** and **flexor digitorum brevis** arise from the medial process.

- **Abductor digitiminimi** arises from medial and lateral processes both.
- **Flexor digitorum accessorius** medial head arises from the medial surface of the calaneus while the lateral head arises from the lateral margin of its plantar surface.

Navicular

- **Tibialis posterior** is inserted mainly into the tuberosity of the navicular. Accessory slips pass to all the tarsal

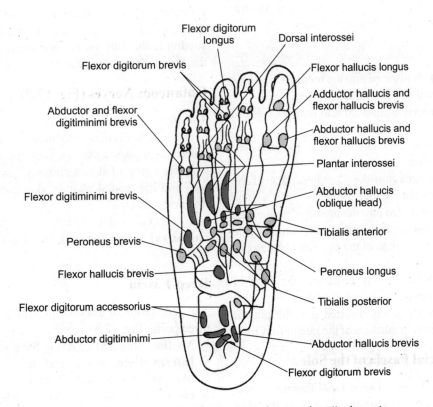

Fig. 17.1: Sole of foot: Skeletal framework muscular attachments

bones except the talus and to all the metatarsal bones except the first and the fifth.

Cuboid

*   **Flexor hallucis brevis** arises from the plantar surface.

Cuneiformis

*   **Tibialis anterior** is inserted into the antero-inferior part of the medial surface of medial cuneiform and the adjacent part of the first metatarsal bone.
*   **Peroneus longus** is inserted into the antero-inferior part of the lateral surface.

Metatarsals

*   **Flexor digitiminimi brevis** takes origin from the medial part of the plantar surface of the fifth metatarsal bone.
*   **Adductor hallucis (oblique head)** arises from the plantar aspect of the bases of the second, third and fourth metatarsals.
*   **Tibialis anterior** gives a slip of insertion to the plantar aspect of the medial surface of the first metatarsal.
*   **Peroneus longus** also gives a slip of insertion to the first metatarsal, on the plantar aspect of the lateral surface of its base.
*   The **plantar interossei** take origin from the ventral aspect of the lateral three metatarsal bones.

Phalanges

*   **Abductor hallucis** is inserted into the medial side of the base of the proximal phalanx of the big toe.
*   **Flexor hallucis brevis** is inserted into the two sides of the proximal phalanx of the big toe.
*   **Adductor hallucis** into the lateral side of the proximal phalanx of the big toe.
*   **Flexor hallucis longus** into the plantar surface of the terminal phalanx of the big toe.
*   The **interossei** are inserted into the proximal phalanges.
*   **Abductor** and **flexor digitiminimi brevis** are inserted on the lateral side of the base of the proximal phalanx of the little toe.
*   **Flexor digitorum brevis** is inserted into the sides of the middle phalanges of the lateral four toes.
*   **Flexor digitorum longus** is inserted into the plantar surface of the terminal phalanges of the lateral four toes.

Skin and Superficial Fascia of the Sole

The skin is supported by tough superficial fascia which is continuous around the sides of the foot with the thin

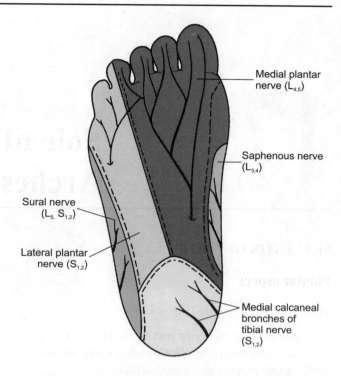

Fig. 17.2: Sole of foot: Cutaneous nerves

subcutaneous tissue of the dorsum of the foot. Traversing the superficial fascia there are tough, fibrous bands which subdivide the fatty tissue into small lobules and connect the skin with the deep fascia.

Cutaneous Nerves (Fig. 17.2)

The plantar surface of the foot is supplied by the tibial nerve which divides into **medial** and **lateral plantar nerves** as it passes into the foot; the lateral plantar nerve supplies a strip of skin corresponding to one and one-half toes and the medial plantar, skin corresponding to three and one-half toes.

The skin under the heel is supplied by the **medial calcaneal branches** arising directly from the tibial nerve.

Deep Fascia

The deep fascia of the sole (plantar fascia) is divided into three parts (Fig. 17.3):
*   **Medial:** Thin part covering the abductor hallucis.
*   **Intermediate:** Strong and dense part and known as **plantar aponeurosis**. It covers the flexor digitorum brevis. Morphologically, it is regarded as the degenerated part of plantaris muscle.

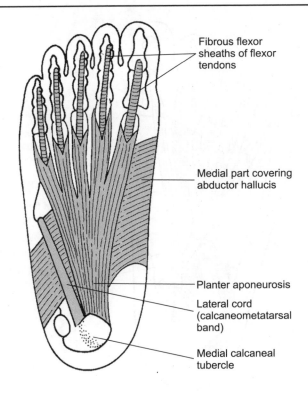

Fig. 17.3: Sole of foot: Plantar fascia

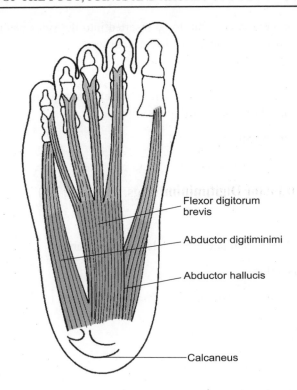

Fig. 17.4: Sole of foot: First layer (consists of muscles only)

- **Lateral:** Thin but stronger than the medial part due to a strong band stretching between the lateral process of the calcaneus and the base of the fifth metatarsal bone **(calcaneometatarsal band).**

Plantar aponeurosis is triangular in shape. Its apex is attached to the medial tubercle of the calcaneus. The base divides into five slips. Each slip divides into two slips which diverge to enclose the flexor tendons and get attached to the plantar ligament of the metatarsophalangeal joint and to the deep transverse ligament of the sole. They also blend with the fibrous flexor sheaths of the flexor tendons.

MUSCLES OF SOLE

There are four musculotendinous layers in the sole with vessels and nerves lying between the first and second layers and the third and fourth layers.

LAYER 1

There are three muscles (Fig. 17.4):
- **Abductor hallucis** medially.
- **Flexor digitorum brevis** in the middle.
- **Abductor digitiminimi** laterally.

Abductor Hallucis (Figs. 17.1 and 17.4)

Origin

- Medial tubercle of calcaneum.
- Flexor retinaculum.

Insertion

- Medial side of the base of proximal phalanx of great toe.

Action

- Abduction of great toe from second toe.

Nerve Supply

- Medial plantar nerve.

Flexor Digitorum Brevis (Figs. 17.1 and 17.4)

Origin

- Medial tubercle of calcaneum.

Insertion

- The muscle forms four tendons each tendon splits,

unites, splits again to be inserted into the sides of the middle phalanx of the lateral four toes.

Action

- Flexion of proximal interphalangeal and metatarsophalangeal joints.

Nerve Supply

- Medial plantar nerve.

Abductor Digitiminimi (Figs. 17.1 and 17.4)

Origin

- Medial and lateral tubercles of calcaneum.

Insertion

- Lateral side of the base of proximal phalanx of the little toe.

Action

- Abductor of little toe.

Nerve Supply

- Lateral plantar nerve.

LAYER II

It consists of two tendons and two muscles:

Tendons

- Tendon of flexor hallucis longus.
- Tendon of flexor digitorum longus.

Muscles

- Flexor digitorum accessorius.
- Lumbricals.

Flexor Digitorum Accessorius (Figs. 17.1 and 17.5)

Origin by Two Heads

- Lateral head from lateral tuberosity of calcaneum.
- Medial head from medial surface of calcaneum.

Insertion

- Lateral border of flexor digitorum longus tendon.

Action

- Corrects the obliquity of flexor digitorum longus and straightens the direction of its pull.

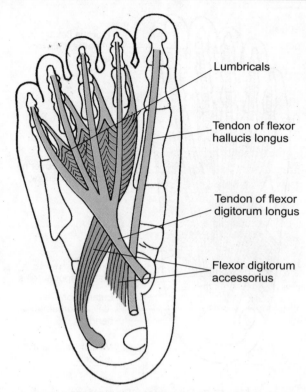

Fig. 17.5: Sole of foot: Second layer (consists of tendons and muscles)

Labels:
- Lumbricals
- Tendon of flexor hallucis longus
- Tendon of flexor digitorum longus
- Flexor digitorum accessorius

Nerve Supply

- Lateral plantar nerve (main trunk).

Lumbricals (Figs. 17.1 and 17.5)

They are four in number.

Origin

- First lumbrical (unipennate) from the medial aspect of first flexor digitorum longus tendon.
- Second, third and fourth lumbricals (bipennate) from the adjacent sides of flexor digitorum tendons for second, third and fourth toes.

Insertion

- Extensor expansion of the lateral four toes after crossing the medial side of the metatarsophalangeal joints of the toes.

Action

- Flex proximal and extend distal interphalangeal joints.

Nerve Supply

- First lumbrical by medial plantar nerve.

- Second, third and fourth lumbricals by lateral plantar nerve (deep branch).

Tendons

- **Flexor hallucis longus tendon** crosses the tendon of flexor digitorum longus to reach its insertion into the distal phalanx of great toe. It gives slips to flexor digitorum longus tendon where it crosses it. These slips are called **"Turner's Slips"**.
- **Flexor digitorum longus tendon** divides into four tendons, which get inserted into the base of the terminal phalanx of lateral four toes. The tendon receives the insertion of **flexor digitorum accessorius**.

Medial and lateral plantar nerves and arteries are derived from the tibial nerve and the posterior tibial artery under cover of the flexor retinaculum. Both the nerves along with their respective arteries enter the sole deep to abductor hallucis muscle. The arteries are marginal, so that the medial plantar artery is medial to the nerve and the lateral plantar artery is lateral to the lateral plantar nerve (Fig. 17.8).

The lateral plantar artery and nerve cross the sole obliquely just deep to the first layer of muscles.

LAYER III

Consists of three short muscles of the great and little toes confined to the metatarsal region of the foot (Fig. 17.6).
- Flexor hallucis brevis medially.
- Adductor hallucis in the middle.
- Flexor digitiminimi brevis laterally.

Flexor Hallucis Brevis (Figs. 17.1 and 17.6)

Origin

- Plantar surface of cuboid.

Insertion

- Medial and lateral side of proximal phalanx of big toe in common with the abductor hallucis and adductor hallucis respectively.

Action

- Flexion of metatarsophalangeal joint of big toe.

Nerve Supply

- Second digital branch of medial plantar nerve.

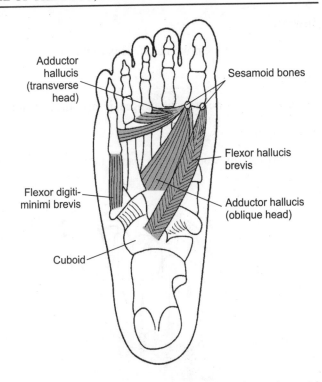

Fig. 17.6: Sole of foot: Third layer (consists of muscles only)

Adductor Hallucis (Figs. 17.1 and 17.6)

Origin by two Head

- **Oblique head** from bases of second, third and fourth metatarsals.
- **Transverse head** from plantar ligaments of the lateral four metatarsophalangeal joints.

Insertion

- Lateral side of the proximal phalanx of the big toe by a common tendon.

Action

- Adduction of big toe.

Nerve Supply

- Deep division of lateral plantar nerve.

Flexor Digitiminimi Brevis
(Figs. 17.1 and 17.6)

Origin

- Base of the fifth metatarsal bone.

Insertion

• Lateral side of the proximal phalanx of the little toe.

Action

• Flexion of the metatarsophalangeal joint of the little toe.

Nerve Supply

• Superficial division of lateral plantar nerve.

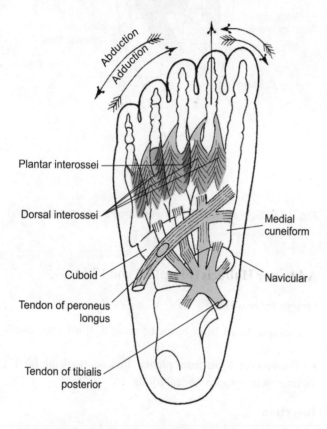

Fig. 17.7: Sole of foot: Fourth layer (consists of muscles and tendons)

LAYER IV

Consists of two tendons and two groups of muscles.

Tendons

• Tibialis posterior.
• Peroneus longus.

Muscles

• Three plantar interossei.
• Four dorsal interossei.

Tibialis posterior tendon divides into a medial part and a lateral part. The medial part is inserted into the tuberosity of the navicular and medial cuneiform. The lateral part is inserted into all the tarsal bones except talus and into the bases of second, third and fourth metatarsals.

Tendon of peroneus longus lies in the groove in the cuboid bone and crosses the sole to get inserted into the base of the first metatarsal bone and the adjoining part of the medial **cuneiform**.

Plantar Interossei are three in Number
(Figs.17.1 and 17.7)

Origin

• Medial aspect of the third, fourth and fifth metatarsal bones.

Insertion

• Medial sides of the bases of the proximal phalanx of the third, fourth and fifth digits.
• Additional attachment into the dorsal extensor expansion.

Action

• Adduction of the toes (PAD-Plantar adduct) towards the second toe through which the axial line of the foot passes.

Nerve Supply

• Lateral plantar nerve: First and second by deep branch and the third by the superficial branch.

Dorsal Interossei are Four in Number

Origin

• By two heads from the adjacent sides of the two metatarsals between which they lie.

Insertion

• First and second are inserted into the two sides of the proximal phalanx of the second toe on which they act.
• Third and fourth are inserted into the lateral side of the proximal phalanx on the third and fourth toes respectively.

Action

• Abduction of the toes (DAB-Dorsal abduct) away from the line of the second toe.

Nerve Supply

- Lateral plantar nerve.

PLANTAR ARTERIES (FIG. 17.8)

Medial Plantar Artery

It is the smaller terminal division of the posterior tibial artery. It is accompanied by the medial plantar nerve on its lateral side. It ends at the medial side of the big toe to join the digital branch of the first plantar metatarsal artery.

Branches

- Cutaneous to medial side of sole.
- Muscular.
- Digital branches—variable to about 3½ toes.

Lateral Plantar Artery

It is the larger of the two terminal division of the posterior tibial artery. The lateral plantar nerve lies on its medial side

as it runs across the sole between the first and second layers towards the base of the fifth metatarsal bone. It then changes direction to pursue a recurrent course medially, between the third and fourth layers of sole as the **plantar arch**.

The arch ends in the first intermetatarsal space by joining the **deep plantar branch of the dorsalis pedis** artery.

Branches of the Plantar Arch

- Articular branches to the adjoining joints.
- Perforating arteries, which pass to the dorsum through the intermetatarsal spaces to join dorsal metatarsal branches of the arcuate artery.
- Four or five plantar metatarsal arteries, which divide distally into digital arteries which supply the flexor aspects of the digits. The first plantar metatarsal artery bifurcates to supply the medial side of the big toe and the first interdigital cleft.

Medial Plantar Nerve (L_4 and L_5; S_1) (Fig. 17.9)

It is the larger terminal division of the tibial nerve, which

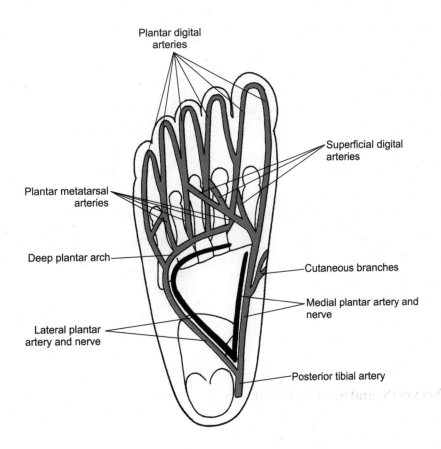

Fig. 17.8: Sole of foot: Plantar arteries

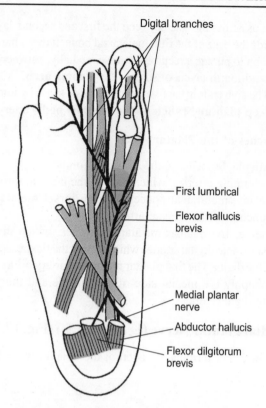

Fig. 17.9: Sole of foot: Medial plantar nerves

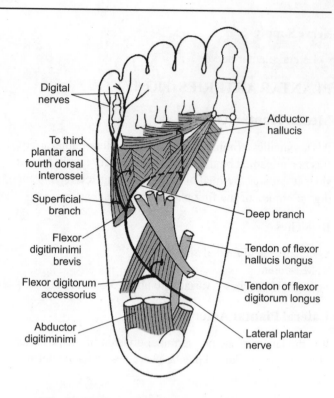

Fig. 17.10: Sole of the foot: Lateral plantar nerves

passes from undercover of the flexor retinaculum and the abductor hallucis to appear in the interval between the abductor hallucis and the flexor digitorum brevis. It is accompanied by the medial plantar vessel on the medial sides (Fig. 17.8).

Branches

- **Cutaneous:** Medial part of sole (Fig. 17.2)
- **Digital:** Plantar surface of the medial three and a half toes and also the dorsum of the terminal phalanges (Fig. 15.13).
- **Muscular:**
  From trunk :
  – Abductor hallucis.
  – Flexor digitorum brevis.
  From first digital:
  – Flexor hallucis brevis.
  From second digital:
  – First lumbrical.

Lateral Plantar Nerves (S₁ and S₂) (Fig. 17.10)

It is the smaller terminal division of the tibial nerve. It runs anterolaterally towards the base of the fifth metatarsal bone between the first and second layers of the sole. The lateral

plantar vessels lie lateral to it (Fig. 17.8). It terminates into a superficial and deep branch.

Branches from Trunk

- **Cutaneous:** To lateral part of sole (Fig. 17.2).
- **Muscular to:**
  – Abductor digiti minimi.
  – Flexor digitorum accessorius.

From Superficial Branch

- **Cutaneous:** To lateral part of sole.
- **Digital:** Plantar surface of the lateral one and a half toes.
- **Muscular:**
  – Flexor digitiminimi brevis.
  – Interossei of the fourth intermetatarsal space (3rd plantar and fourth dorsal.)

From Deep Branch

This branch pursues a recurrent course medially lying between the third and fourth layers of the soles and supplies:
- Two heads of adductor hallucis.
- The lateral three lumbricals on their deep surface.
- The medial two plantar interossei.

- The medial three dorsal interosei.
- Articular: Intertarsal and tarsometatarsal joints.

Summary

The lateral plantar nerve supplies all the intrinsic muscles of the foot except the following, which are supplied by the medial plantar nerve.

- Abductor hallucis and flexor digitorum brevis (in first layer)
- First lumbrical (in second layer).
- Flexor hallucis brevis (in third layer).

JOINTS OF THE FOOT

There are numerous synovial joints in the foot. They are classified as follows (Fig. 17.11):

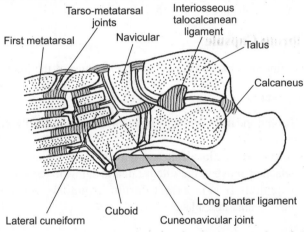

Fig. 17.11: Joints of the foot: An oblique section showing the synovial cavities of intertarsal and tarsometatarsal joints

- **Intertarsal:** Between the tarsal bones.
- **Tarsometatarsal:** Between the lateral bones and the bases of the metatarsals.
- **Intermetatarsal:** Between the bases of the metatarsals.
- **Metatarsophalangeal:** Between the heads of metatarsals and bases of proximal phalanges.
- **Interphalangeal:** Between the proximal intermedial and distal phalanges.
  Most of these joints have the following features:
- They are of plane, synovial variety.
- The cartilage covered joint surfaces are more or less flat, thereby allowing very little movement.
- The capsule is thickened on the plantar aspect of the joints as the weight is transmitted downwards and the foot is arched.

- The interosseous ligaments, wherever present are nearer the concavity of the sole.

Ligaments of the Sole

There are three strong ligaments in the sole of the foot. Two on the lateral side.

- Long plantar.
- Short plantar (plantar calcaneocuboid).
  One on the medial side.
- Spring ligament (plantar calcaneonavicular).

Long Plantar Ligament (Fig. 17.12)

- Posteriorly, it is attached to the plantar surface of the calcaneus in front of the tuberosity.
- Anteriorly, it is attached to the bases of the third, fourth and fifth metatarsal bones. As it passes forwards over the groove in the cuboid for the tendon of peroneus longus, it is attached to both the lips of the groove, thereby forming a tunnel for that tendon.

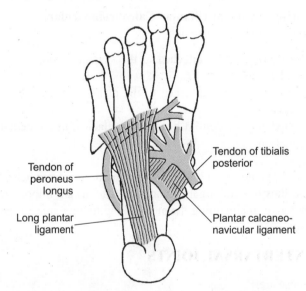

Fig. 17.12: Sole of the foot: Long plantar ligament

Short Plantar Ligament (Plantar Calcaneocuboid) (Fig. 17.13)

Short plantar ligament is placed undercover of the long plantar ligament. It is broader and so can be seen as its medial border.

- Posteriorly, it is attached to plantar surface of the calcaneus in front of the attachment of the long plantar ligament.
- Anteriorly, it is attached to the ridge on the cuboid behind the groove for the tendon of peroneus longus.

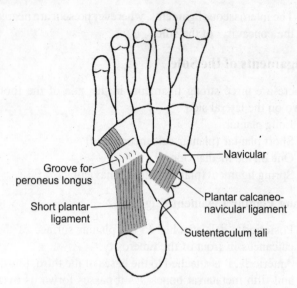

Fig. 17.13: Sole of the foot: Short plantar and plantar calcaneonavicular (spring) ligament

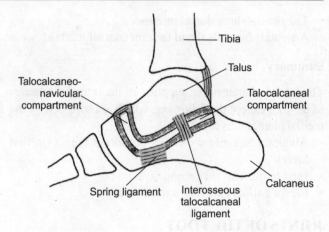

Fig. 17.14: Joint of the foot: Subtalar joint

Spring Ligament (Plantar Calcaneonavicular) (Fig. 17.13)

- Posteriorly, it is attached to the sustentaculum tali of calcaneus.
- Anteriorly, it is attachéd to the plantar surface of the navicular.
- Medially the deltoid ligament is attached to its medial margin.

The tendon of tibialis posterior supports it from below and thus both the ligament and the tendons are important factors in maintaining the medial longitudinal arch of the foot.

INTERTARSAL JOINTS

These are:
- Subtalar (posterior talocalcanean).
- Talocalcaneonavicular.
- Transverse tarsal consisting of talonavicular and calcaneocuboid.
- Cuneonavicular.

Subtalar Joint (Fig. 17.14)

It is a synovial joint of the plane type:

Articular Surfaces

- Concave facet on the inferior surface of the talus.

- Convex posterior facet on the back of the upper surface of the calcaneus.

Fibrous Capsule

The fibrous capsule is attached to the edges of the joint.

Ligaments

- Lateral and medial ligaments are thickenings in the fibrous capsule.
- Interosseous talocalcanean ligament, in the sinus tarsi, attached above to the sulcus tali and below to the sulcus calcanei. It acts as a fulcrum around which the movements take place.

Talocalcaneonavicular joint

It is a synovial joint of ball and socket type:

Articular Surfaces (Fig. 17.15)

- Head of the talus with the navicular.
- The inferior surface of the neck and the adjacent part of the body of the talus with the socket formed by the middle and anterior facets on the upper surface of the calcaneus, the superior surface of the spring ligament and the proximal surface of the navicular.

Ligaments

The fibrous capsule is strengthened by:
- Medial ligament of the ankle joint medially.
- Calcaneonavicular (medial limb of bifurcate ligament) on lateral side. Bifurcate ligament is a strong ligament on the dorsum of the foot, it is attached proximally to the dorsal surface of the calcaneus anterolateral to the

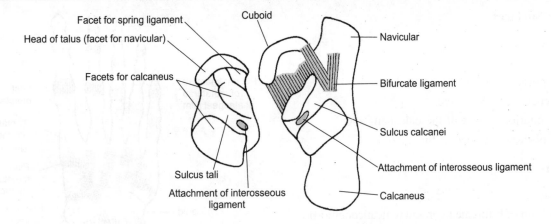

Fig. 17.15: Joints of the foot: Talocalcaneonavicular joint

head of the talus and distally, after bifurcating, to the dorsal surfaces of the cuboid and the navicular.
- Part of the interosseous talocalcanean ligament posteriorly.
- Talonavicular ligament superiorly.
- Plantar calcaneonavicular (spring ligament) on the inferior aspect. It has a fibrocartilage for articulation with a special facet on the inferior surface of the head of the talus.

Movements

These are inversion and eversion. The axis of movement is oblique like that of radioulnar joint. It runs upwards and medially from the back of the calcaneum through the sinus tarsi to the medial side of the neck of talus.
- **Inversion** which involves movement of the foot on the talus so that the sole is turned inwards and the medial border of the foot moves medially as well as upwards. Inversion is maximum with the foot plantar flexed. In inversion, the navicular rotates clockwise with a downward movement of cuboid over calcaneum. The muscles producing inversion are:
  - Tibialis anterior which is supplied by the deep peroneal nerves (L_4 and L_5).
  - Tibialis posterior which is supplied by the tibial nerves (L_4 and L_5).
- **Eversion** causes the sole to turn outwards with the lateral border moving laterally as well as upwards. It is maximum with the foot dorsiflexed. In eversion the navicular rotates anticlockwise with an upward movement of cuboid over calaneum. The muscle involved are:
  - Peroneus longus and peroneus brevis supplied by superficial peroneal nerves (L_4 and L_5).

- Peroneus tertius supplied by the deep peroneal nerve (L_4 and L_5).

Transverse Tarsal (Midtarsal) Joint (Fig. 17.16)

It is the name given to the combined joints.
- **Talonavicular** medially and
- **Calcaneocuboid** laterally.

They do not communicate with each other and do not take part in the movements of eversion and inversion.

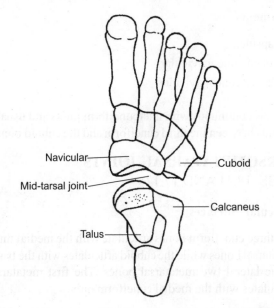

Fig. 17.16: Joints of the foot: Transverse (midtarsal) joint
(Bones are shown separated at the joint)

Articular Surfaces

- Talonavicular is between:
  - The head of talus and;
  - The posterior surface of navicular.
- Calcaneocuboid is between:
  - The anterior surface of the calcaneus and;
  - The posterior surface of the cuboid.

Ligaments

- Capsular.
- Lateral limb of bifurcate ligament (calcaneocubiod).
- Long plantar ligament.

The transverse tarsal joint is the line of division between the forepart of the foot and the hindpart.

Movements

The forepart moves on the hindpart in plantar flexion and dorsiflexion, inversions and adduction and eversion and abduction.

Cuneonavicular Joint (Fig. 17.11)

Its articular surfaces are:
- Anterior articular surface of navicular.
- Posterior articular surfaces of the three cuneiforms.

Ligaments

- Capsule.
- Dorsal cuneonavicular.
- Plantar cuneonavicular.

It is continuous with intercuneiform joints and usually extends between the third cuneiform and the cuboid bones.

TARSOMETATARSAL JOINTS
(FIGS. 17.11 AND 17.17)

Articular Surfaces

The three cuneiform bones articulate with the medial three metatarsal bones while the cuboid articulates with the bases of the lateral two metatarsal bones. The first metatarsal articulates with the medial cuneiform only.

Ligaments

All are synovial joints and are provided with plantar interosseous and dorsal tarsometatarsal ligaments.

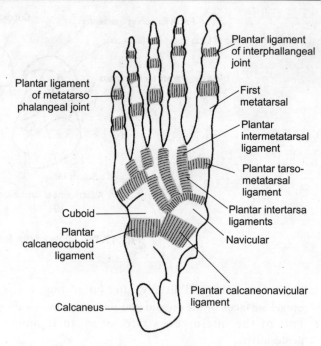

Fig. 17.17: Joints of the foot: Intertarsal, tarsometatarsal, intermetatarsal, metatarsophalangeal and interphalangeal

Movements

The tarsometatarsal joint of the big toe is separate, so it permits slight amount of gliding and rotator movements.

INTERMETATARSAL JOINTS
(FIGS. 17.11 AND 17.17)

They are present only between the adjacent surfaces of the lateral four metatarsal bones.

METATARSOPHALANGEAL JOINTS
(FIG. 17.17)

They are ellipsoid synovial joints.

Articular Surfaces

- Convex head of metatarsal.
- Concave bases of the proximal phalanges.

Ligaments

- **Fibrous capsule** which is thickened on the plantar surface in the lateral four toes and is grooved for the flexor tendons. In the big toe there are two sesamoid bones embedded in the capsule.
- **Deep transverse metatarsal ligaments** join the plantar parts of the capsule. They separate the

interossei from the lumbrical muscles and digital nerves and vessels.

- **Collateral ligaments** pass from the sides of the metatarsal heads to the sides of the bases of the phalanges in the plantar direction.

Movements

- Plantar flexion.
- Dorsiflexion which is much more extensive than plantar flexion.
- Abductor is the movement of the toes away from the second toe.
- Adduction is the movement of the toes towards the second toe.

INTERPHALANGEAL JOINTS (FIG. 17.17)

The structure of proximal and distal interphalangeal joints in the lateral four toes is similar to those in the digits of the hand.

Movements

- Dorsiflexion.
- Plantar flexion is much more extensive than dorsiflexion.

ARCHES OF THE FOOT

Examination of a normal footprint shows that the foot is arched anteroposteriorly and transversely and is described as forming half a dome (Fig. 17.8). The anteroposterior curve is most marked on the medial side is called the **medial longitudinal arch**. The **lateral longitudinal arch** much flatter than the medial, lies along the lateral border of the foot and is almost non-existent. The **transverse arch** is really half an arch and is most marked in the region of the cuneiforms and the bases of the metatarsals. Although it is convenient to describe the arches separately, but they are so interlocked with each other that they form a functionally single arch of complex form.

The arches of the foot are present nearly as soon as the skeletal elements are in their definitive form during intrauterine life. Prenatally, fat is distributed throughout the sole of the foot and forms the sole pad which is responsible for the convexity of the sole of the foetal foot. At birth and during infancy, the sole pad still masks the arches of the skeleton and the sole of the foot may appear flat. Later in life the encapsulated pockets of subcutaneous fat thin out in areas that are not in contract with the ground. Hence, in most adults, the medial arch can be recognized in footprints.

Factors Involved in the Maintenance of an Arch (Fig. 17.9)

- Segmentation of the arch which also facilitates movement.
- Shape of the segments forming the arch.
- Intersegmental ties which must be particularly strong on the under surface of the arch.
- Tie beam or bowstring between the supporting pillars of the arch. This is the most efficient means of maintaining an arch as it ties the two pillars of an arch together.
- Strap or sling on the under surface of the highest point suspending the arch from below.
- Suspension of the arch from above.

Medial Longitudinal Arch

It is apparent as the medial side of the foot does not touch the ground during weight bearing and walking.

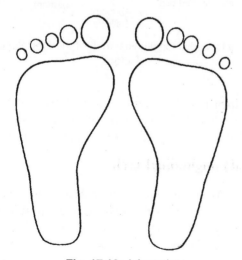

Fig. 17.18: A footprint

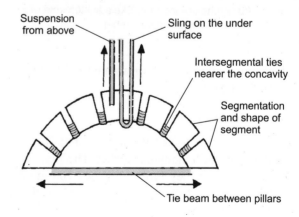

Fig. 17.19: Factors involved in the maintenance of an arch

The bones forming the arch are (Fig. 17.20):
• Calcaneus behind.
• Talus at the summit is the mortise bone between the leg and foot.
• Navicular.
• Cuneiform.   } in front
• Medial three metatarsals.
• The **pillars of the arch** are the tuberosity of the calcaneus posteriorly and the heads of the medial three metatarsal bones anteriorly.
• The **key stone** of this arch is the head of the talus which forms the region of maximum convexity of the arch.

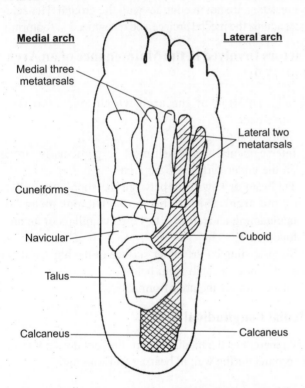

Fig. 17.20: Arches of the foot: Skeletal elements of the longitudinal arches

Factors Supporting and Maintaining the Medial Longitudinal Arch

Shape of the Segments

The shape of the bones do not contribute to the maintenance of the longitudinal arches. The bones fit into each other, so that they form an arched configuration. The rounded head of the talus in the centre of the arch acts as the key stone.

Intersegmental Ties

These are formed by all the interosseous ligaments. Those which are nearer the concavity of the arch are stronger and prevent the collapse of the arch. The most important ligament is the spring ligament (plantar calcaneonavicular), whose upper surface supports the head of the talus.

Tie beams or **bowstrings** between the anterior and posterior pillars are provided by:
• Medial part of plantar aponeurosis.
• Short superficial muscles (abductor hallucis and flexor digitorum brevis).
• Tendon of flexor hallucis longus is overwhelmingly efficient as a tie beam.

Sling or **strap** is provided by:
• The tendon of tibialis posterior and its slips to the plantar aspects of the various tarsal and metatarsal bones of the medial arch help to support the arch from below.

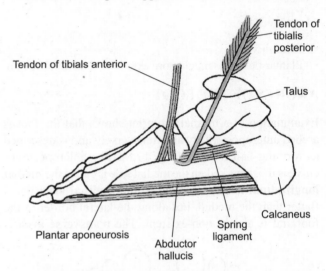

Fig. 17.21: Medial longitudinal arch of the foot: Supporting factors

Suspension of the arch from above is done by:
• The tendon of tibialis anterior which is attached to the medial cuneiform and the first metatarsal bones.

Lateral Longitudinal Arch

This less pronounced arch is noticeable when the foot simply rests on the ground without supporting any weight. The bones forming this arch are (Fig. 17.20):
• Calcaneus behind.

- Cubiod: Its posterior part forms the key stone or summit.
- Lateral two metatarsal in front.

Factors Supporting and Maintaining the Lateral Longitudinal Arch (Fig. 17.22)

Shape of the Segments

The shape of the bones do not contribute to the maintenance of the longitudinal arches. The articulation between calcaneum and cuboid may help to maintain the arch.

Intersegmental Ties

The long and short plantar ligaments are the most significant of the intersegmental ties for the lateral arch. They play more important role than in the case of medial longitudinal arch.

Tie beams or **bowstrings** between the anterior and posterior pillars are provided by:
- Lateral part of the plantar aponeurosis.
- Tendons of flexor digitorum longus to the fourth and fifth toes assisted by flexor digitorum accessorius.
- Muscles of the first layer of sole (lateral half of flexor digitorum brevis and abductor digiti minimi).

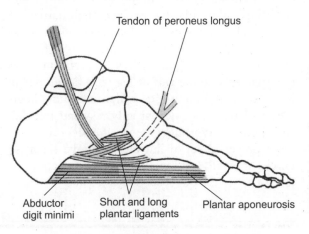

Fig. 17.22: Lateral longitudinal arch of the foot: Supporting factors

Sling or **strap** is provided by:
- Tendon of peroneus longus, by winding round the lateral border of the foot and passing below the cuboid is the most important single factor in the sustentacular mechanism.

Suspension of the arch from above is done by:
- Peroneus brevis.
- Peroneus tertius tie, the lateral border of the foot from above.

Transverse Arch

The transverse arch is only half an arch being completed as an arch by that of the other foot. It is most pronounced about the region of the tarsometatarsal joints. Its constituent bones are (Fig. 17.23):
- Cuboid.
- Three cuneiforms.
- Bases of the five metatarsals.

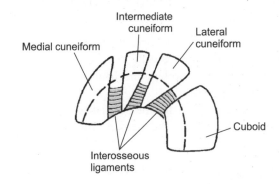

Fig. 17.23: Arches of the foot: Skeletal elements of transverse arch

Factors Supporting and Maintaining the Transverse Arch

Shape of the Segments

The cuneiforms, the cuboid and the bases of the metatarsals are all wedge-shaped, being narrower on the plantar aspect except for the medial cuneiform. This arrangement gives the plantar surface of the bones a much smaller radius of curvature than their dorsal surfaces and forms a transverse arch.

Intersegmental Ties

- Strong interosseous ligaments binding the cuneiforms and the five metatarsals prevent the bones from splaying out.
- The oblique and transverse heads of adductor hallucis.

Tie beam or **bowstring** is provided by:
- The tendon of peroneus longus as it passes from the lateral to the medial border of the foot.

Sling or **Strap**
- The peroneus longus supports from below.

Suspension from above is done by:
- The tendon of peroneus tertius.

Function of Arches of Foot

From the functional point of view, the foot consists of two parts:
- The **fibular sided static portion** lying flat on the ground, that provides a big weight bearing area and gives stability and balance to the foot.
- The **tibial part which is arched** away from the supporting surface and constitutes an elastic lever that may be used for propelling the body forwards during movement.

Apart from the above two functions the arches have the following functions as well:
- To act as shock absorbing mechanism during walking, jumping, running, etc.
- To provide a space for the soft parts of the sole and protect them and the nerves and vessels from compression.

CLINICAL APPLICATION

When the medial longitudinal arch is low it results in **flat foot (pes planus)**.

Weakness of the muscles cause the condition known as **fallen arches,** because the ligaments alone cannot support the arches over a long period of time. As the arch becomes inefficient, the head of talus is no more supported. It drops and forces its way between the medial malleolus and the tubercle of the navicular bone. There is loss of plantar concavity as the arches get flattened. The plantar vessels and nerves are compressed and this produces pain in the metatarsal region of the foot. The condition is known as **metatarsalgia**.

Talipes equinus: The heel is raised, the foot points downwards and is fixed in plantar flexion. The patient walks on toes.

Talipes calcaneus: The heel is weight bearing and the toes are upturned due to fixed dorsiflexed position of the ankle. Patient walks on heels.

Talipes varus: The foot is fixed in inverted position. Patient walks on lateral border of foot.

Talipes valgus: The foot is fixed in everted position. Patient walks on medial border of foot.

The anterior pillar of the arches of foot stretches from the summit or pay stone to the pad of foot or fulcrum. The posterior pillar projecting as the heel extends from summit to the point at which the muscular power is applied. A foot with short anterior pillar and long posterior pillar or heel is the one designed for power and not for speed; it serves a hill climber or a heavy corpulent man. The opposite kind–the one with short heel and long pillar in front is well adopted for running and sprinting. Some like the dark skinned natives of Africa and West Indies, have long heels while others have short stumpy heels like the natives of Europe and China. For long heels less powerful muscles are required and the calf or leg is ill developed in dark races as the muscles which move the heels are small, but their gait is usually easy and graceful. Europeans have short heels, hence require a more powerful set of muscles to move them, so calves are well developed but the gait is apt to be jerky.

18

The Venous and Lymphatic Drainage and Segmental Innervation of Lower Limb

THE VENOUS DRAINAGE OF LOWER LIMB

The veins of the lower limb are (Fig. 18.1):

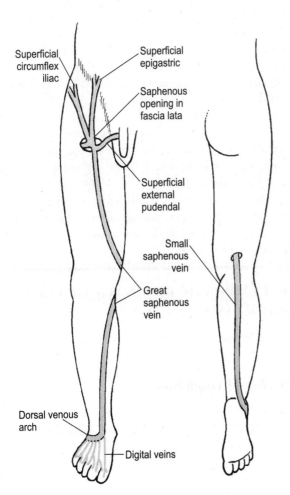

Fig. 18.1: Superficial venous drainage of lower limb

Superficial Veins viz.

- Great saphenous vein.
- Small saphenous vein.

They drain the superficial fascia and skin of the whole lower limb.

Deep Veins

- Medial and lateral plantar veins.
- Anterior and posterior tibial veins.
- Popliteal vein.
- Femoral vein.

SUPERFICIAL VEINS

They are equipped with numerous valves which direct the blood flow upwards.

Great Saphenous Vein

It is formed by the union of the medial digital vein of the big toe with the medial side of the dorsal venous arch. It passes anterior to the medial malleolus and ascends on the medial subcutaneous surface of the tibia. It enters the thigh by passing posterior to the medial condyle of the femur. In the thigh it ascends on the medial side to reach the saphenous opening where it pierces the cribriform fascia and opens into the femoral vein by hooking over the inferior crescentic margin of the opening. There is a constant valve at the saphenofemoral junction. The great saphenous vein lies in the superficial fascia throughout its course and is usually covered by a thin condensed layer of this fascia, which has to be incised for a satisfactory exposure of the vein. It has following tributaries:

- A number of tributaries in the leg and thigh.

- Superficial circumflex iliac, superficial epigastric and superficial external pudendal before it passes through the saphenous opening.

Small Saphenous Vein

It is formed by union of dorsal digital vein of the little toe with the lateral end of the dorsal venous arch. It runs behind the lateral malleolus in company with the sural nerve and ascends along the midline of the calf to the lower part of the popliteal fossa where it pierces the popliteal fascia to enter the popliteal vein. Its tributaries are:
- Tributaries from the lateral side of the leg.
- Superficial communication with the great saphenous vein.

The two saphenous veins are connected with each other by a profuse plexus of smaller veins, so that they cannot be regarded as having exact areas of drainage. They are both connected to the deep veins by communicating vessels known as **perforators** which pierce the deep fascia. These connections are most numerous with the deep veins of the flexor compartment of the leg. The valves in the communicating veins are so placed that they direct the blood flow from the superficial to the deep veins.

THE DEEP VEINS

- **Lateral and medial plantar veins** begin as digital and metatarsal veins of the sole.
- **Anterior tibial veins** which are vena comitantes of the anterior tibial artery begin as upward continuation of the veins associated with dorsalis pedis artery. They pass backwards through the upper part of the interosseous membrane and join the posterior tibial veins to form the popliteal vein.
- **Posterior tibial veins** which are venae comitantes of posterior tibial artery are formed by the union of the lateral and medial plantar veins. They join the anterior tibial veins to form the popliteal vein.
- **Popliteal vein** passes upwards through the popliteal fossa and through the opening in the adductor magnus to form the femoral vein.
- **Femoral vein** becomes the external iliac vein deep to the inguinal ligament. Its main tributaries are the profunda femoris vein, the great saphenous vein, medial and lateral circumflex femoral veins and several muscular veins.
- **Superior and inferior gluteal veins** and **obturator veins** accompany the corresponding arteries and drain into the internal iliac vein.

Mechanism of Venous Return

The venous blood is squeezed upwards along the deep veins by the following factors:
- Contraction of the **'calf muscle pump'** (peripheral heart) within the closed fascial compartment of the leg.
- Pulsations of the adjacent arteries.
- Competency of the valves in the perforating veins does not allow the blood to go into the superficial veins.
- Tension created in the overlying skin created by joint movements squeezes the superficial veins against the underlying deep fascia or bone.

CLINICAL APPLICATION

Dilated, lengthened and tortuous veins are called **varicose veins**. Any of the veins of the lower limb may be subject to dilatation and consequent valvular incompetence, because of the high pressure which they have to withstand. The incompetency of the valves in the perforating veins, allows the blood to leak in, the wrong direction (from deep to superficial veins) particularly in the standing position, which leads to dilation of the superficial veins, the valves of which are then inadequate to function normally. Incompetency of the saphenofemoral valve is specially serious, as it throws great strain on the more distal valves causing the whole great saphenous vein to become varicose.

The great saphenous vein is removed when a length of vein is required as a graft in a limb or as a coronary bypass graft to improve blood supply to myocardium in cases of angina.

THE LYMPHATIC DRAINAGE OF THE LOWER LIMB (FIG. 18.2)

The lymph nodes draining the lower limb comprise two groups:

Superficial Lymph Nodes

These are divided into **horizontal sets,** lying between the layers of the superficial fascia a short distance below the inguinal ligament. These drain the lining membrane of the lower half of the anal canal the external genitalia excepting the glans penis, lateral part of the gluteal region and the skin over the anterolateral abdominal wall below the umbilicus.

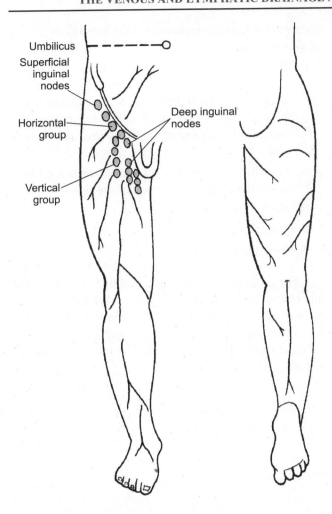

Fig. 18.2: Lower limb: Superficial lymphatic drainage

Vertical set lying along the upper end of the great saphenous vein. It receives lymph vessels from the skin of the whole of lower limb except the lateral part of the foot and the posterior and lateral aspects of the leg (**"the great saphenous area"**).

Deep Lymph Nodes

One anterior tibial node, a small node situated near the upper end of the anterior tibial vessels adjoining the interosseous membrane.

Popliteal lymph nodes, 6-7 in number are distributed alongside the popliteal vessels in the fat occupying the popliteal fossa. They receive lymph vessels which accompany the anterior and posterior tibial arteries and also from the lateral part of the foot and posterior and lateral aspect of the leg (**"the small saphenous area"**).

Deep inguinal lymph nodes which are situated on the medial side of the femoral vein. They receive lymphatics from the popliteal nodes as well as those accompanying the profunda femoris artery. The lymphatics from the glans penis or clitoris and in the female from the lateral angle of the uterus (through vessels which run with the round ligament) also drain into the deep inguinal nodes.

It should be noted that the lymphatics of the testis do not drain into the inguinal nodes, but go to the para-aortic nodes in relation to the origin of the testicular arteries from the abdominal aorta.

THE SEGMENTAL INNERVATION OF THE SKIN OF THE LOWER LIMB (FIG. 18.3)

The area of skin supplied by a single spinal nerve is called a **dermatome**. The skin that envelops a limb is drawn out over the developing limb from the trunk, so a good deal of skin is 'borrowed ' from the trunk and it is all borrowed on the cranial side (from T_{12}; L_1 to L_3) except for a small area of perineal skin which may be considered caudal.

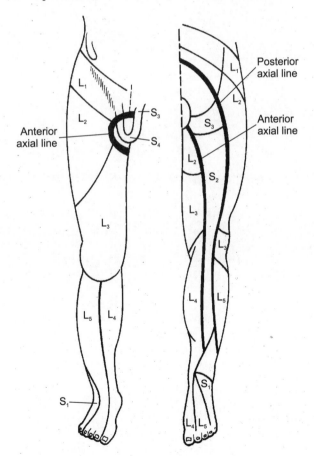

Fig. 18.3: Lower limb: Dermatomes and axial lines

The posterior axial line runs from the fourth lumbar interspace in a bold convexity to the back of thigh down to the head of the fibula and thence half way down the lateral side of the calf. In broad terms the segmental innervation of the lower limb is as under:

The lumbar segments are associated with successive skin areas down the lower the front of the limb.
- L_1: Immediately below the centre of the inguinal ligament.
- L_2: Middle of the front of the thigh.
- L_3: Immediately above the patella.
- L_4: Middle of the medial side of leg.
- L_5: Middle of the lateral side of leg.

Dermatomes near the root of a limb show that here many of the dermatomes are missing; they lie out along the limb. The line of junction of two dermatomes supplied from discontinuous spinal levels is known as the **axial line** and such axial lines extend from the trunk onto the limbs. The skin of the lower limb is innervated by the lumbosacral nerves (T_{12} – S_3 spinal segments)which are situated opposite to the developing limb bud. Considerable distortion occurs to the dermatomes pattern of the lower limb because of two reasons:

- The limb, from the fetal position of flexion, is medially rotated and extended, so that the anterior axial line is made to spiral from the root of penis or clitoris across the front of the scrotum or labium majus around to the back of thigh and calf in the midline almost to the heel.
- The first three sacral segments are placed with successive areas up the back of the limb.
- S_1: Back of the heal.
- S_2: Over the popliteal fossa.
- S_3: Over the gluteal fold.

The genital organs are innervated by S_3 and S_4. Dorsal and plantar aspects of the foot are innervated by L_4, L_5 and S_1 from medial to lateral side. The skin areas supplied by the ventral and dorsal rami of L_1, L_2 and S_3 are continuous with each other. This relationship does not exist with other nerves.

Index

A

Abdomen, 13
  cavity, 56
    peritoneum, 48
    position of viscera, 65, 77, 99
  regions, 65
  walls
    anterior, 13
      bony framework, 13
      cutaneous arteries, 17
      cutaneous nerves, 16
      lymphatics, 17
      muscles, 17–24
    posterior, 29
      bony framework, 29
      fascia, 40
      lymphatics, 46
      muscles, 31
      nerves, 35
      vessels, 41
Abduction,
  at hip joint, 262
  at metatarsophalangeal joints, 310
Abscess,
  anal, 162
  horseshoe, 164
  ischiorectal, 164
  liver, 103-105
  pelvic, 130
  psoas, 41
  renal, 72
  subphrenic, 89
Acetabulum, 198, 260
Adduction,
  at hip joint, 264
  at metatarsophalangeal joints, 310
Ala,
  of sacrum, 30
Ampulla,
  of ductus deferens, 118, 144
  hepticopancreatic (of Vater), 85
  of rectum, 127
  of uterine tube, 154
  of Vater, 85

Anastomosis, Anastomoses,
  arterial,
    around knee joint, 292
    of back of thigh, 256
  portal-systemic, 96, 103
Angle(s),
  of neck of femur, 227, 263
Antrum,
  pyloric, 78
Anus, 159, 160
  digital examination, 144
  fistula-in-ano, 164
Aorta
  abdominal, 41
  aneurysm of, 46
Apex,
  urinary bladder, 130, 131, 134
Aponeurosis, Aponeuroses,
  obliquus abdominis,
    externus, 19
    internus, 19
  plantar, 300
  of transversus abdominis, 20
Appendages,
  of epididymis, 178, 179
  of testis, 178, 179
Appendices epiploicae, 88
Appendicitis, 89
Appendix vermiform, 88
  arterial supply, 88
  development, 89
  lymphatic drainage, 88
  nerves supply, 88
  position, 88
Arch(es)
  of foot,
    lateral longitudinal, 311, 312
    medial longitudinal, 311, 312
    transverse, 311, 313
  plantar arterial, 305
  Rolan's, 94
Artery, Arteries,
  arteria pancreatica magna, 110
  appendicular, 88, 93

  arcuate, of foot, 273
  to bulb, 167
  caecal, 93
  circumflex,
    femoral,
      lateral, 230, 243, 257
      medial, 230, 243, 257
    iliac,
      deep, 18
      superficial, 18, 228
  to clitoris,
    deep, 181
    dorsal, 181
  coeliac (trunk), 43, 78
  colic,
    left, 94
    middle, 93
    right, 93
  cremasteric, 175
  cystic, 80, 106
  deep, of penis, 167, 171
  digital,
    dorsal, 273
    plantar, 306
  dorsal of penis, 167, 171
  dorsalis pedis, 272
  to ductus deferens, 144
  epigastric,
    inferior, 17
    superficial, 17, 228
    superior, 17
  femoral, 230, 241
    circumflex, 230, 243, 257
    femoral deep (profunda), 243
  artery of foregut, 80
  gastric,
    left, 79
    right, 79
    short, 80
  gastroduodenal, 79, 102
  gastro-epiploic,
    left, 80
    right, 80

genicular,
    descending, 242
gluteal,
    inferior, 122, 251
    superior, 123, 251
gonadal, 43
hepatic,
    common, 79
    proper, 79
of hindgut, 43, 93
ileal, 93
ileocolic, 93
iliac,
    circumflex, deep, 17
    circumflex, superficial, 17, 228
    common, 43
    external, 241
    internal, 122
iliolumbar, 122
jejunal, 93
labial,
    lateral, 167
    medial, 167
lumbar artery, 43
marginal (Drummond's), 94
mesenteric,
    inferior, 43, 93
    superior, 43, 92
metatarsal,
    dorsal, 273
    plantar, 305
of midgut, 92
obturator, 122, 172
    abnormal, 233
ovarian, 43, 148
pancreaticoduodenal,
    inferior, 93, 110
    superior, 110
    of thigh, 243
perineal, 167, 170
phrenic, inferior, 43
plantar,
    arch, 305
    lateral, 305
    medial, 305
popliteal, 258
profunda femoris, 231, 242, 257
pudendal,
    deep external, 229
    internal, 122, 167,
    superficial external, 17, 229
rectal,
    inferior, 167
    middle, 122
    superior, 123
renal, 43
    aberrant, 72
sacral,
    lateral, 122
    median, 43, 123
scrotal,
    lateral, 167
    medial, 167

sigmoid, 94
splenic, 80, 113
supraduodenal (of Wilkie), 85
suprarenal,
    inferior, 43
    middle, 60
    superior, 59
testicular, 43, 117
tibial,
    anterior, 283
    posterior, 283
umbilical, 122
    obliterated, 27
utreteric, 74
uterine, 122, 150
vaginal, 122, 157
vesical,
    inferior, 122
    superior, 123
Axes of pelvis, 115
Axial lines,
    of lower limb, 318

B
Band, calcaneometatarsal, 301
Bartholin's cyst, 182
Bile passages, 105
Bladder, urinary, 131
    automatic, 137
    blood supply, 134
    cystocele, 137, 158, 184
    cystoscopy, 137
    cystostomy, 137
    form, 131
    development, 134
    diverticula, 137
    interior, 134
    ligaments, 133
    lymphatic drainage, 134
    nerve supply, 137
    and peritoneum, 125
    relations, 131
    rupture, 137
    sphincters, 173
    structure, 134
    surfaces, 130
    trigone, 134
Body(ies)
    anococcygeal, 160
    perineal, 159
Bones,
    calcaneum, 222, 266, 277, 299
    cuboid, 223, 266, 277, 299
    cuneiform, 224, 266, 277, 299
    Medial, 224
    Intermediate, 224
    Lateral, 224
    femur, 227, 237, 285
    fibula, 214, 265
    hip, 13, 89, 226
    ilium, 13, 30, 226
    metatarsus, 224, 266, 277, 299
    navicular, 223, 266, 277, 299

ostrigonum, 298
patella, 206, 227, 286
of pelvic wall, 115
phalanges, 266, 277, 299
pubis, 9, 15, 227
sacrum, 30
talus, 266, 277
tarsus, 220, 266, 277
tibia, 207, 265, 278, 286
twelfth rib, 30
Bony framework,
    abdominal walls,
        anterior, 13
        posterior, 29
    compartments of leg,
        anterior, 265, 267
        lateral, 273
        posterior, 278
    compartments of thigh,
        anterior, 227
        medial, 237
        posterior, 253
    foot, 299
    gluteal region, 246
Brodel's white line, 69, 72
Bulb(s) of vestibule, 181
Bursa(e)
    of gastrocnemius, 291
    infrapatellar, 290
    of knee joint, 290, 292
    omental, 181
    prepatellar, 290
    psoas, 262
    suprapatellar, 290
Bursitis,
    infrapatellar (Clergyman's knee), 294
    prepatellar (house maid's knee), 294
    suprapatellar, 294

C
Caecum, 87
    blood supply, 93
    interior, 88
    lymphatic drainage, 96
    relations, 87
    sub-hepatic, 54
Calcaneus, 266, 300
Calices, renal, 72
Calot's triangle, 107
Canal(s),
    adductor (of Hunter), 240
    anal, 159
        blood supply, 161
        development, 162
        lining, 160
        lymphatic drainage, 162
        muscles, 160
        nerves, 160
    cervical, of uterus, 147
    femoral, 233
    inguinal, 24
        boundaries, 24
        contents, 26

defensive mechanism, 26
obturator, 116, 120
pleuroperitoneal, 49
pudendal (Alcock's), 163
subartorial, see adductor, 240
Cap, duodenal, 82
Capsule,
of kidney, 68
of liver (Glisson's), 49, 105
of spleen, 113
Caput medusae, 96, 104
Cartilage(s)
semilunar, of knee joint, 289
bucket handle tear, 293
Cavity(ies),
abdominal, 13
pelvic, 125
peritoneal, 56
Cervix of uterus, 146
Cisterna chyli, 46
Clitoris, 181
Cloaca, 135
Coccyx, 8, 116
Colic,
renal, 74, 140
ureteric, 74, 140
Colon,
ascending, 89
blood supply, 93, 95
descending, 91
flexures,
right (hepatic), 90
left (splenic), 91
lymphatic drainage, 96
nerve supply, 97
sigmoid (pelvic), 91
transverse, 90
Colpotomy, 158
Column(s)
anal, 160
renal, 71
Compartments,
of leg,
anterior, 265, 268, 273
lateral, 273
posterior, 280
of thigh,
anterior, 236
medial, 237
posterior, 252, 253
Condyle(s)
of femur, 227
of tibia, 30
Cord(s)
spermatic, 157
Corona glandis, 171
Corpus, Corpora,
cavernosum,
of clitoris, 181
of penis, 168, 171
spongiosum of penis, 168, 171
Cortex,
of kidney, 71

of suprarenal gland, 76
Crest, Crista,
iliac, 30
intertrochanteric, 227, 236
medial, of fibula, 278, 279
pubic, 15
urethral, 142, 182
Crus, Crura,
of clitoris, 181
of diaphragm, 33
of penis, 170
of superficial inguinal ring, 24
Cryptorchidism, 179
Cuboid bone, 266, 299, 312
Cuneiform bones, 266, 299, 312
Curvatures,
of rectum, 127
of stomach, 79
Cyst, Bakers, 294
Bartholins, 182
Cystocele, 137, 158, 187
Cystoscopy, 136
Cystostomy, 137

D

Dermatomes,
of lower limb, 317
Diaphragm, 33
development, 35
function, 34
nerve supply, 34
openings, 34
parts, 33
pelvic, 123, 124
urogenital, 165
Diverticulum, ileal (Meckel's), 87
Dorsal digital expansion, 277
Dorsiflexion,
at ankle joint, 297
Dorsum,
of foot, 271
Duct(s), Ductus,
bulbo-urethral, 168
common bile, 107
cystic, 105
deferens, 144, 145
vasectomy, 145
ejaculatory, 141, 142, 144
of epididymis, 178
of Gartner, 153
hepatic, 105
longitudinal, of epoophoron, 153
mesonephric (Wolffian), 72, 135, 153
pancreatic,
main (of Wirsung), 110
accessory (of Santorini), 110
paramesonephric, (Mullerian), 152
para-urethral, 182
prostatic, 142
of seminal vesicle, 145
Duodenum, 81
blood supply, 84
cap, 82

interior, 85
lymphatic drainage, 84
papilla, 85
subdivisions, 82
suspensory muscle (ligament) of Treitz, 84

E

Ejaculation, 145, 172
Enteromata, 87
Epicondyles,
of femur, 286, 287
Epididymis, 148
Episiotomy, 182
Epoophoron, 152
Eversion of foot, 309
Exampholas, 54
Extension,
at ankle joint (dorsiflexion), 298
at hip joint, 262
at knee joint, 293
Extravasation of urine, 16, 174, 228

F

Fabricius, bursa of,
Fascia, superficial(e),
of abdominal wall,
anterior, 16
posteior, 40
anal, 164
Camper's, 15, 228
Colle's, 16, 168, 175
cremasteric, 20
of Denonvillers, 129, 130
diaphragmatic, 40
iliac, 40, 231
inferior, of urogenital diaphragm,
lata, 228
of levator ani, 123, 124
obturator, 164
pectineal, 228
pelvic,
parietal, 120
visceral, 121
of penis (bucks), 171
perineal, superficial (Colle's), 16
psoas, 40
renal (Gerotas), 67
of sole of foot, 281
Scarpa, 15, 55, 175, 228
spermatic,
external, 175
internal, 175
superior, of urogenital,
diaphragm, 166
of thigh, 228
thoracolumbar, 40
transversalis, 24, 231
of Waldeyer, 129
Fat,
pararenal, 66
perirenal, 68
retropubic, 142
Femur, 227
Fibula, 265, 278

Fimbria(e), 154
  ovarica, 154
  of uterine tube, 154
Fissure(s)
  for ligamentum teres, 99, 102
  for ligamentum venosum, 99, 102
Fissure-in-ano, 162
Fistula-in-ano, 161, 164
  umbilical, 87
Flexon,
  at ankle joint (plantar flexion), 297
  at hip joint, 262
  at knee joint, 293
  a midtarsal joint, 309
Flexure(s),
  of colon, 90, 91
  dudenojejunal, 84, 85
Floor, pelvic,
  muscles, 123
Fold(s),
  alar, of knee joint, 290
  infrapatellar, 290
  interureteric, 134
  peritoneal, 59
  of rectum, 128
Follicles, aggregated lymph, 86
Foot, 266, 271
  arches, 311
  flat (pes planus), 314
  joints, 307
  skeleton, 266, 299
  sole, 290
Foramen, Foramina
  of Bochdalek, 35
  epiploic (Winslow), 55, 61, 63
  obturator, 116
  of Morgagani, 35
  sacral, 117
  sciatic,
    greater, 247
    lesser, 247
Fornices, vaginal, 147, 157
Fossa(e),
  iliac, 29, 31
  ischiorectal, 163
  ovarian, 154
  paraduodenal, 62
  peritoneal, 60
  popliteal, 258
Fourchette, 182
Frenulum,
  of clitoris, 182
  of prepuce, 141
Fundus,
  of gall bladder, 105
  of stomach, 78
  of uterus, 146

G

Gall bladder, 105
  blood supply, 106
  interior, 106
  lymphatic drainage, 106

relations, 105
subdivisions, 105
Ganglion, ganglia,
  aorticorenal, 39
  coeliac, 39
  hypogastric, 39, 120
  lumbar sympathetic, 37
  mesenteric,
    inferior, 39
    superior, 39
  parasympathetic, 39
  parasympathetic nerves, 39, 135, 152
  pelvic sympathetic, 120
Genitalia,
  external,
    female, 11
    male, 170
Gland(s),
  adrenal, (suprarenal), 74
  bulbo-urethral (Cowper's), 168
  greater vestibular (Bartholin's), 181, 182
  para-urethral (Skene's), 182
  prostate, 140
  suprarenal, 74
  urethral,
    in female (Skene's), 182
    in male (Littre's), 173
  vestibular,
    greater (Bartholin's), 181, 182
Glans,
  of clitoris, 182
  of penis, 171
Gluteal region, 246
Gubernaculum,
  ovary, 154
  testis, 178
Gut, rotation of, 51
Gutter, paracolic, 58-60

H

Haemorrhoids (piles), 103, 130, 162
Haustrations, 87
Hepatico-portal system, 95
  relations, 95
  tributaries, 95
Hernia,
  diaphragmatic, 35
  femoral, 233
  inguinal,
  direct, 28, 37
  indirect, 27, 179
  ischiorectal, 124
  obturator, 124
  sciatic, 124
Hiatus,
  oesophageal, 35
  of Schwalbe, 124
Hilum (Hilus),
  of kidney, 69
  of spleen, 112, 113
Hip bone, 13
  ilium, 13, 30
  ischium, 13

pubis, 13, 14
Hydatid of Morgagni, 179
Hydrocele, 179
Hymen, 182

I

Ileum, 86
  blood supply, 86
  differences with jejunum, 86
  extent, 86
  lymphatic drainage, 96
  mesentery, 86
  nerve supply, 40
  relations, 86
Ilium, 13
Incisions,
  McBurney's Gridiron, 24
  median, 23
  paramedian, 23
  pfannenstiel's, 24
  subcostal, right (Kocher's), 23
  transrectus, 23
Incontinence overflow, 137
  stress, 183
  urine, 137
Infundibulum,
  of uterine tube, 155
Innominate (hip) bone, 13
Intestine, 81, 87
  large, 87
    appendices epiploicae, 87
    blood supply, 93, 94
    comparison with small, 87
    haustra (sacculations), 87
    lymphatic drainage, 96
    megacolon (Hirschsprung's disease), 97
    nerve supply, 40
    parts, 87
    rotation, 51
    taenia coli, 87, 89
  small, 81
    blood supply, 86, 93
    comparison with large, 87
    enteromata, 87
    intussusception, 87
    lymphatic drainage, 84, 96
    mesentery, 86, 114
    nerve supply, 40
    rotation, 51
Intussusception, 87
Inversion of foot, 309
Ischium, 15
Islets of Langerhan's, 111
Isthmus,
  of uterine tube, 155
  of uterus, 146

J

Jejunum, 86
  blood supply, 86
  differences with ileum, 86
  extent, 86
  lymphatic drainage, 96
  mesentery, 54, 86
  nerve supply, 40
  relations, 86

Joints(s),
    ankle (talocrural), 295
        articular surfaces, 295
        ligaments, 295
        movements, 297
        relations, 295
        synovial membrane, 298
    calcaneocuboid, 307, 309
    cuneo-navicular, 310
    hip, 260
        articular surface, 260
        blood supply, 262
        capsule, 260
        ligaments, 260
        movements, 263
        nerve supply, 262
        relations, 262
        synovial membrane, 262
    intermetatarsal, 307, 310
    interphalangeal, 307, 311
    intertarsal, 307, 308
    knee, 285
        articular surfaces, 285
        Bursae around, 291
        capsule, 286
        ligament, 286
        locking mechanism, 293
        movements, 293
        relations, 292
        semilunar cartilages (menisci), 288, 289
        stability, 292
        synovial membrane, 289
    lumbo-sacral, 184
    metatarsophalangeal, 307, 310
    midtarsal, 309
    patellofemoral, 285
    sacro-coccygeal, 184
    sacro-iliac, 183
        articular surfaces, 183
        ligaments, 183
        nerve supply, 184
    subtalar, 308
    symphysis pubis, 184
    talocalcaneonavicular, 308
    talocrural (ankle), 295
    talonavicular, 310
    tarsometatarsal, 307, 310
    tibiofemoral, 285
    tibiofibular,
        inferior, 295
        middle, 295
        superior, 294
    transverse tarsal (midtarsal), 309

K
Kidney, 66
    blood supply, 69
    capsule, 66
    development, 71
    floating, 72
    hilum, 69
    hydronephrosis, 74
    lymphatic drainage, 71

    nerve supply, 71
    polycystic, congenital, 72
    position, 66
    relations, 68
    segments, 69
    structure, 69
    variations, 72, 73

L
Labia,
    majora, 181
    minora, 181
Labrum,
    acetabular, 260
Ligament(s), Ligamentum,
    acetabular, transverse, 260, 261
    arcuate popliteal, 287
        lateral, of knee joint, 287
        medial, of knee joint, 287
        oblique posterior, of knee joint, 287
        posterior of knee joint, 288
    bifurcate, 308
    of bladder, 133
    broad, of uterus, 148
    calcaneocuboid, plantar, 308
    calcaneonavicular, plantar, 309
    cardinal, of uterus, (Mackenrodt's), 148
    cervical, lateral, of uterus (Mackenrodt's), 147
    collateral,
        lateral (tibular), 286
        medial (tibial), 280
    of toes, 311
    coronary, 49, 58, 99
    of knee, 287, 288
    of liver, 100
    cruciate, of knee joint, 287, 288
    deltoid, 295
    falciform, of liver, 49, 58, 98, 100
    false, of bladder, 133
    fibular collateral (lateral) of knee joint, 287
    gastrophrenic, 49, 58
    gastrosplenic, 55, 58, 113
    of head of femur, 261
    iliofemoral (of Bigelow), 260
    iliolumbar, 186
    inguinal (Poupart's), 233
    lacunar (Gimbernat's), 233
    lieno-renal, 55, 58, 113
    lumbosacral, 186
    reflected part, 19
    interosseous,
        of foot, 306
        sacro-iliac, 183
        talocalcanean, 297, 309
        tibiofibular, 295
    ischiofemoral, 261
    lacunar (Gimbernat's), 233
    lateral,
        of ankle joint, 297
        of knee joint, 287
        of bladder, 132
        of rectum, 128
    lienorenal, 55, 58, 113

    medial,
        of ankle joint, 296
        of knee joint, 286
    oblique popliteal, 287
    ovarian, 148
    patellar, 236
    pectineal (of Cooper), 233
    phrenicocolic, 91
    plantar,
        long, 307
        short (calcaneo cuboid), 307
    pubic,
        anterior, 184
        inferior, 184
        superior, 27
    pubocervical, 149
    pubofemoral, 261
    puboprostatic, 133
    pubovesical, 133
    round, of uterus, 148
    sacro-iliac,
        dorsal, 184
        interosseous, 183
        ventral, 183
    sacrospinous, 115, 247
    sacrotuberous, 115, 247
    spring, 308
    calcaneonavicular (spring), 308
    supraspinous, 186
    suspensory,
        of duodenum (Treitz), 85
        of ovary, 147
    talofibular, 297
    teres, 98
    tibial collateral (medial) of knee joint, 286
    tibiofibular,
        anterior, 295
        inferior, 295
        transverse, 295
    triangular, of liver,
        left, 100
        right, 100
    umbilical,
        lateral, 133
        medial, 122
        median, 133
    uterosacral, 149
    of uterus, 148
    venosum, 99
Line(s), Linea
    alba, 18
    arcuate,
        of pelvis, 14
        of rectus sheath, 22
    aspera, 227, 236, 253
    axial,
        lower limb, 318
        Brodel's, 69, 72
    gluteal, 246
    intercondylar, 287
    intertrochanteric, 227
    pectinate, of anal canal, 160
    pectineal, 15

semilunaris, 31
soleal, 278
supracondylar, of femur, 236, 237, 253
terminalis, 31
Liver, 98
    bare area, 105
    blood vessels, 102
    capsule (Glisson's), 98
    cirrhosis, 103
    development, 103
    ligaments, 99
    liver bed, 102
    lobes, 98
    lymphatic drainage, 103
    nerve supply, 38
    peritoneum, 100
    porta hepatis, 99
    position, 98
    relations, 100
    segments, 102
    subdivisions, surgical, 99
    subphrenic spaces, 103
    surfaces, 100
Lobes(s),
    caudate, 99
    of kidney, 69
    of liver, 98
    of prostate, 141
    quadrate, 99
    Reidel's, 105
Lower limb,
    axial lines, 318
    lymphatic drainage, 316
    segmental innervation, 318
    venous drainage, 315
Lymph nodes,
    arotic, 46
    coeliac, 81
    colic, 96
    diaphragmatic, 103
    gastric,
        inferior, 81
        superior, 81
    hepatic, 81, 99, 103
    ileocolic, 96
    iliac, 47
        common, 47
        external, 46, 173
        internal, 173
    inguinal,
        deep, 171, 173
        superficial, 171, 228, 316
    mesenteric, 96
    pancreaticoduodenal, 84
    pancreaticolienal, 114
    pancreaticosplenic, 81
    popliteal, 257
    pre-aortic, 84
    portal, 102
    rectal, 96
    regional,
        of abdomen, 46

of lower limb, 316
    retrosternal, 102
    sigmoid, 96
    subpyloric, 81
    venacaval, 102
Lymph trunks,
    intestinal, 47
    lumbar, 47

M
Malleolus,
    lateral, 266
    medial, 265
Maralgia paraesthetica, 37
McBurney's point, 24
Meatus(es),
    urethral, 134, 182
Meckel's,
    diverticulum, 54, 86
Mediastinum,
    testis, 176
Medulla,
    of kidney, 71
    of suprarenal gland, 76
Megacolon (Hirschsprung's disease), 97
Membrane(s), Membrana
    anal, 129, 135
    interosseous of leg, 295
    obturator, 116
    perineal, 164, 166
Menisci of knee joint, 288
Mesentery,
    dorsal, 48, 51
    ventral, 48
Meso-appendix, 88
Mesocolon,
    pelvic, 93
    transverse, 49
Mesoduodenum, 50
Mesogastrium,
    dorsal, 49
    ventral, 48
Mesometrium, 148
Mesonephros, 72
Mesosalpinx, 148
Mesovarium, 149
Metatarsal bones, 266, 300
Metatarsalgia, 314
Micturition, 137
Mons pubis (Veneris), 181
Morison's pouch, 59, 63
Muscle(s),
    abductor,
        digiti minimi, 301
        hallucis, 301
    adductor,
        brevis, 239
        hallucis, 303
        longus, 239
        magnus, 239, 256
    articularis genu, 237
    biceps,
        femoris, 253

bulbospongiosus,
        in female, 181
        in man, 169
    coccygeus, 124
    cremaster, 175
    dartos, 175
    detrusor, 134
    diaphragm, 33
    extensor,
        digitorum,
            brevis, 272
            longus, 269
        hallucis,
            brevis, 272
            longus, 269
    flexor,
        digitiminimi brevis, 303
        digitorum,
            accessorius, 302, 303
            brevis, 301
            longus, 280, 282, 302, 303
        hallucis,
            brevis, 303
            longus, 280, 282, 302, 303
    gastrocnemius, 281
    gemelli, 250
    gluteus,
        maximus, 248, 250
        medius, 248
        minimus, 250
    gracilis, 237
    hamstring, 253
    iliacus, 33
    iliococcygeus, 123
    interossei,
        dorsal, 277, 304
        plantar, 304
    ischiocavernosus,
        in female, 181
        in male, 169
    levator,
        ani, 123
        prostate, 123
    lumbrical, 301, 302
    oblique,
        external, 18
        internal, 19
    obturator,
        externus, 240
        internus, 116, 249
    pectineus, 237
    peroneus,
        brevis, 274
        longus, 274, 304
        tertius, 270
    piriformis, 118, 250
    plantaris, 281
    popliteus, 281, 283, 289
    psoas,
        major, 33
        minor, 33
    pubococcygeus, 123

puborectalis, 123
pubovaginalis, 123
pyramidalis, 21
quadratus,
    femoris, 250
    lumborum, 31
quadriceps femoris, 235, 250
recto-urethralis (of Roux), 130
rectus,
    abdominis, 20
    femoris, 235
sartorius, 234
semimembranosus, 254
semitendinosus, 254
soleus, 281, 282
sphincter,
    ani, 160
    pyloric, 78
    urethral, 134, 168, 182
    vaginal, 123
    vesicae, 173
suspensory of,
    duodenum, 84
tensor, fasciae latae, 237, 251
tibialis,
    anterior, 268
    posterior, 281, 283, 304
transversus,
    abdominis, 20
    of perineum,
        deep, 168
        superficial, 169, 181
vastus,
    intermedius, 236
    lateralis, 236
    medialis, 236

N
Navicular, 266, 299
Nerve(s),
    coccygeal, 120
    cutaneous,
        of anterior abdominal wall, 16
        of thigh, 229
        femoral, 171
            intermediate, 228
            lateral, 36, 37, 228, 231, 247
            medial, 229
            posterior, 120, 174, 253, 279
        lateral of calf, 267
    erigentes, 120, 135, 145
    femoral, 36, 37, 231, 233, 243
    gastric, 34
    genitofemoral, 35, 229, 231
    gluteal,
        inferior, 118, 251
        superior, 118, 251
    to hamstrings, 255
    hypogastric, 120, 135
    iliohypogastric, 36, 248
    ilio-inguinal, 36, 229
    to levator ani, 120, 124
    labial, posterior, 166, 181

lumbar, 35
lumbosacral trunk, 36, 37
obturator, 36, 37, 120, 229, 233, 244
    accessory, 36, 245
to obturator internus, 120,
parasympathetic nerves, 39, 152
pelvic splanchnic, 39, 120
of penis,
    dorsal nerve, 166
perforating cutaneous, 118, 247
perineal,
    of fourth sacral, 120
    of pudendal, 166, 169, 181
    of posterior femoral cutaneous, 164,
    253
peroneal,
    common, 118, 259
    deep, 267, 272
    superficial, 267, 272, 276
to piriformis, 120
plantar,
    lateral, 300, 306
    medial, 300, 305
to popliteus, 259
presacral, 135
pudendal, 120, 166
    block, 164, 252
to quadratus femoris, 120, 252
rectal, inferior, 166
sacral, 118
saphenous, 267, 273, 279
sciatic, 251, 255
scrotal, posterior, 166
splanchnic,
    greater, 35, 39
    lesser, 35, 39
    lowest (least), 35
    pelvic, 39, 120
subcostal, 243
sural, 259, 267, 273, 280
tibial, 120, 233, 259
Nodules,
    aggregated lymphoid, of ileum, 86
Notch,
    acetabular, 245, 260, 261
    sciatic,
        greater, 247
        lesser, 247

O
Oesophagus,
    abdominal, 77
Omentum,
    gastrocolic, 58
    greater, 49, 58
    lesser, 49, 54, 58, 101
Openings,
    in diaphragm, 34
    saphenous, 228
Organ of Giraldes, 179
Orifice,
    cardiac, of stomach, 78
    ileocaecal, 88

pyloric, 78
ureteric, 131, 134
urethral,
    external,
        in female, 134, 182
        in male, 172
    internal, 134, 182
Os of uterus, 147
Ovary, 155
    accessory, 156
    congenital absence, 156
    development, 156
    lymphatic drainage, 156
    maldescent, 156
    nerve supply, 156
    relations, 155

P
Pad(s) of fat,
    infrapatellar, 291
    retropubic, 141
Pancreas, 107
    annular, 89
    blood supply, 110, 111
    development, 110
    ducts of, 110
    islets of Langerhans, 110
    lymphatic drainage, 110
    nerve supply, 110
    pseudocyst, 112
    relations, 108
    subdivisions, 108
Papilla(e),
    duodenal, 85
    renal, 71
Paralysis of nerves,
    inferior gluteal, 251
    sciatic, 252
    superior gluteal, 252
Parametrium, 146, 148, 152
Parasympathetic nerves,
    of abdomen, 39
    to intestine, 89, 97
    to kidney, 72
    to pancreas, 110
    to prostate, 142
    to rectum, 129
    to stomach, 81
    to urinary bladder, 135
    to uterus and vagina, 152, 157
Paroophoron, 152
Patella, 227, 286
Pecten of anal canal, 160
Pelvic brim, 31
Pelvis,
    aperture,
        inferior (outlet), 159
        superior (inlet, brim), 115
    axes, 115
    bony, 115
    cavity, 115
    diaphragm, 123
    false, 31

fascia, 115, 121
    greater (false), 31, 115
    joints, 183
    lesser (true), 115, 145
    ligaments, 115, 116
    muscles, 116, 123
    true, 31
Pelvis of kidney (ureter), 69, 73
Penis, 170
    blood supply, 171
    coverings, 171
    ligaments, 171
    lymphatic drainage, 172
    nerve supply, 172
    parts, 170, 171
    structure, 171
Perineal body, 123, 157, 159, 169, 180, 181
Perineum, 159
Peritoneum, 48
    arrangement in adult, 55
    cavity, 56
    compartments, 57, 58
    development, 48
    gutters, 58, 60
    ligaments, 48
    mesentery, 48
    pelvic, 125
    pouches,
        recto-uterine (of Douglas), 125
        rectovesical, 125
        uterovesical, 125
    sac,
        greater, 57
        lesser, 60
Pesplanus (flat foot), 314
Peyer's patches, 86
Phalanges,
    of toes, 266, 300
Plane of abdomen, 65
    horizontal,
        intertubercular, 65
        subcostal, 65
        supracristal, 65
        transpyloric, 65
        umbilical, 65
    sagittal,
        median, 65
        midclavicular, 65
Plantar flexion,
    at ankle joint, 297
    of toes, 311
Plexus, Plexuses,
    of nerves,
        aortic, 38
        coccygeal, 120
        coeliac, 39
        hypogastric,
            inferior, 120
            superior, 120
        lumbar, 35
        lumbosacral, 118
        mesenteric, 39
        pelvic, 74, 129, 152

sacral, 118
    ovarian, 156
    of veins,
        uterovaginal, 152
        pampiniform, 177, 179
        prostatic, 140
        rectal, 129
Point, McBurney's, 24
Porta hepatis, 99
Portal hypertension, 96
Portal system of veins, 95
Portal-systemic anastomoses, 103
Pouch,
    Hartmann's, 106
    hepatorenal (or Morison), 59, 63
    perineal,
        deep, 168, 180
        superficial, 168, 180
    recto-uterine (of Douglas), 125, 127, 146
    rectovesical, 125, 126
    uterovesical, 125, 126, 146
Prepuce,
    of clitoris, 182
    of penis, 171
Process(es), Processus,
    caudate of liver, 99
    styloid,
        of fibula, 266
    uncinate,
        of pancreas, 107
    vaginalis of testis, 178
Proctodeum, 161
Prolapse,
    of rectum, 130, 137, 163
    of urethra, 184
    of uterus, 124, 137, 152
Promontory, sacral, 30, 31
Prostate,
    blood supply, 143
    capsules, 141
    development, 143
    examination in living, 144
    lobes, 141
    lymphatic drainage, 143
    nerve supply, 143
    prostatectomy, 143
    relations, 142
    structure, 143
    urethra in, 142
Pubis, 15, 115
Pudendal block, 164, 252
Pudendum, female, 181
Pylorus, 78

R
Ramus, Rami
    ischiopubic, 15, 164, 227
    of ischium, 15, 159, 164, 166
    of pubis, 14, 164, 166
Raphe,
    of scrotum, 175
Recess(es),
    caecal, 60

hepato-enteric, 49
    of lesser sac, 62
    pancreatico-enteric, 49
    paracolic,
        left, 60
        right, 59
    paraduodenal, 60
    pneumato-enteric, 49
    splenic, 63
Rectum, 125
    blood supply, 128
    development, 130
    digital examination, 130
    fascia of, 130
    incontinence, 137
    interior, 128
    lymphatic drainage, 130
    nerve supply, 130
    peritoneal reflection, 127
    prolapse, 130, 137
    rectocele, 158
    relations, 127
    supports, 130
    sphincters, 123
Reflex, cremasteric, 37
Regions,
    of abdomen, 65
    dorsum of foot, 271, 277
    gluteal, 246
    medial aspect of ankle, 283
    medial side of leg, 276
Reidel's lobe, 105
Rete testis, 176
Retinaculum, Retinacula,
    extensor of ankle,
        inferior, 271
        superior, 271
    flexor of ankle, 283
    of hip joint, 260
    patellar, 236
    peroneal, 276
Retroflexion of uterus, 152
Retroversion of uterus, 152
Rib, twelfth, 29
Ridge(s),
    interureteric, 134
Ring(s),
    femoral, 230, 233
    inguinal,
        deep, 23
        superficial, 24
Root(s),
    of mesentery, 86
Rotation,
    of gut, 51

S
Sac,
    of peritoneum,
        greater, 56
        lesser, 56
Sacrum, 30, 118
Saphenous graft, 234

Scrotum, 175
blood supply, 175
layers, 175
lymphatic drainage, 175
nerve supply, 175
Segments,
liver, 102
renal, 69
splenic, 113
Septum, Septa
femoral, 233
intermuscular,
of leg, 265
of thigh, 233
Sesamoid bones,
of great toe, 299
patella, 227
Sheath(s),
femoral, 231
of rectus abdominis, 21, 133
psoas, 40
synovial of ankle tendons, 271
Sign,
Trendelenberg's 250, 252, 264
Sinus, Sinuses,
anal, 160
of epididymis, 178
prostatic, 142
renal, 66, 69, 71
tarsi, 308
Situs inversus viscerum, 54
Skeletal framework of foot, 299
Smegma, 171
Soleal pump, 316
Space(s),
extraperitoneal, 105
perineal, 159
subhepatic, 104
subphrenic, 104
Sphincter,
anal,
external, 162
internal, 162
hepaticopancreatic (of Oddi), 85, 112
pyloric, 78
urethral,
external (vesicae), 174, 183
internal, 134, 174
vesicae, 174, 183
Spine(s), Spina
iliac, 14
ischial, 15
Spleen, 112
accessory, 114
blood supply, 113
development, 114
lymphatic drainage, 114
peritoneal folds, 113
relations, 112
situation, 112
Spondylolisthesis, 186
Stomach, 78
bed, 78

blood supply, 78, 79
cardiac orifice, 78
form, 78
lymphatic drainage, 80
nerve supply, 80
parts, 78
relations, 78
Sulcus,
calcanei, 308
Sympathetic nerves (see also Ganglia),
of abdomen, 37
to intestine, 89, 97
to kidneys, 71
to pelvis, 120
to rectum, 130
to stomach, 81
to urinary bladder, 135
to uterus and vagina, 152, 157
Symphysis pubis,, 184
Synovial sheaths,
of ankle and foot, 271, 276, 283

T
Taeniae coli, 87, 89
Talipes,
calcaneus, 314
equinus, 314
valgus, 314
varus, 314
Talus, 266, 277
Tarsus, 266, 277
Tendo calcaneus (Achillis), 282
Testis, 175
appendices, 178
blood supply, 177
coverings, 176
cryptorchidism, 179
development, 177
descent, 177
anomalies, 179
ectopic, 179
gubernaculum, 178
lymphatic drainage, 177
mediastinum, 176
nerve supply, 177
relations, 176
rete, 176
torsion of, 179
vestigial structures, 178
Tibia, 265, 278
Tract,
iliotibial, 228
Trendelenburg's sign, 249, 252, 264
Triangle,
anal, 159
Calot's, 107
femoral, 230
inguinal (Hesselbach's), 26
urogenital, 164, 166, 168, 180
Trigone of bladder, 134
Trochanters, 227
Trunk(s),
coeliac, 43

lumbosacral, 37
lymph, 35, 47
sympathetic,
lumbar part, 37, 38
sacral part, 120
Tube,
uterine, 152
Tubercle(s), Tuberosity(ies),
adductor, 240
ischial, 184, 253
of navicular bone, 219
peroneal, 275
pubic, 15
quadrate, 249
tibial, 236, 286
Tubules,
seminiferous, 177
Skene's, 182
Tunica,
albuginea, 176
of corpora cavernosa, 171
of testis, 176
vaginalis of testis, 176
vasculosa of testis, 176

U
Umbilicus, 21, 22
Urachus, 132, 134, 135, 137
cysts, 137
lacunae of Luschka, 137
patent, 137
Ureter,
in abdomen, 73
double ureter, 140
hydroureter, 226
in pelvis, 137
Urethra,
in female, 182
in male, 172
membranous, 172
penile (spongiose), 172
prostatic, 141, 172
sphincter, 172
Urine, extravasation of, 16, 174, 228
residual, 144
retention, 144
Uterus,
axis and angulation, 145
blood supply, 150
cavity, 148
cervix, 146
development, 152
isthmus, 146
ligaments, 148, 149
lower segment, 152
lymphatic drainage, 150
masculinus, 179
nerve supply, 152
os, 148
parts, 145
peritoneum, 125
position, 145
prolapse,
relations, 146
supports, 149

surfaces, 145
Utricle,
    prostatic, 143
Uvula,
    vesicae, 134

V

Vagina, 156
    blood supply, 157
    development, 157
    duplicate, 158
    episiotomy, 182
    lymphatic drainage, 157
    nerve supply, 157
    posterior colpotomy, 158
    relations, 157
Vaginal examination, 157
Valve(s),
    anal, 160
    ileocaecal, 88
    spiral, of cystic duct (heister), 106
Vaicocele, 179
Vas deferens, *see* ductus deferens,
Vasectomy, 145
Vein(s), Vena(e)
    adrenal (suprarenal), 120
    azygos, 41, 47
    cava
        inferior, 43
        relations, 43, 44
    circumflex femoral,
        lateral, 231
        medial, 231
    cystic, 96, 106
    deep of leg, 315
    digital dorsal,
        of foot, 266
    dorsal, of penis,
        deep, 171
        superficial, 172
    of clitoris,
        deep, 181
    epigastric, 104
        superficial, 315
    femoral, 243, 316
    gastric,
        left, 80

right, 80
        short, 81
    gastro-epiploic,
        left, 81
        right, 81
    gluteal, 316
        hepatic, 46
        hepatic portal, see portal, 95
        iliac,
            common, 43, 44
            deep circumflex
            external, 242
            internal, 123, 135, 143
            superficial circumflex, 316
        superficial,
            external pudendal, 316
        lumbar, 41, 46
        mesenteric,
            inferior, 95
            superior, 95
        obturator, 316
        ovarian, 46, 70
        phrenic, 46
        popliteal, 259, 279, 316
        portal,
            hepatic, 95
        prepyloric (of Mayo), 80
        profunda femoris, 230
        pudendal,
            superficial external, 171, 316
        rectal,
            inferior, 129
            middle, 129
            superior, 103, 129
            renal, 69
        sacral,
            lateral,
            median, 103
        saphenous,
            great, 266, 315
            small, 279, 316
        splenic, 95, 113
        suprarenal, 57
        testicular, 45, 69
        tibial,
            anterior, 316

posterior, 316
        umbilical, left, 98, 99
        uterine, 150
        vesical, 134
        varicose, 316
Vagotomy selective, 81
Varices, 96
Varicocele, 183
Venacava, inferior, 43
    relations, 45
    tributaries, 45
Venous arch,
    dorsal of foot, 266
Vesicle, seminal, 145
Vestibule,
    of vagina, 180
Volvulus, 54, 88
Vulva, 181

W

Walls,
    abdominal,
        anterior, 13
            blood supply, 17
            bony framework, 13
            incisions, 24
            lymphatic drainage, 17
            muscles, 18
            nerve supply, 17
        posterior, 29
            bony framework, 29
            lymphatic drainage, 46
            muscles, 31
            nerves, 35
            vessels, 41
    pelvic,
        arrangement of
        structures, 115
        fascia, 120
        muscles, 116
        nerves, 118
        vessels, 121

Z

Zona orbicularis of capsule of hip joint, 261